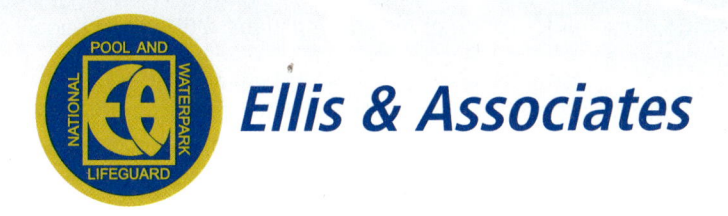

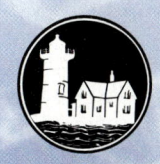

national *Pool* and *Waterpark* lifeguard training second edition

Ellis & Associates

JONES AND BARTLETT PUBLISHERS
Sudbury, Massachusetts
BOSTON   TORONTO   LONDON   SINGAPORE

World Headquarters
Jones and Bartlett Publishers
40 Tall Pine Drive
Sudbury, MA 01776
978-443-5000
info@jbpub.com
www.jbpub.com

Jones and Bartlett Publishers Canada
P.O. Box 19020
Toronto, ON M5S 1X1
CANADA

Jones and Bartlett Publishers International
Barb House, Barb Mews
London W6 7PA
UK

Copyright © 1999 by Jones and Bartlett Publishers, Inc.

All rights reserved. No part of the material protected by this copyright notice may be reproduced or utilized in any form, electronic or mechanical, including photocopying, recording, or by any information storage and retrieval system, without written permission from the copyright owner.

The procedures and protocols in this book are based on the most current recommendations of responsible medical sources. Ellis & Associates, the National Safety Council, and the publisher, however, make no guarantee as to, and assume no responsibility for the correctness, sufficiency or completeness of such information or recommendations. Other or additional safety measures may be required under particular circumstances.

This textbook is intended solely as a guide to the appropriate procedures to be employed when rendering emergency care to waterpark or lakefront guests. It is not intended as a statement of the standards of care required in any particular situation, because circumstances and the patient's physical condition can vary widely from one emergency to another. Nor is it intended that this textbook shall in any way advise lifeguards concerning legal authority to perform the activities or procedures discussed. Such local determinations should be made only with the aid of legal counsel.

Library of Congress Cataloging-in-Publication Data
Ellis, Jeff.
National Pool and Waterpark Lifeguard Training / Jeff Ellis, Jill White.
     P. cm.
    "Ellis & Associates, Inc."
    ISBN 0-7637-0793-7
    1. Lifeguards—Training of—Handbooks, manuals, etc.
I. White, Jill E., II. Ellis & Associates. III. Title.
GV838.72.E45   1999
797.2'0028'9—dc21   98-21019
                                                               CIP

Production Credits

Chief Executive Officer: Clayton Jones
Chief Operating Officer: Don Jones, Jr.
Publisher: Tom Walker
Vice President, Sales and Marketing: Tom Manning
Managing Director: Judith H. Hauck
Marketing Director: Rich Pirozzi
Emergency Care Marketing Manager: Kimberly Brophy
Publisher, EMS & Aquatics: Larry Newell
Project Editor: Kathryn Twombly

Production Director: Anne Spencer
Senior Production Editor: Cynthia Knowles Maciel
Manufacturing Director: Therese Bräuer
Manufacturing Buyer: Kristen Guevara
Design and Composition: Studio Montage
Illustrations: Network Graphics
Photography: Ellis & Associates
Printing and Binding: Banta Company

Printed in the United States of America
02 01 00 99 98   10 9 8 7 6 5 4 3 2 1

Contents

Preface v

Acknowledgements vii

Part 1: Lifeguarding Responsibilities

Chapter 1:
Lifeguard Accountability and Professionalism 2

Chapter 2:
Awareness and Recognition 8

Chapter 3:
Reaction 26

Part 2: Responding to an Emergency

Chapter 4:
Guest on the Surface—Breathing 38

Chapter 5:
Rescue Breathing 52

Chapter 6:
Supplemental Oxygen 62

Chapter 7:
CPR and Airway Obstruction 74

Chapter 8:
Guest on the Surface—Not Breathing 90

Chapter 9:
Spinal Injury Management 102

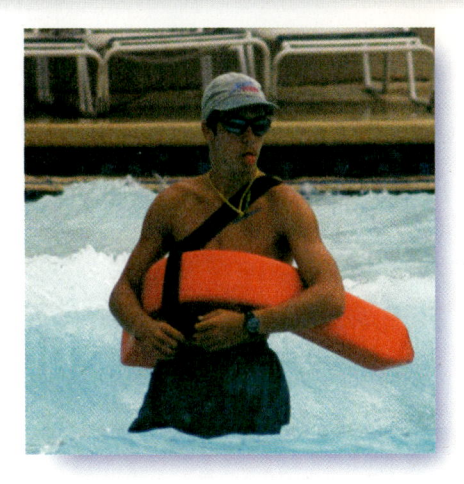

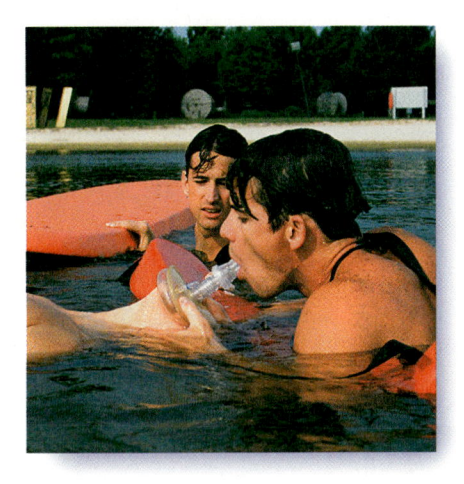

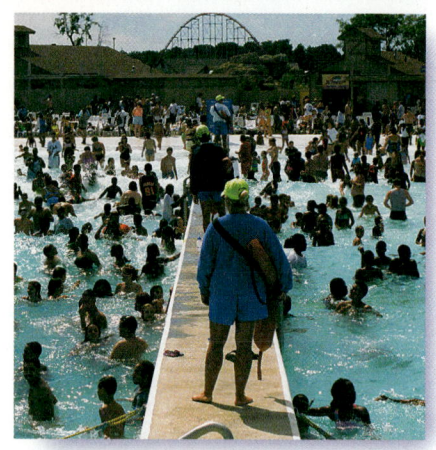

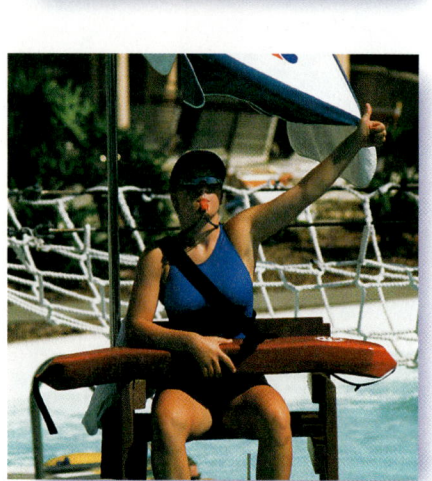

Chapter 10:
Submerged Guest—Within Reach 120

Chapter 11:
Submerged Guest—Beyond Reach 126

Part 3: Lifeguard First Responder

Chapter 12:
Lifeguarding—Dealing with Risks 134

Chapter 13:
Medical Emergencies and Injuries 142

Chapter 14:
Additional Responsibilities 164

Chapter 15:
Automated External Defibrillation 172

Chapter 16:
Waterfront Lifeguarding 186

Part 4: Appendixes

Appendix A:
Sample Rescue Flow Charts 204

Appendix B:
Glossary of Key Terms 206

Index 210

Preface

Congratulations on your decision to become an Ellis & Associates (E&A™) certified lifeguard. Following successful completion of our National Pool and Waterpark Lifeguard Training Program (NPWLTP), you will join a select group of aquatic professionals who apply proven state-of-the-art aquatic injury prevention practices in emergency incidents. As a result of E&A's emphasis on prevention, professionalism, and accountability, our safety record is unsurpassed in the aquatic industry.

The NPWLTP was originally developed in 1983 to address waterpark safety issues. Since then, because of the demand for this quality program by aquatic professionals, it has expanded into waterfront safety. This program has been credited by national and international agencies for revolutionizing the standards of the aquatic safety industry.

Specifically, the NPWLTP has led the industry in:

- Elevating professional lifeguard standards.
- Using operational safety audits for lifeguard accountability.
- Developing the "10/20 Protection Rule" as the standard of care.
- Introducing body substance isolation precautions to protect lifeguards from disease transmission.
- Introducing the use of supplemental oxygen, resuscitation masks, bag-valve-masks, manual suction devices, and automated external defibrillation to enhance resuscitation efforts.
- Eliminating body contact rescues and advocating the exclusive use of the rescue tube.
- Establishing a national database for injury prevention.

The E&A "Make It Work" Philosophy

Lifeguard rescue skills are best learned in the water, under the watchful eye of an E&A instructor. Once you have gained competency in these basic skills, you will apply what you have learned to real-life simulated incidents. This is where the E&A objective – driven curriculum and "Make It Work" philosophy become apparent. This curriculum and philosophy stress that it is not as important to execute "textbook perfect" rescues, which seldom occur in real life, as it is for lifeguards to problem solve to overcome adverse situations that might arise during a rescue effort. As long as the techniques used always provide maximum safety for both the victim and the lifeguard and the rescue is conducted effectively, the rescue is a success. In this respect, the E&A rescue philosophy differs significantly from that of other nationally recognized lifeguard training programs.

The NPWLTP emphasis is on effectively preventing aquatic accidents by scanning zones, consistently monitoring swimmers, and enforcing rules, rather than on achieving "textbook perfect" skills. The NPWLTP also emphasizes lifeguard teamwork for the successful management of catastrophic incidents. Unlike other national lifeguard training curricula, the NPWLTP focuses upon team lifeguarding concepts rather then emphasizing "perfect" individual rescue skills.

Another unique component of the NPWLTP is that lifeguard candidates learn to lifeguard while participating in class activities. In this way, they gain "hands on" lifeguarding experience before they complete the course. E&A is the only national lifeguard training agency to mandate "hands on" or apprentice lifeguard experience in its training curriculum.

About This Manual

The contents of this book are your guide to becoming an E&A lifeguard. The contents reflect the educational and technological advances that the NPWLTP has made, which continue to position it as the industry leader in the reduction of aquatic injuries.

The parameters of the fundamental concepts of professional lifeguarding are included in this book. However, the responsibility for mastering these concepts is the responsibility of each individual. Each lifeguard candidate should practice and customize his or her personal aquatic rescue skills from the information contained here and developed in the NPWLTP, to gain confidence and become a truly proficient lifeguard.

This manual has 16 chapters, separated into four sections. The first section, Lifeguard Responsibilities, presents the basics of accountability, professionalism, recognition of an emergency, and reaction. The second section, Responding to an Emergency, focuses on the rescue and management of a guest who is submerged or on the surface, conscious or unconscious, breathing or non-breathing, with or without a pulse, and with or without possible spinal injury. The third section, Lifeguard First Responder, addresses ways to minimize risks, the need for first aid skills, the importance of automated external defibrillation in saving lives, and special situations involving waterfront lifeguarding. The Appendices include easy-to-use flow charts for responding to emergency situations, and the glossary of key terms.

As you read, you will notice that some photographs may not show lifeguards executing a "textbook perfect" rescue. This is because the photos were taken during actual rescues. While these photographs may not depict a perfect rescue, they do depict realistic events in which our program objectives and philosophy enabled lifeguards to execute a safe and effective rescue.

National Pool and Waterpark Lifeguard Training attempts to present the knowledge required of E&A's professional lifeguards as accurately, clearly, and concisely as possible. However, each aquatic facility is unique, and it is beyond the scope of this manual and our National Pool and Waterpark Training Program to address all of the differences. To this end, you must rely on the management personnel at your aquatic facility to provide facility-specific information to supplement your training.

Jeff Ellis
President
Ellis & Associates

Acknowledgements

The task of writing, editing, reviewing, and producing a manual of this size and quality is complex. Many talented people were involved in the original development of this manual, as well as this second edition. We are proud to be associated with so many dedicated professionals. To name everyone would be an impossible task, so we trust that they all recognize our sincere appreciation for their assistance by this notation.

There are, however, several individuals, agencies, and organizations whose contributions to our program and publications over the years warrant special attention:

First Edition Contributors

We wish to thank the professionals listed below who played an important role in the development of the first edition of this manual, published in 1994:

- DoAnn Geiger
- Rosemary Umenhofer
- Mel Umenhofer
- Betty Street
- John Hunsucker
- Richard Allen
- Lamar Parker
- Gene Weeks
- Joe Martinez
- Bob Billie
- Gary Henry
- Jeff Henry
- Jana Faber
- Rick Faber
- Ron Sutula
- J.P. Moss
- Gary Maurek
- Steve Loose
- Greg Mastriona
- Tim Demke
- Dennis Mattey
- Ray Landers
- Steve Cable
- Brenda McVitty
- Christine Crutcher
- Coy Jones
- Vera Solis
- Jack Waterman
- Turk Waterman
- Dr. Robert Clayton
- Janis (Carley) Keim
- Dean Cerdan
- Tom Werts

We also wish to gratefully acknowledge the following groups for their assistance during the development of the first edition of this manual:

- Wet N' Wild – Orlando
- Schlitterbahn
- City of Portland
- Hyland Park and Recreation District
- Rockford Park District
- Columbia Association
- Deer Park Independent School District
- Dorney Park Wildwater Kingdom
- College Station Parks and Recreation Department
- Noah's Ark
- City of Cape Coral Parks and Recreation
- Walt Disney World

A special thanks to Louise Priest and Grant Gould for their professional expertise and contributions, and to our partners, Walter Johnson and his staff of the National Recreation and Park Association/ Aquatic Section, and Donna Siegfried and Neil Boot of the National Safety Council.

Second Edition Contributors

We wish to thank the advisory committee members listed below for their technical review, guidance, and specific contributions to this second edition:

Craig Aman, Hewlett Packard/Heartstream Corporation

Richard Carroll, Splish Splash Water Park, Riverhead, New York

Tabor Cowden, Ellis & Associates – Walt Disney World, Orlando, Florida

Michael Friscia, Walt Disney World, Florida

Linda D. Frizzell, Ph.D.

Heather Hill, Paramount's Canada's Wonderland, Ontario, Canada

Robert Hollerbach, St. Paul Parks and Recreation, Minnesota

Eric Johnson, City of Pico Rivera, California

Tim Kopka, Oakland County Parks and Recreation, Michigan

Brenda Lloyd, Walt Disney World, Orlando, Florida

Jeremy Malone, Ellis & Associates

Denise McCoy, Everett Parks and Recreation, Washington

Eric McGinnis, Walt Disney World, Florida

Larry Newell, Ed.D., NREMT-P, Ellis & Associates

Emily Nolte, Ellis & Associates

Mark Oostman, Ellis & Associates

Mike Oostman, Ellis & Associates

Joe Pecoraro, Chicago Parks and Recreation

Gayle Strange, Rockford Park District, Rockford, Illinois

Kelly Werts, Sun Splash Water Park, Cape Coral, Florida

Lynn Waldorf, St. Paul Parks and Recreation, Minnesota

Norm Matzl for his contributions as leader, mentor, and manager of the advisory committee.

Tom Werts, Aquatic Consulting, Inc. who served as an advisory committee member and a writer for this second edition.

Carol Fick and Louise Priest for their significant editorial contributions.

And last, but not least, we gratefully acknowledge the thousands of NPWLTP lifeguards and instructors who have unselfishly given their time and expertise to help make this manual practical for new lifeguard candidates.

Introduction

COURSE OVERVIEW

Professional lifeguards prevent people from drowning. If lifeguards don't perform, people will die.

In 1998, Ellis & Associates (E&A) served over 500 client facilities including waterparks, public and private pools, and lakefront environments. E&A lifeguards protected over 60 million guests visiting these facilities and performed over 30 thousand rescues. In each of these situations, if the lifeguard had not intervened, a guest would have drowned.

Ellis & Associates' National Pool and Waterpark Lifeguard Training Program (NPWLTP) provides professional lifeguard training as one of the components of a comprehensive aquatic safety system. This program and system, developed and managed by E&A, protects guests and lifeguards from catastrophic injury and drowning.

The NPWLTP is designed for highly skilled and responsible individuals. This course will help you prepare for one of the most challenging jobs you will ever have. Few other positions carry the responsibility to guard, protect, and save human lives.

The purpose of the NPWLTP is to equip you with the skills and technical knowledge to become an effective member of your aquatic facility's Emergency Response Team.

Your National Pool and Waterpark Lifeguard (NPWL) license will show that you have participated in levels of training beyond a reasonable standard.

For waterpark personnel, your training will include rescue techniques specifically designed for use in moving water.

It is intended that the material in this textbook will be taught by an approved National Pool and Waterpark Lifeguard Instructor, or by an official instructor in an educational institution. Use of this manual by anyone untrained in NPWL teaching methods could result in injury to participants practicing rescue techniques.

The National Pool and Waterpark Lifeguard Training Program is divided into the following training courses:

- Shallow water lifeguard training
- Pool lifeguard training
- Special facilities lifeguard training

Your NPWLTP course is unlike any other lifeguard training course. Some of the skills you will learn in the NPWLTP course will be how to:

- Anticipate how and where incidents will occur
- Recognize incidents
- Effectively manage the incident with skills that work
- Think critically about complications that might be present in real situations
- Act in a professional manner
- Protect your safety and well-being

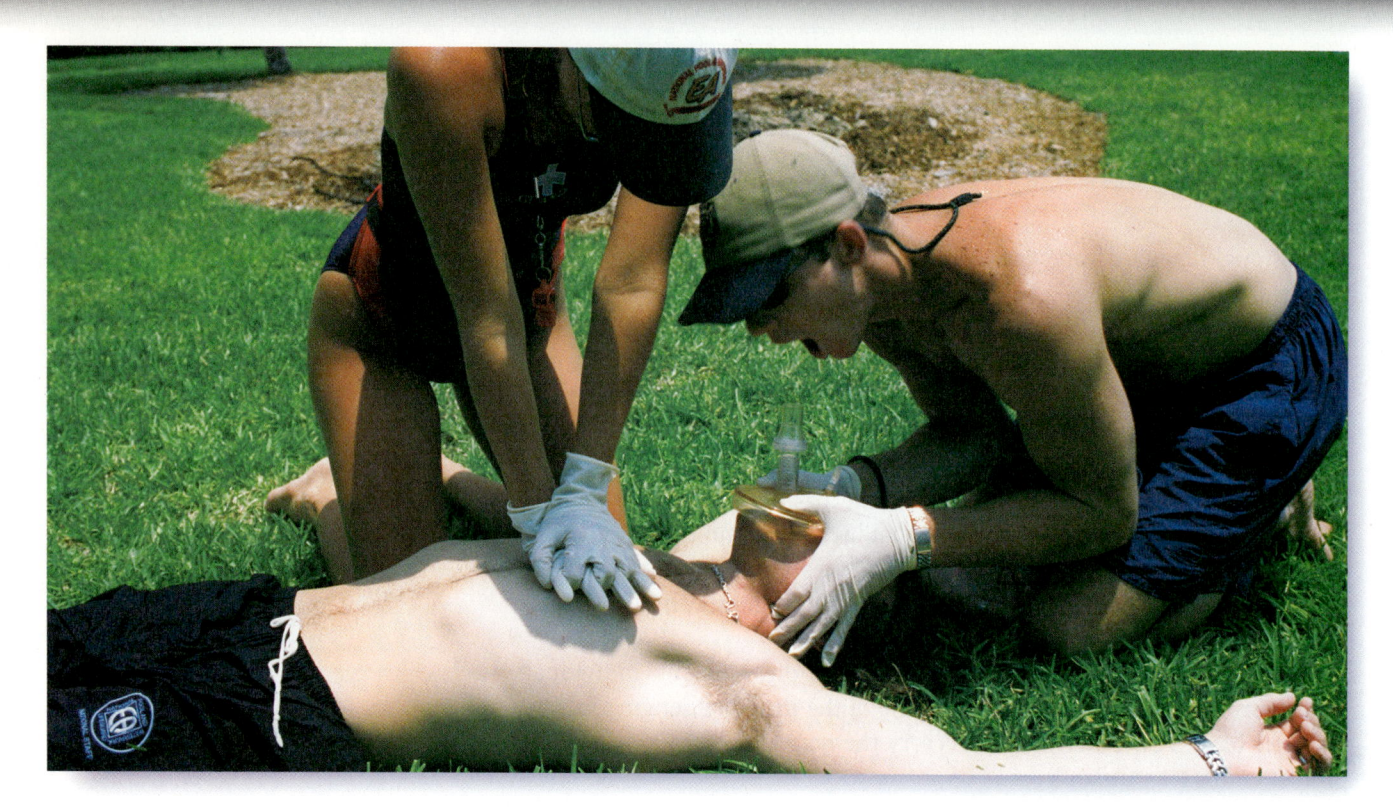

You must be able to react and make a rescue work without *stopping* to think about how to perform the various parts of a skill. *This course will help you build that confidence.* In class you will learn how to manage situations by "simulating" reality as closely as possible. You will learn skills that are safe, practical and that work.

As a professional lifeguard, you will have two primary responsibilities:

- Prevent aquatic emergencies
- Provide rescue and emergency care

At this point, *you should examine what you really think about lifeguarding.*

- *How do you view the job of lifeguarding?*
- *Is it "fun in the sun" all day?*

If you believe lifeguarding is a fun job that offers time to "take it easy" and "get a beautiful tan," you may want to select another job. Many lifeguards are athletic, physically attractive, active and young. It is fair to say that the public has this image of today's lifeguard.

Having a job with such "status" among your peers could tempt you to concentrate on the wrong people and places while you are lifeguarding. If you think a lifeguarding job will give you the opportunity to watch many good looking people, you are right. However, if you let yourself become *distracted* by such interests while you are supposed to be *protecting guests in your facility*, it could be the most tragic mistake you ever make. It is common for the glamour associated with lifeguarding to wear off two or three days after you begin working, and you discover what lifeguarding is truly about.

If you decide to proceed, and if you successfully complete the training and are employed as a lifeguard, it will undoubtedly become one of the most challenging and rewarding jobs you will ever experience.

COURSE INFORMATION

The following information outlines the various National Pool and Waterpark Lifeguard course requirements:

Minimum age to obtain license and validity period:

>Shallow water lifeguard: 15 / 1 year
>Pool Lifeguard: 15 / 1 year
>Special facilities lifeguard: 16 / 1 year

Prerequisite skills:

Swim distance using crawl or breaststroke without resting

>**Shallow water lifeguard:** 50 yards
>**Pool lifeguard:** 100 yards
>**Special facilities lifeguard:** 200 yards

Feet first surface dive, retrieve 10-pound brick and bring it to the wall from a depth of:

>**Shallow water lifeguard: 4 feet (must also swim a distance of 10 feet underwater)**
>**Pool lifeguard: 8 feet**
>**Special facilities lifeguard: 8 feet**

Treading water without using arms for:
>**Shallow water lifeguard:** None
>**Pool lifeguard:** 1 minute
>**Special facilities lifeguard:** 2 minutes

Facility where license is valid:
>**Shallow water lifeguard:** At any client facility where water is 4 feet deep or less.
>**Pool lifeguard:** Any client facility where the pool has not been classified as a "special facility" by Ellis & Associates.
>**Special facility lifeguard:** Any client facility that has been classified as a "special facility" by Ellis & Associates.

Qualifications for license renewal:

All courses:
- Meet all prerequisites for the regular course.
- Attend review/update class.
- Pass written and water practical examinations.

Course Rules:

All courses:
- Enter the water feet first at **ALL TIMES**.
- When using a rescue tube, keep it between the guest and yourself.
- Wear hat, sunscreen, and sunglasses when you are outdoors.

General Course Information:

1. All courses include Lifeguard First Responder first aid skills and National Safety Council CPR certification for adults, children and infants.
2. If you do not pass all the requirements for **any** class you are taking, you must take the **entire course** again to be eligible for a license.

General information about the NPWLTP license:

1. Your license becomes valid only when you:
   - Meet prerequisites
   - Demonstrate proper attitude, maturity and judgement
   - Pass all practical (water and CPR) examinations
   - Pass all written examinations with an 80% score
   - Complete site-specific training at your facility

Your license may be revoked for cause at any time. Read the license agreement carefully before you sign it to be sure you understand your responsibilities.

2. Educational Market:

    Students successfully completing a training course taught by an Ellis & Associates approved instructor in an educational institution (high school, vocational/technical, college and university) are eligible to receive a license as National Pool and Waterpark Lifeguards. Students can obtain a license request form from their instructor. This form must be completed by the student and verified by the instructor. The completed form should be submitted to the following address for processing:

    License Request Department
    Ellis & Associates
    3506 Spruce Park Circle
    Kingwood, Texas 77345

Please allow three to four weeks for processing.

part ONE
1

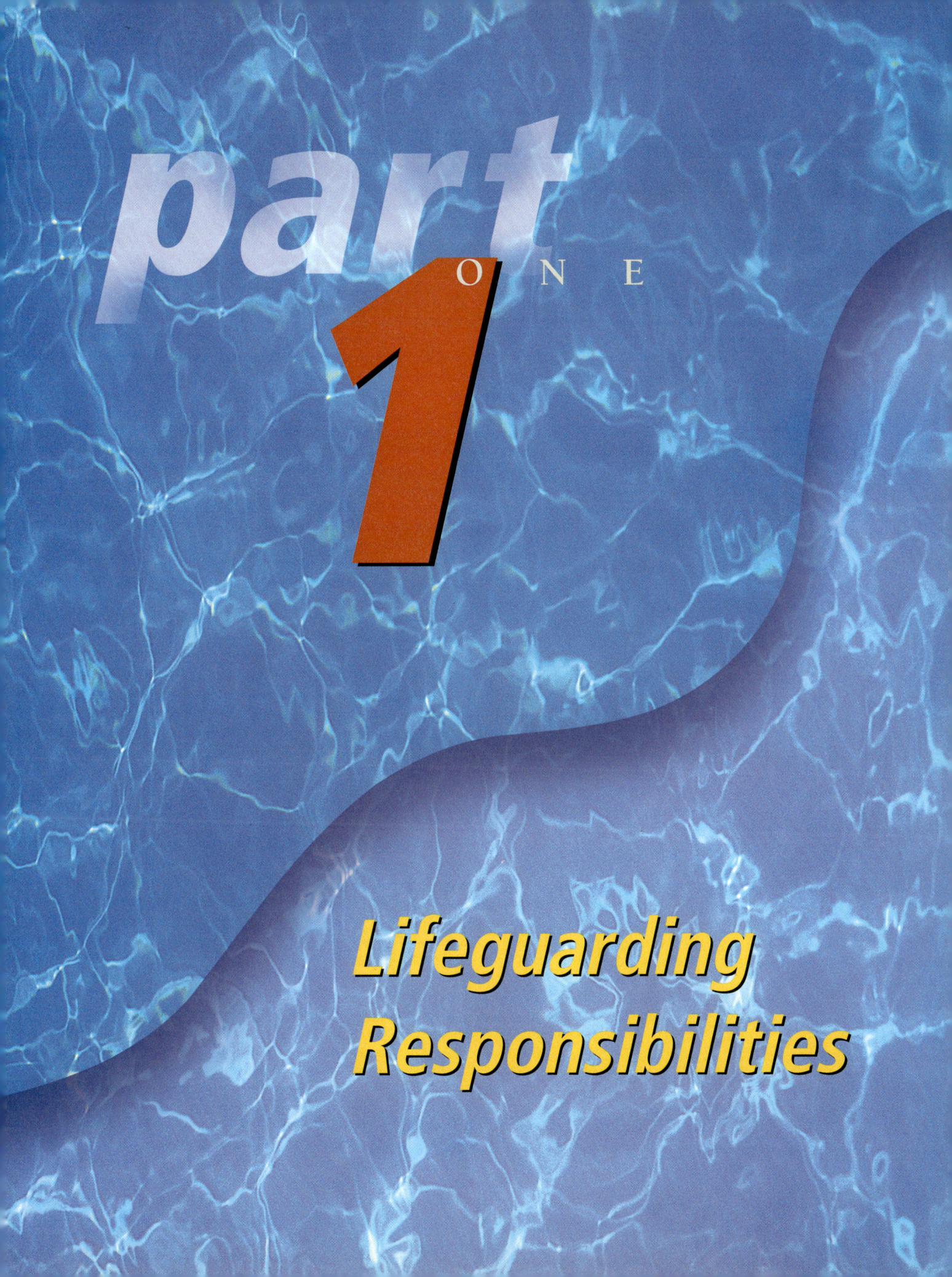

Lifeguarding Responsibilities

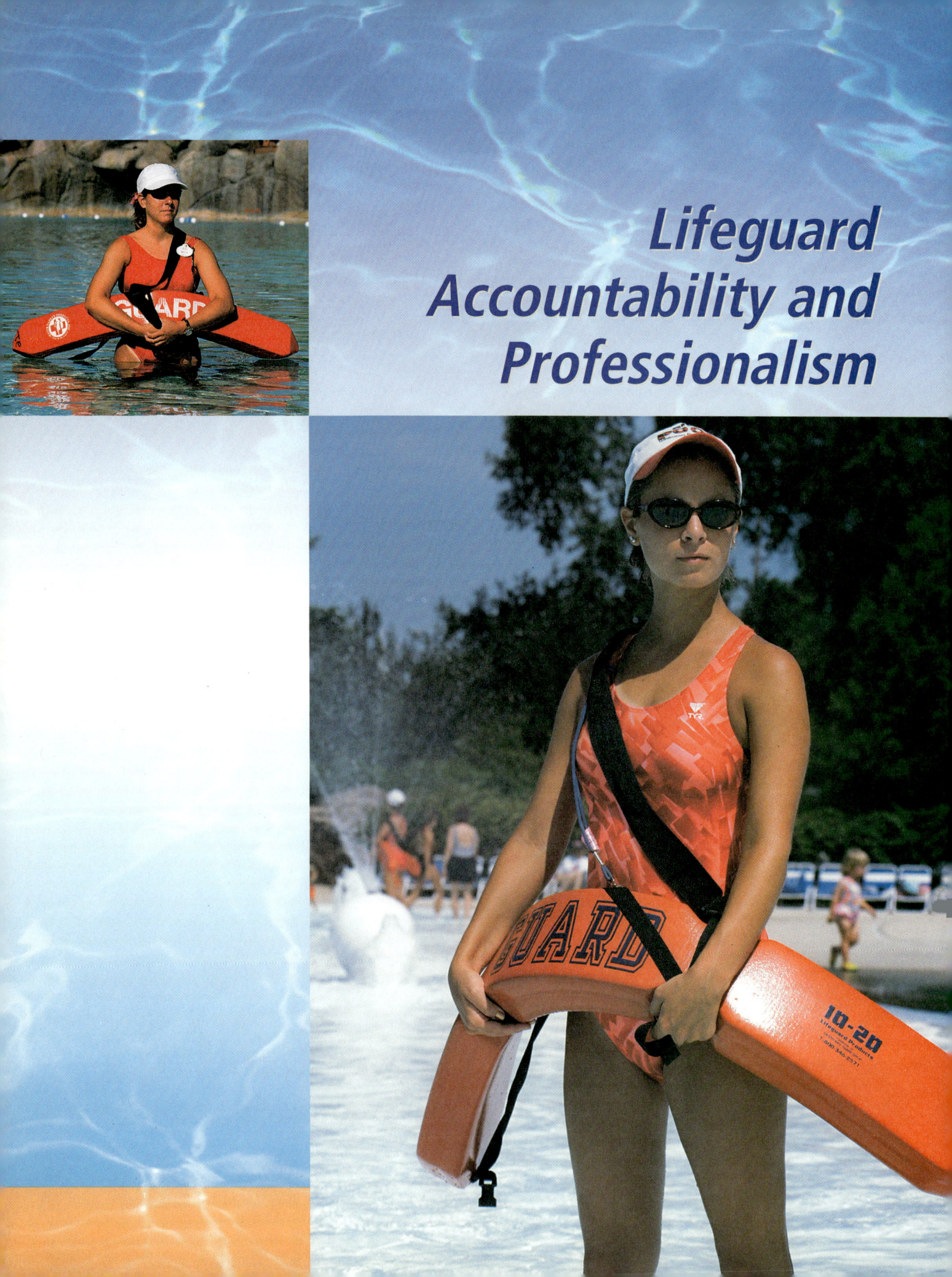

Lifeguard Accountability and Professionalism

chapter 1

OBJECTIVES

After reading this chapter and completing the related course work, you should be ab le to:

1. Identify ways to project a professional lifeguard image.
2. Explain the "Golden Rule" of guest relations.
3. Understand the concept of and the reason for the auditing process.
4. Describe how an audit is conducted.
5. Identify ways to ensure a successful audit.

The National Pool and Waterpark Lifeguard Training Program (NPWLTP) teaches you how to act and respond as a professional lifeguard. You will learn how to anticipate, recognize, and manage an aquatic emergency. **You** are the critical, frontline component in a comprehensive, professional water safety and risk management system coordinated by Ellis & Associates.

You will receive a National Pool and Waterpark Lifeguard license following your successful completion of this program that has become the "Standard of Care" in the aquatic industry. Our safety records and statistics document that Ellis & Associates' client facilities provide **the highest standard of care for their guests**.

Ellis & Associates, along with your facility's management, and insurance company are interested in preventing losses and providing a safe environment. They work together in the total risk management program.

As an Ellis & Associates lifeguard, you are stating that you are willing to accept the responsibility and accountability that go along with the job. This means you will look and behave as a professional at all times when you are working. You also will maintain your personal skills and knowledge at a "test-ready" level. Whether your job is part time, seasonal, or full time, you will be judged as a *professional*, one who is able to provide the "Standard of Care" required for the safety of your guests. You will be compared with lifeguards at facilities across the country.

As a professional lifeguard, you are accountable on three levels:

- **You are accountable to the GUESTS who use your facility**.
  This means that you will provide a safe environment for them when they come into your facility. You will protect the guests, minimizing hazardous situations whenever possible. You will respond appropriately to emergency situations and provide the necessary care. You will be friendly and courteous at all times.

- **You are accountable to your EMPLOYER.**
  You will be expected to perform the duties of your job. You will adhere to the objectives established by your organization. You will give your employer the time, energy, and dedication it takes to do the job. You will perform at or above your employer's expectations.

- **You are accountable to YOURSELF.**
  You have to believe in yourself. You are responsible for human life. You have to be sure of yourself and your actions. You have to know all of the responsibilities of your position, and must maintain your knowledge and skill levels. You must recognize, respond to, and manage aquatic emergencies quickly and effectively.

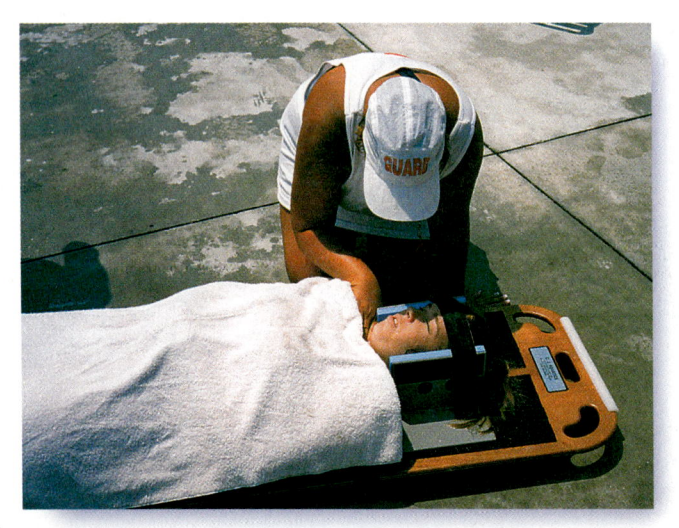

FIG 1.1 Provide proper care to guests when needed.

CHAPTER 1 • LIFEGUARD ACCOUNTABILITY AND PROFESSIONALISM 5

You will be evaluated as a *professional lifeguard* on a daily basis, by both the guests and your employer, while you are at work. You should also evaluate yourself on a continuous basis. Ask yourself: Am I the type of person with whom I would entrust the lives of my family?

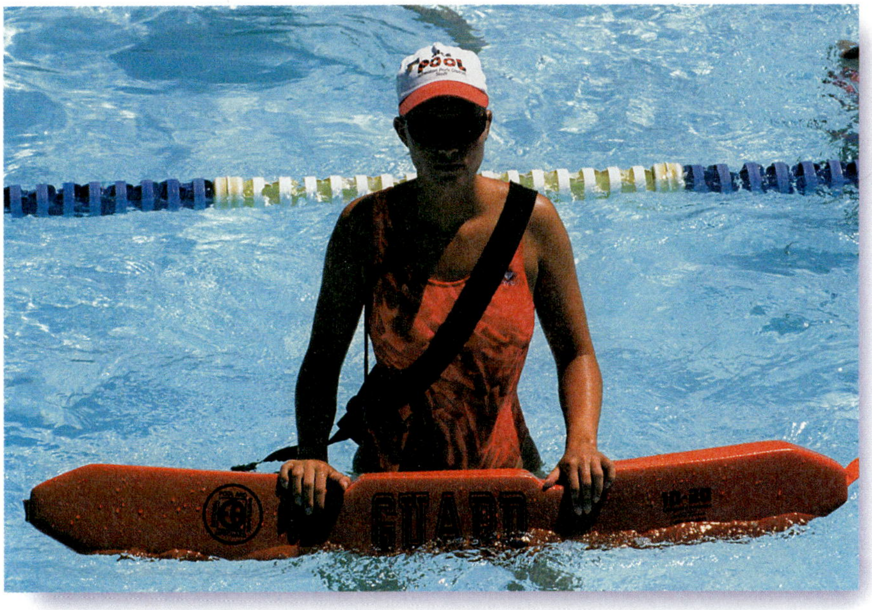

PROFESSIONAL IMAGE

As a lifeguard, you are part of the facility's team. You contribute to the total operation. If you look and act like a professional, the facility looks like a professionally run facility.

Guests at the facility will constantly be watching you. You are "on stage." Do you look and act "the part"? If they view you as a professional, they will respond to your requests and directions because they believe in you. If they have no respect for you or your position, they will disregard your requests.

FIG 1.2 As a lifeguard, you need to look professional and be easily recognizable.

You can establish and maintain your professional image by being:

- **Punctual**—arrive at work ahead of time.
- **In full uniform**—look neat and clean, easily identified as a lifeguard.
- **Prepared**—bring the items you need to do the job (whistle, sun protection, etc.).
- **Pleasant**—cordial to guests and co-workers at all times.
- **Attentive**—keep your eyes on the guests and avoid distractions.

GUEST RELATIONS

Part of your responsibility is to make the guests feel welcome at your facility. Base your actions on the *Golden Rule: Treat people like you would like to be treated.*

The guests who visit your facility may be of diverse cultures. You must be sensitive to their beliefs and customs. Be open to the ideas and input of guests and co-workers from various cultures. Avoid being biased or judging others by their background.

Remember, dealing with people—the public, co-workers, and supervisors—becomes easier with experience. There are many styles and approaches for dealing with people that are equally effective. You must use a style and approach that suit both your personality and scope of responsibility.

LIFEGUARD AUDITS

A major component of the Ellis & Associates total risk management program is the independent audit. Ellis & Associates staff will visit your facility unannounced to conduct these audits. During the visit, the auditor will observe you and other lifeguards in the normal day-to-day operation of your facility. You will be evaluated on several aspects of your professionalism. You will be asked to manage simulated aquatic emergencies, during which your ability will be observed and documented. You will also be evaluated on how well you participate as a member of your emergency response team.

The purpose of an audit is to evaluate your job performance during a specific time of observation. It is not the job, nor the intent of the auditor to catch you doing something wrong. The auditor must determine whether you and your team would be able to anticipate, recognize, and manage an aquatic emergency if one did occur. Your activity, including scanning skills, posture, and use of rescue equipment will be observed and documented. Your professionalism and diligence will be evaluated, along with your personal rescue skills.

Your performance will be documented in both written and video form. This information will become part of your facility's risk management documentation. Professional lifeguards perform well during audits because they are committed to preventing, recognizing, and managing aquatic emergencies; they are always on the job.

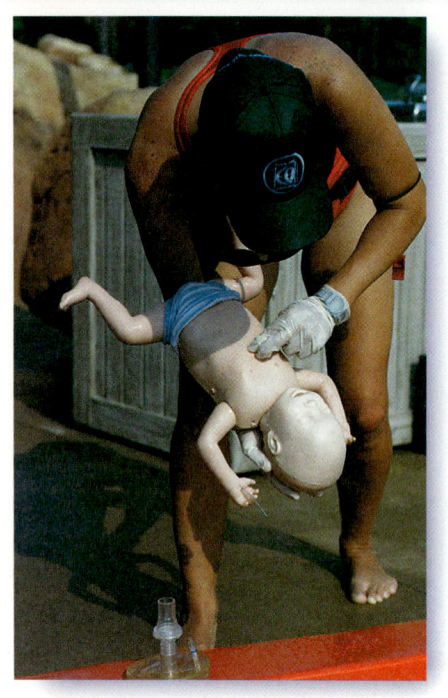

FIG 1.3 Lifeguard demonstrating personal skill during an audit.

REVIEW QUESTIONS

1. (T) (F) The National Pool and Waterpark Lifeguard License has become the standard of care in the aquatic industry.

2. (T) (F) As a lifeguard, you are one component in a total risk management program at your facility.

3. When an auditor visits your facility, he or she will document if you could (a) _____,

   (b) _____,

   and (c) _____
   an aquatic emergency during that specific time of observation.

4. Part of an audit will also include reevaluating your _____ and _____ , along with your rescue skills.

5. (T) (F) Professional lifeguards perform well during audits, because they perform well every minute they are on the job.

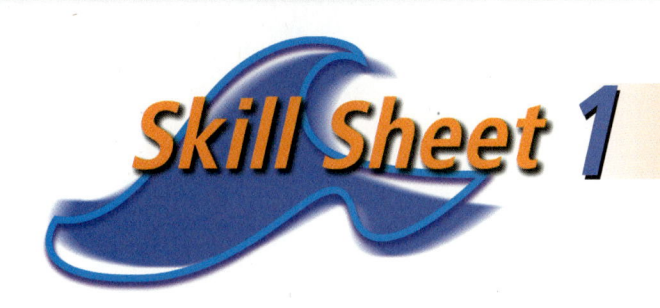

CHAPTER 1 • LIFEGUARD ACCOUNTABILITY AND PROFESSIONALISM 7

Skill Sheet 1

AUDIT PERFORMANCE

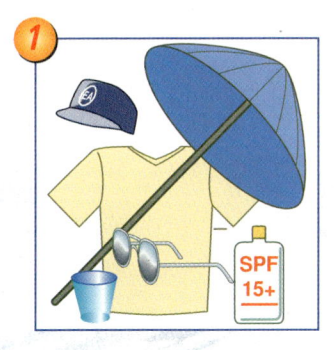

1. Sun Protection
Sunglasses, hydration, and shade.

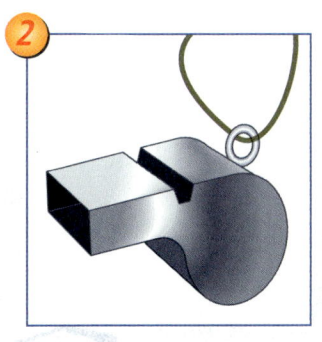

2. Whistle
Blow firmly; no twirling.

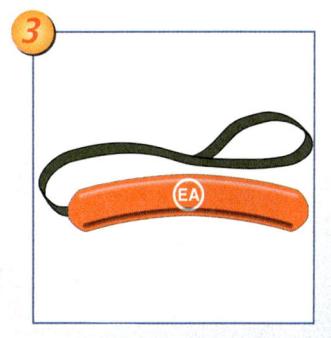

3. Rescue Tube
Hold professionally; gather strap.

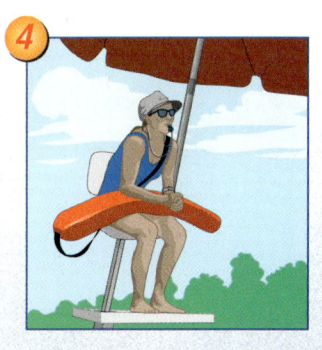

4. Posture
Feet flat; anticipatory.

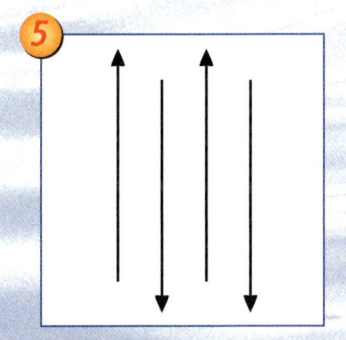

5. Scanning
10/20 Protection Rule; have a pattern; know your zone.

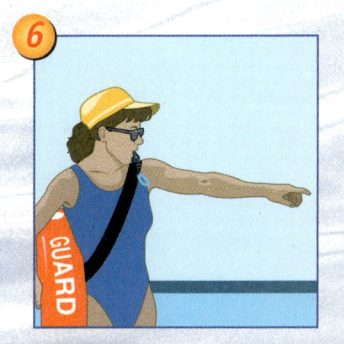

6. Communication
Golden Rule.

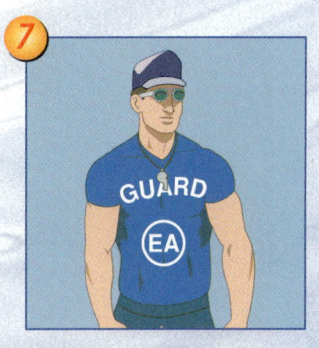

7. Professionalism and Uniform
Easily recognizable.

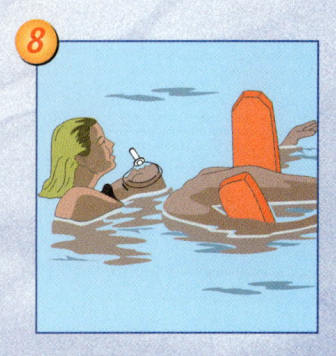

8. Rescue Skills
Attend frequent in-services. Always be "rescue ready."

KEY POINTS:

- Practice skills.
- Be responsible.
- Be mature.
- Do your job well.
- Be a professional lifeguard.

CRITICAL THINKING:

For each of the categories above, what would you consider:

- Exceeding the standard?
- Meeting the standard?
- Failing to meet the standard?

Awareness and Recognition

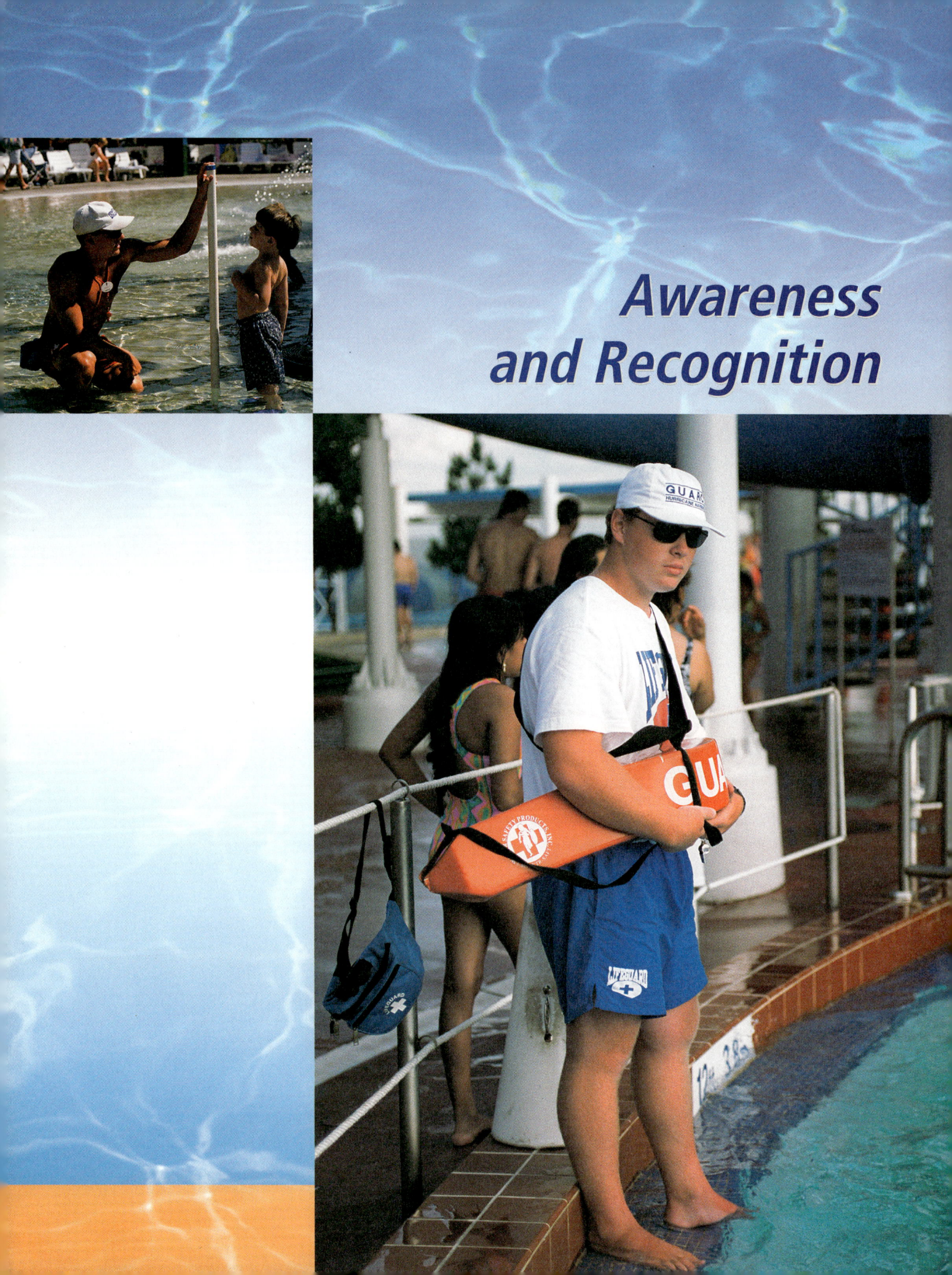

chapter 2

OBJECTIVES

After reading this chapter and completing the related course work, you should be able to:

1. Explain and implement the 10/20 Protection Rule.

2. Explain the importance of diligence while scanning your zone.

3. Demonstrate proper scannning techniques.

4. Describe the different behavior patterns of a guest in distress and a guest who is near-drowning.

5. Explain the various phases of the drowning process.

6. Describe the different types of drowning.

7. Explain the different situations that lifeguards should be aware of in order to anticipate potentially hazardous situations.

8. Demonstrate the proper procedure for conducting a lifeguard rotation.

10/20 Protection Rule means that:

- The lifeguard has 10 seconds to recognize that a guest is in distress.

- The lifeguard then has 20 seconds to reach the guest and begin to render aid.

10/3 Minute Protection Rule:

The 10/3 Minute Protection Rule states that the entire designated lakefront swimming area must be able to be searched within 3 minutes.

Consider how you will actually spend your time as a lifeguard. You will not always be making rescues and caring for the guests. Instead, most of your time will be spent lifeguarding—preventing potentially hazardous situations, watching people, and protecting them.

THE 10/20 PROTECTION RULE

The National Pool and Waterpark Lifeguard Training Program is based on the 10/20 Protection Rule. Studies have shown that if you can manage a guest in distress within the first 30 seconds, you can minimize the danger in a hazardous situation and possibly prevent a guest from drowning.

The *10/20 Protection Rule* can help facilities determine appropriate lifeguard stations and zones.

Each zone will have its own unique scanning problems. Each scan of the zone should be completed within a time frame that allows the lifeguard to recognize that someone is in distress and react to the situation. Ask yourself the question: "Can the 10/20 Protection Rule be followed in this situation?"

You may need to continually adjust your scanning pattern to accommodate certain situations in your zone. For example, you may have several different groups of guests in your zone. You will want to return your focus to those areas more frequently, or pause a little longer on certain individuals in those areas.

The only facilities not required to use the 10/20 Protection Rule are protected lakefronts and other open water areas that have been granted a variance by Ellis & Associates. These special areas can be protected following a *10/3 Minute Rule*, which states that the entire lakefront area must be able to be searched within 3 minutes.

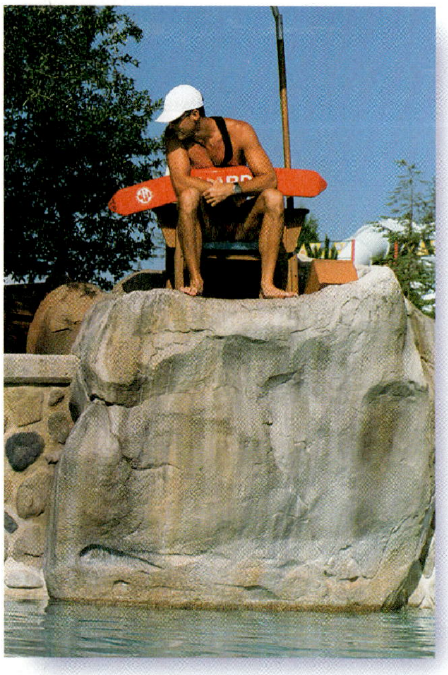

FIG 2.1 Understand and implement the 10/20 and 10/3 Protection Rules.

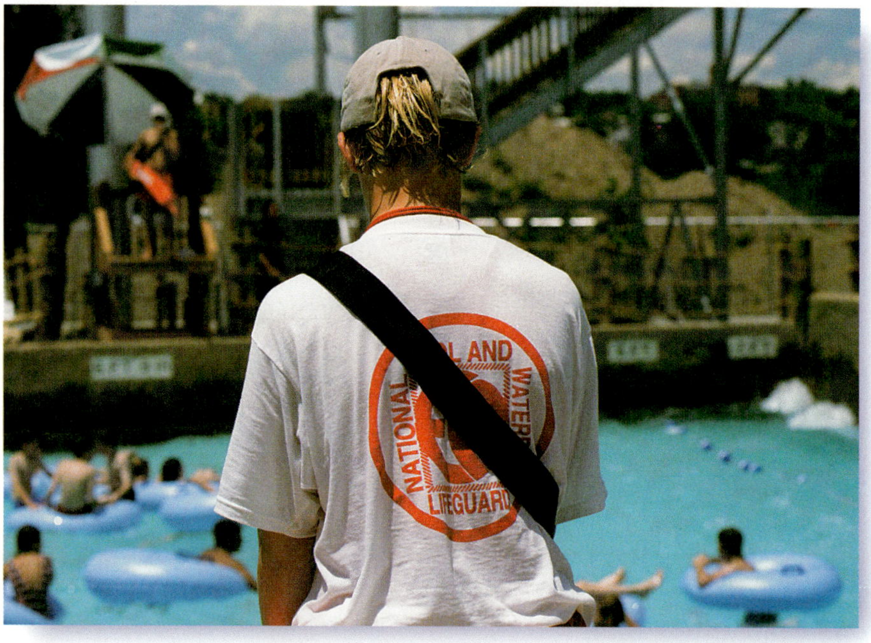

FIG 2.2 Remember the 10/20 rule at all times so you can be ready for any situation.

CHAPTER 2 • AWARENESS AND RECOGNITION 11

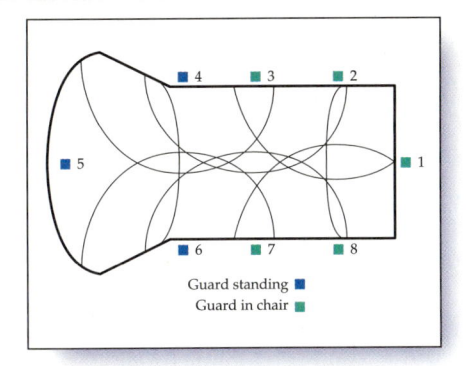

FIG 2.3a Lifeguard zone coverage.

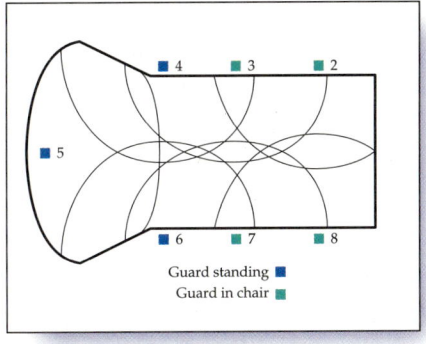

FIG 2.3b Lifeguard zone coverage with no lifeguard in position 1.

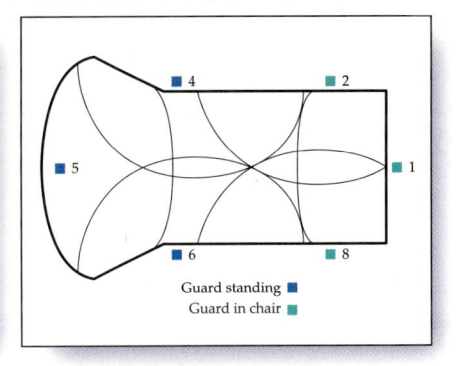

FIG 2.3c Lifeguard zone coverage, no lifeguards 3 and 7.

ZONES

Each lifeguard station, or position, is assigned a specific area of responsibility, or *zone*.

In a multiple lifeguard facilty, the zone will be different for each position at your facility. You must be able to clearly see every part of your zone. In order to physically do this you:

- Cannot allow yourself to be distracted, even for a second, or some part of your zone will not be scanned.

- Must continually move your head. You cannot just move your eyes.

- Must be able to swim to the farthest part of your zone within 20 seconds.

- Must be able to identify the problem areas or blind spots and take corrective measures to insure that these areas are being protected.

Every facility should have a chart showing the zones for each lifeguard position. Depending on the number of guests in the pool, these zones may be adjusted. As a lifeguard, it is your responsibility to know the exact area you are accountable for when you are in your station. This means you could be responsible for knowing several lifeguard zones, depending on your location, the design of the pool, and the number of guests in the pool.

Figures 2.3a-c show a standard wave pool with lifeguard positions on each side, a shallow water position and a position on the head wall. Each zone is indicated by an arc, showing the proper coverage for a normal load of guests. Notice that every area of the pool is scanned by at least one lifeguard. Most of the pool is scanned by two lifeguards. And in some areas, three zones overlap.

If positions are eliminated, as they sometimes are when there are few guests, the coverage would be shifted to other lifeguards.

Focus...

Keep your eyes on the water, even if:

There is a large grassy area on the other side of the pool where a lot of people are sunbathing.

There are several attractive guests in brief bathing suits, lying on the grass.

The crowd is noisy, there is music playing, and you can barely hear yourself talk.

A guest walks up to you and starts complaining that there are not enough lounge chairs.

There is a blazing hot summer sun and you have a dry throat.

DILIGENCE

You must avoid being distracted while you are lifeguarding. Staring at the water is not particularly exciting; in fact, it can become routine and boring. Even if a pool has guests in it, the job can be as bad as sitting and staring at a bathtub full of water. When there are no guests in the pool—just flat, calm water—you must continue to scan because guests may enter the pool at any moment.

You cannot become distracted, even for a few seconds. It only takes a second for a person to slip under the water. The job is tough and demanding. There can be no compromise.

Diligence is the constant and careful attention to your area of responsibility. Do not compromise the safety of the guests, no matter what the circumstances. Diligence is one of the most important characteristics you can develop as a professional lifeguard.

SCANNING

As you diligently watch your zone, your head and eyes need to move in regular patterns.

This movement is known as *scanning*.

There are several scanning patterns that are commonly used by lifeguards. These include the six paterns shown in figures 2.4a-f.

Up and Down (Figure 2.4a)

Side to Side (Figure 2.4b)

Circular (Figure 2.4c)

Double Triangle (Figure 2.4d)

Figure Eight (Figure 2.4e)

Alphabet (Figure 2.4f)

The shape of your zone is not important. It could be a rectangle or a semicircle, or it could be defined by the shape of your facility. The important point is to be sure that zones overlap, so that no part of the facility is left uncovered. You can develop a scanning pattern that works for you. You may also find that changing your scanning pattern occasionally is helpful in maintaining your diligence and attention.

If there is a glare on the surface, you need to physically change your position so that you can see the entire zone.

With experience, you will develop your own scanning technique. Here are some suggestions to help you begin:

1. Know the exact area to be scanned and develop a pattern that covers all of it.

2. Know where your area overlaps with another lifeguard's area. You should know the overlapping regions for each lifeguard position in your facility.

3. Be sure that you check your entire zone each time you scan, regardless of guest concentration.

CHAPTER 2 • AWARENESS AND RECOGNITION   13

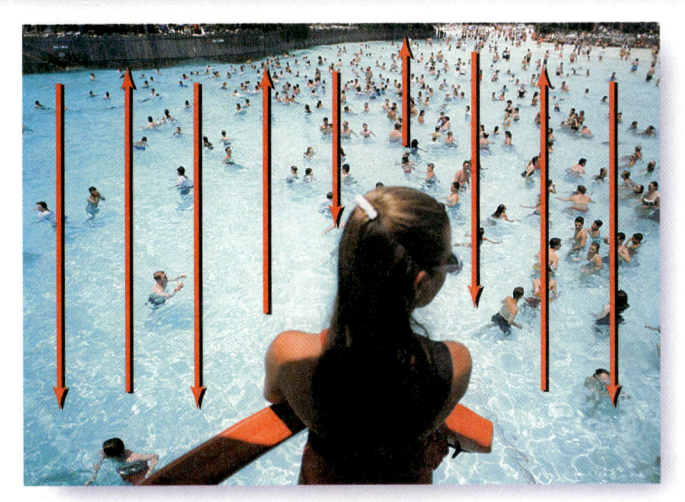

FIG 2.4a Scanning pattern: Up and Down.

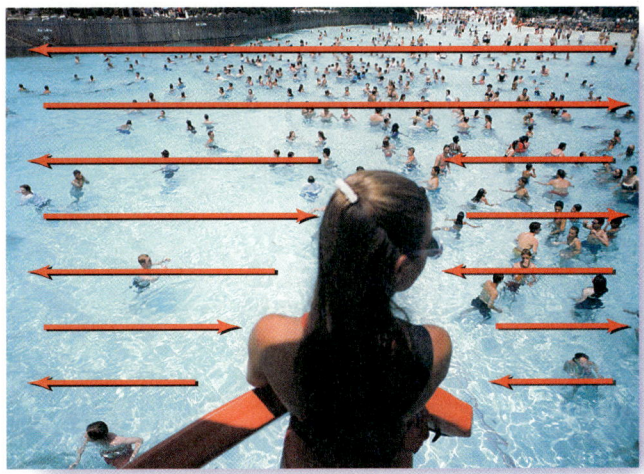

FIG 2.4b Scanning pattern: Side to Side.

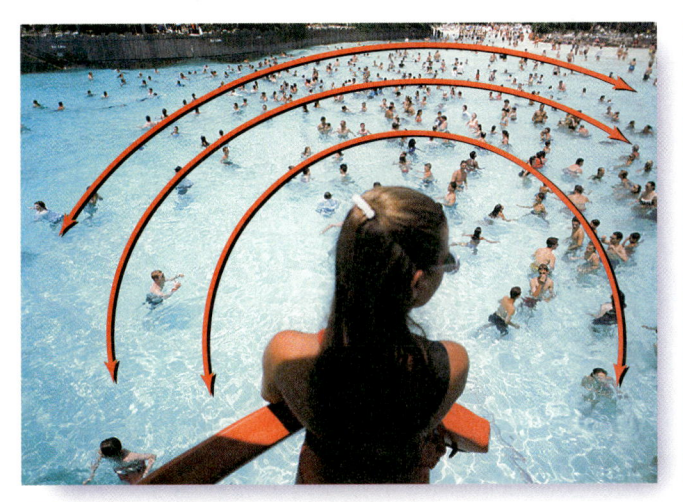

FIG 2.4c Scanning pattern: Circular.

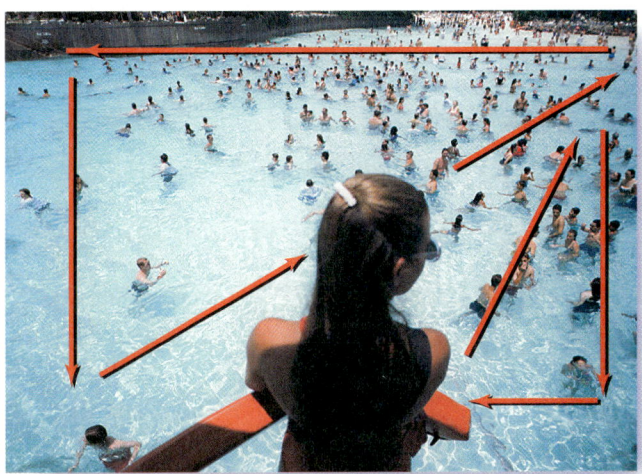

FIG 2.4d Scanning pattern: Double Triangle.

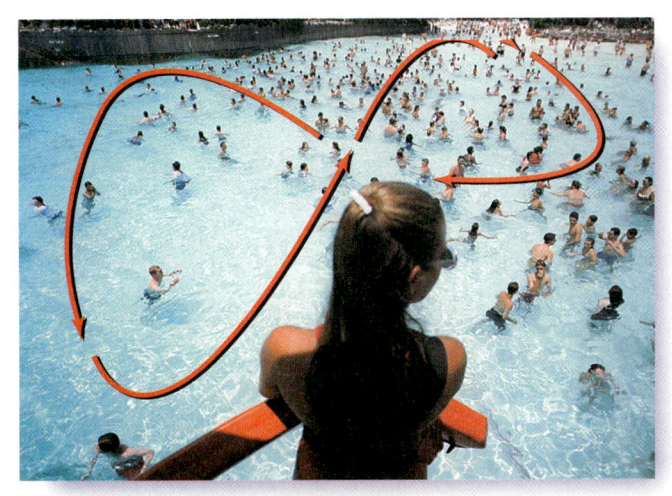

FIG 2.4e Scanning pattern: Figure Eight.

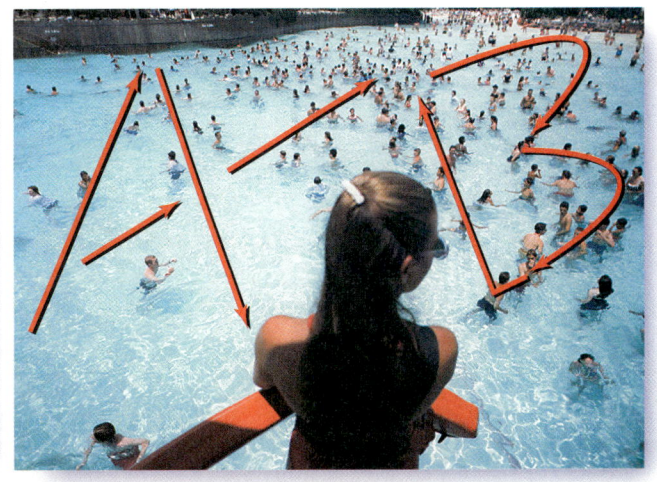

FIG 2.4f Scanning pattern: Alphabet (A, B, C)— progress through the alphabet and change your patterns.

**Guard from the bottom up—
IF YOU DON'T KNOW—GO!**

4. Know the "high risk" areas and blind spots in your zone. You may need more time to scan these areas.
5. Ask the lifeguard you are relieving if there are any special circumstances you should know about.
6. Don't forget that the pool is three-dimensional—view the surface, the middle water, and the bottom.
7. Periodically check the lifeguard that would back you up and the lifeguard that you would back up.
8. Don't forget to scan directly beneath your stand and to the sides.
9. Be active—move your eyes and your head.
10. Maintain good posture. It helps to both stay alert and maintain a professional appearance.

RECOGNITION OF A GUEST IN DISTRESS

A guest in distress in the water will be in one of three locations:

1. On the surface.
2. Below the surface, within arms' reach.
3. Below the surface, beyond arms' reach.

In all three of these locations, the guest will either be breathing or not breathing. There are certain behavior patterns that a guest in distress will usually exhibit:

- **Body position**—The body will come to a diagonal or vertical position. There is no kick and the arms are extended out to the side. It may look like the guest is trying to reach or grab for something. The guest may have turned toward safety (a lifeguard position, a wall, or a lane line).
- **Movement**—There will be little or no forward movement.
- **Appearance**—Long hair may be covering the face. All effort is expended to stay above the water. The eyes may be tightly closed or opened very wide.
- **Breathing**—In an attempt to breathe, the head will usually be back in order to get the mouth as high as possible. The guest is attempting to concentrate only on breathing while on the surface. The mouth will be kept closed when underwater. There will be little or no calling out for help.

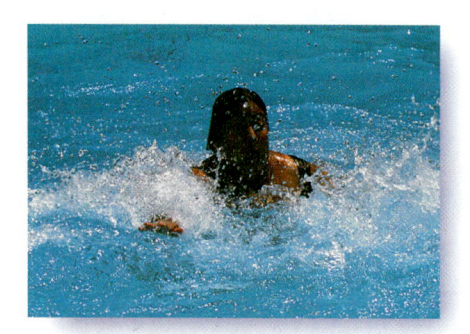

FIG 2.5 A guest in distress on the surface.

It is easier to recognize a guest in distress on the surface than one who is under the surface. That is why it is important to scan dimensionally. Even in a clear pool, it may be difficult to recognize a body under water. The number of guests in the water, water movement, glare, or reflection may make it almost impossible to see under the surface.

A body on the bottom of the pool may look only like a blurred spot. When water clarity and crowd conditions allow—guard from the bottom up. If you notice anything on the bottom of the pool and can't identify it, **GO!—IF YOU DON'T KNOW—GO!**

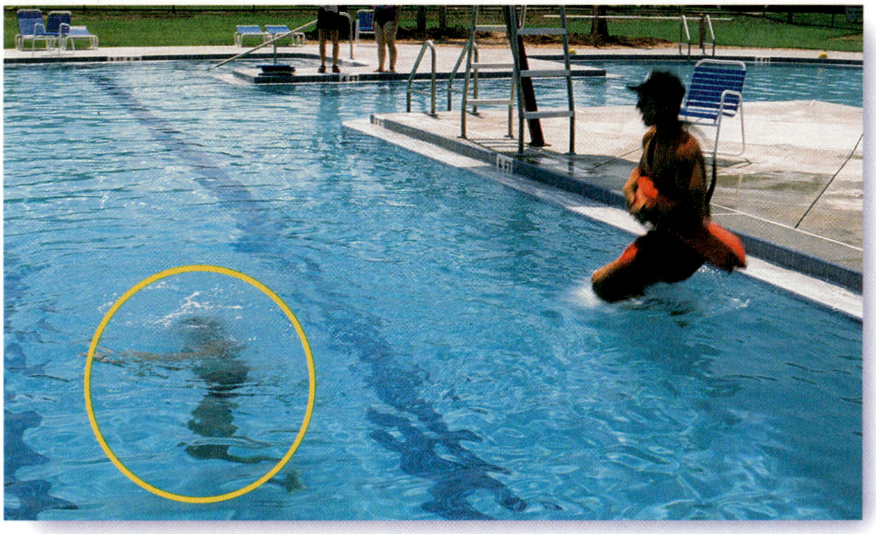

CHAPTER 2 • AWARENESS AND RECOGNITION   15

FIG 2.6 A body on the bottom may be difficult to see.

Any **lack of movement** demands your immediate attention, quick evaluation, and appropriate response. The faster you recognize a guest in distress, the more effective you will be in handling the incident.

You should be prepared for all types of situations. For example, a guest who has lost his balance may be unable to regain his footing, even in shallow water. An inexperienced swimmer who becomes tired in moving deep water could panic and grab another guest. These situations could easily turn into drownings. Your diligence, attention to detail, and scanning patterns could prevent such drownings.

THE DROWNING PROCESS

An understanding of the drowning process will help you recognize a guest who needs immediate assistance. A more thorough discussion of the physiology of drowning will be covered in later chapters.

A guest who is drowning can slip beneath the surface in as little as 20 seconds. There is a recognized pattern to the drowning process. The time span for the complete process may vary from seconds to minutes. Children seem to move through the drowning process more quickly than adults. Their pattern of distress may include a slight struggle once completely submerged, followed immediately by unconsciousness. A child may appear to be "bobbing" in the water. This is an attempt to get to the surface. Recognition, reaction, and treatment by the lifeguard may be the difference between life and death. Following are the stages of a drowning.

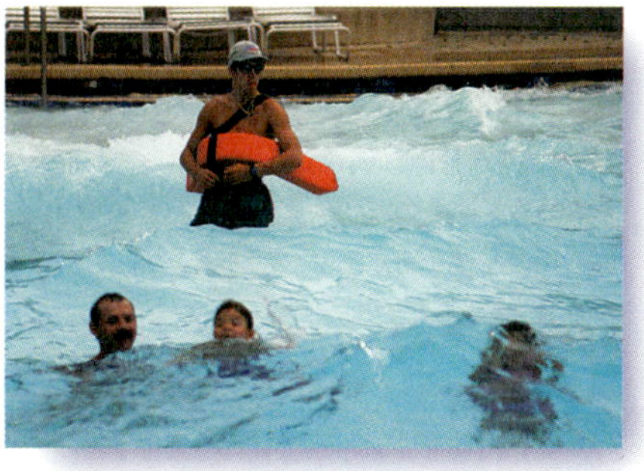

FIG 2.7 An inexperienced swimmer in water over his head, or unable to regain his footing, could panic.

Surprise

Initially, the guest recognizes the danger and is afraid.

What you will see, as a lifeguard:

- The guest is in a vertical or diagonal body position.
- There is little or no leg movement.

- The arms are at or near the surface, making random "grasping" or "flapping" motions.
- The head is tilted back, with face upward.
- The guest may, or may not be making any sounds. This guest is more concerned with getting air than with calling out for help.

Involuntary Breath Holding

During the drowning process, water enters the mouth and causes the *epiglottis* to close over the airway.

What you will see, as a lifeguard:

- There may be a continued attempt to struggle.
- Usually, there is no sound.
- The guest is not breathing.

This guest is not getting oxygen and will become unconscious.

Unconsciousness

The guest will not move. The guest is in **Respiratory Arrest**. The breathing process has stopped.

What you will see, as a lifeguard:

- There is no movement.
- The guest may sink to the bottom, either slowly or rapidly, depending on factors such as the amount of air left in the lungs, body weight, and muscle mass.

The guest will remain unconscious (and die) unless breathing is reestablished.

Hypoxic Convulsions

Because of the lack of oxygen in the brain, the guest may look as if he or she is having a convulsion.

What you see, as a lifeguard:

- The skin turns blue, especially in the lips and the beds of the fingernails.
- The guest may appear to be rigid or stiff.
- There may be violent jerking.
- There may be frothing at the mouth.

The guest will remain unconscious (and die) unless breathing and circulation are reestablished by rescue breathing and/or CPR, after the convulsions have subsided.

Clinical Death

Normally, **Clinical Death** occurs when breathing and circulation have stopped. The guest is in **Cardiac Arrest**. The heart has ceased to pump blood and function. The vital organs are no longer receiving oxygen-rich blood.

CHAPTER 2 • AWARENESS AND RECOGNITION

What you will see, as a lifeguard:
- The lack of oxygen causes the skin to turn blue, particularly in the lips and the beds of the fingernails.
- The pupils of the guest's eyes will dilate (widen).
- The pulse will be absent.
- The guest will not be breathing.

If you begin cardiopulminoary resuscitation (CPR) within the first 4 minutes of when the guest's heart stops, and provide difibrillation (electric shock) quickly thereafter, there is a good chance that he will not have permanent brain damage.

After 4 minutes without oxygen, brain cells will begin to die, and irreversible brain damage occurs. This is called *Biological Death*.

As a lifeguard, you must realize that even if CPR efforts are successful at the scene, many drowning victims die later as a result of secondary complications. This is another reason why it is so important to activate the Emergency Medical Services System. The drowning guest needs to get advanced life support as quickly as possible.

TYPES OF DROWNING

Silent Drowning

Lifeguards are given no warning signs of *silent drownings*. The guest does not struggle on the surface. This can be caused by various physical conditions or situations, such as:

- Heart attack
- Head Injury
- Stroke
- Shallow water blackout
- Alcohol or other drugs
- Epileptic seizure

Wet Drowning

Research indicates that approximately 80% of all drownings are *wet drownings*. Wet drownings occur when the epiglottis relaxes because of lack of oxygen, and opens the airway, allowing water to enter the lungs.

Dry Drowning

Dry drowning, or asphyxiation, is caused when water makes contact with the epiglottis and causes it to close over the airway. This prevents air from entering the air passages, and the dry drowning guest suffocates.

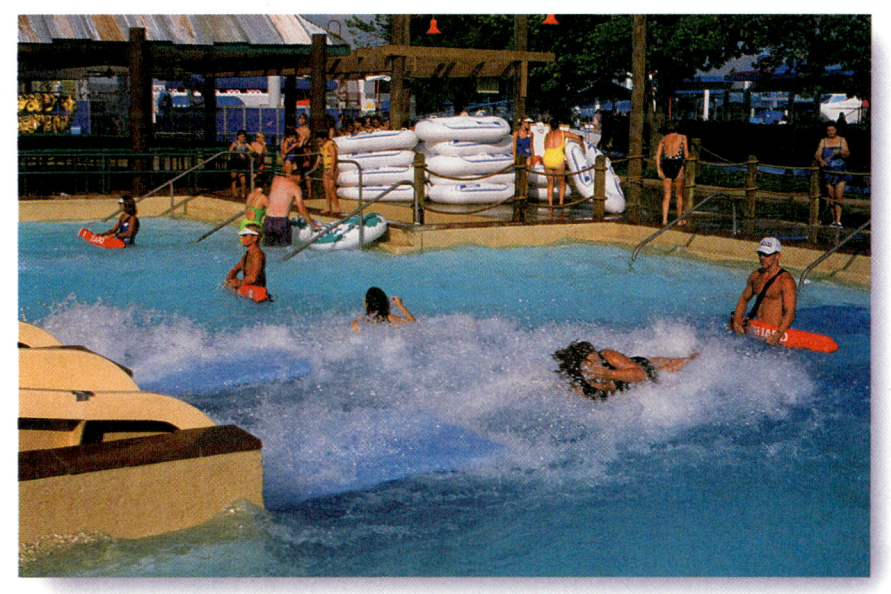

FIG 2.8 High velocity activities, such as water slides, have a potential for dry drowning.

Drowning Comparison

Wet Drowning	Dry Drowning
• Accounts for approximately 80% of drownings.	• Accounts for approximately 20% of drownings.
• Water enters the guest's lungs.	• The guest suffocates from lack of oxygen.
• Usually causes death within 3 to 6 minutes from immersion.	• Usually occurs within 6 to 10 minutes after water forces the epiglottis to close over the airway.

Dry drownings generally occur during activities which involve the use of speed slides, diving boards, or slides that end in a free-fall from a height.

As a lifeguard, you may see the guest choking or having a gagging reaction. You should immediately remove the guest from the water. After the reactions have stopped, and the guest is breathing without any difficulty, he may be released.

SPECIAL CONCERNS

Now you know what signs to look for to identify that a guest is in distress. You must also be aware that there are certain situations that will allow you to anticipate potential incidents before they occur.

There are three categories of concern:

1. **GUESTS**—everyone who enters your facility has the potential for becoming distressed.
2. **LOCATION**—places where guests are most likely to become distressed.
3. **TIMES**—times of the day that statistically have had high rescue rates.

All of these categories have been determined by actual rescue statistics involving millions of guests and thousands of documented rescues compiled by Ellis & Associates.

Guests—Who Are They?

The guests who enter your facility can be grouped according to their potential for becoming distressed:

1. **Children between the ages of 7 and 12**—Smaller individuals, who are not very strong, may have less skill in the water, and are less aware of danger.
2. **Parents with small children**—They may not have the swimming skill to support both themselves and their children.
3. **Intoxicated guests**—Even one drink can slow down reaction times, as well as impair the ability to control movement and balance.
4. **Extreme body proportions**—Guests with unusual or extreme body proportions will react differently in the water than an average person's physique.

5. **Guests wearing lifejackets**—Lifejackets usually suggest that a guest is not confident in the water. Many guests are not used to the feel of a lifejacket. It may not fit properly, or it may not hold them up at a level they feel comfortable with. A guest may easily panic or attempt to take the jacket off.

6. **Elderly guests**—These guests may tire easily. Also, they may have physical conditions that limit their strength or mobility.

7. **Disabled guests**—Their ability to move may be limited because of their condition. They may have trouble regaining their balance or turning over in the water.

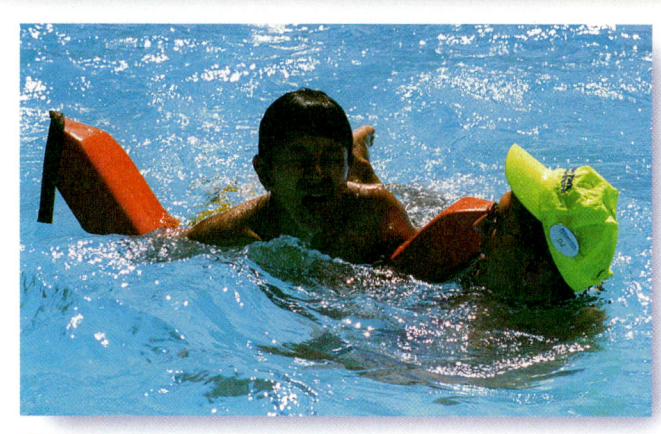

FIG 2.10 Rescuing a high risk guest.

8. **Guests wearing clothes**—Clothing absorbs water, and can become very heavy and restrict movement. If a guest does not have a bathing suit, this may indicate a low level of skill.

Locations

There are several areas of your facility that have greater numbers of rescues.

1. **Deep water**
   Guests may find themselves in water over their heads when they fall off a tube, land in water that is deeper than they imagined, or inadvertantly float or swim into water over their heads.

2. **Wave pools**
   - These are especially dangerous at the point where the waves break. Also, guests have a tendency to gather there.
   - The return currents along the sides of the pool may pull a guest into deep water.

3. **Activity pools**
   Slide exits into activity areas may put guests into deep water.

4. **Slide catch pools**
   Although the water may be less than 4 feet deep, guests may lose their footing and be unable to stand up.

5. **Hydraulic currents**
   On rides with currents, the force of the water may hold a guest in one place, in or out of his tube.

6. **Diving tanks**
   Any type of deep water pool where guests are in water over their heads.

7. **Pool exits**
   Guests may gather around stairs, ladders, drop-off areas or slides.

8. **Lakes**
   The regions outside of marked swimming areas, around or between piers and docks are the most dangerous. Even inside swimming areas, the visibility in the water may be limited.

Times

The times when most guests become distressed are:

1. **Midday**
   Between noon and 4 p.m.
2. **Unusually crowded conditions**
   Holiday seasons and warm weather usually indicate an increase in the numbers of guests in a facility.

As a professional lifeguard, you now know where to look, what to look for, and how to look. While you are on duty, remember the importance of diligence and maintaining the 10/20 Protection Rule at all times.

LIFEGUARD ROTATIONS

A *Rotation* is when you are relieved by another lifeguard, and you move to another location or go on a break. During a rotation it is very important that the 10/20 Protection Rule be maintained. It is very easy to become distracted during the rotation.

As you rotate, you should:

1. Always walk to the next location.
2. Be on time.
3. Limit your conversation with the other lifeguard.
4. Remember that the guests are aware of your movements and the way you conduct yourself.
5. Rotate professionally with no loss of eye contact to the zone. Proactively scan the zone before you rotate. Confirm with the other lifeguard that the bottom is clear.
6. Be sure that the incoming lifeguard is ready and has assumed responsibility for the area before you leave. Proactively scan the zone after you rotate. Confirm with the other lifeguard that the bottom is clear.

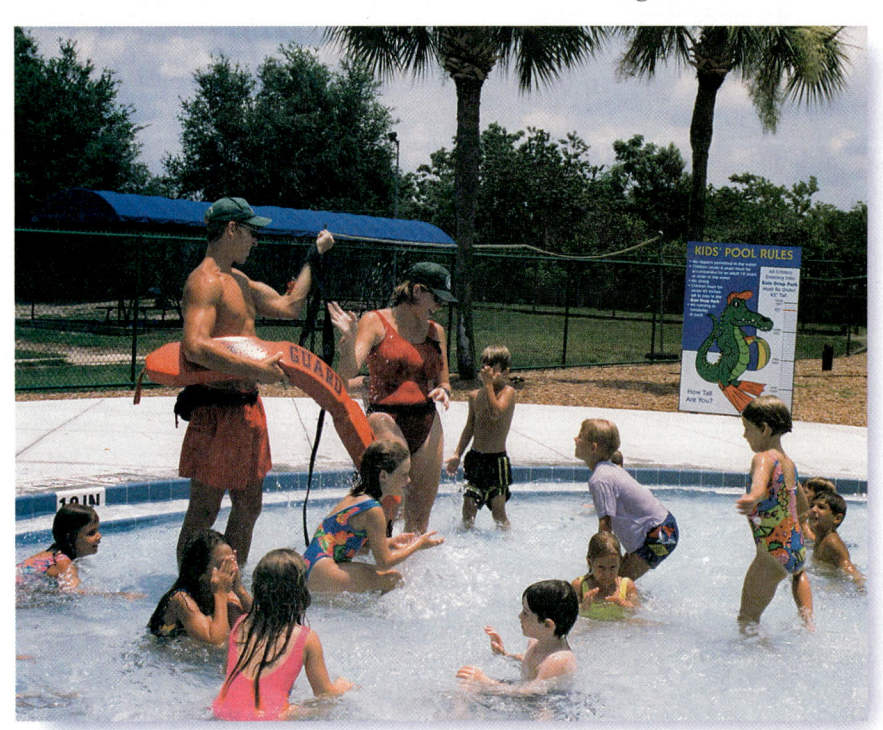

The actions of the lifeguards during the rotation will be determined by whether each lifeguard has a rescue tube. For maximum protection and professionalism, you should conduct your rotation in the following manner:

FIG 2.11 Rotate stations without losing eye contact with the zone.

CHAPTER 2 • AWARENESS AND RECOGNITION   21

Incoming Lifeguard Has No Rescue Tube
Figure 2.12

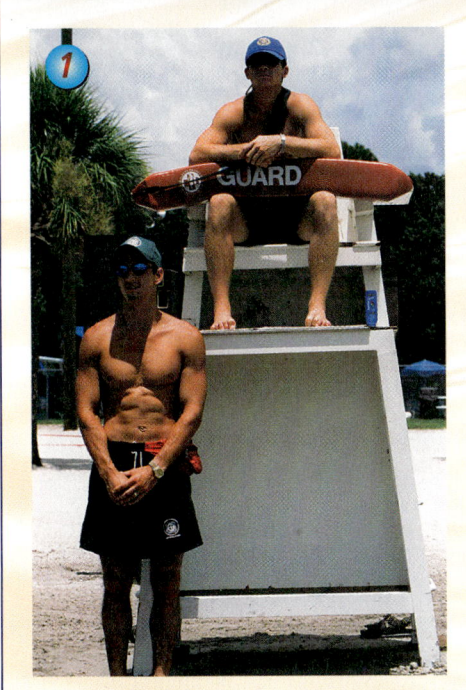

1. Incoming lifeguard reports and begins scanning the area.

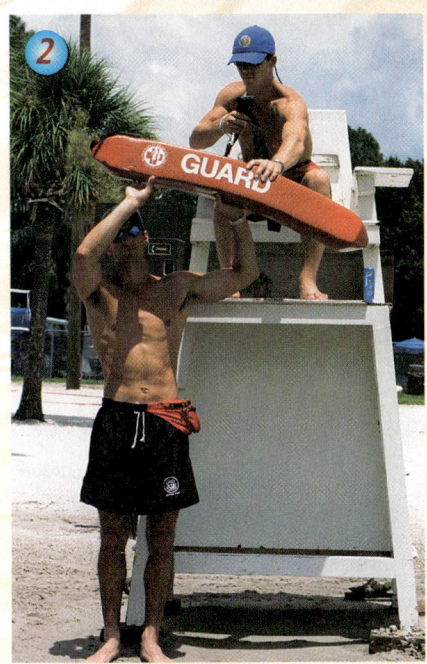

2. Lifeguard equipment is transferred to incoming lifeguard.

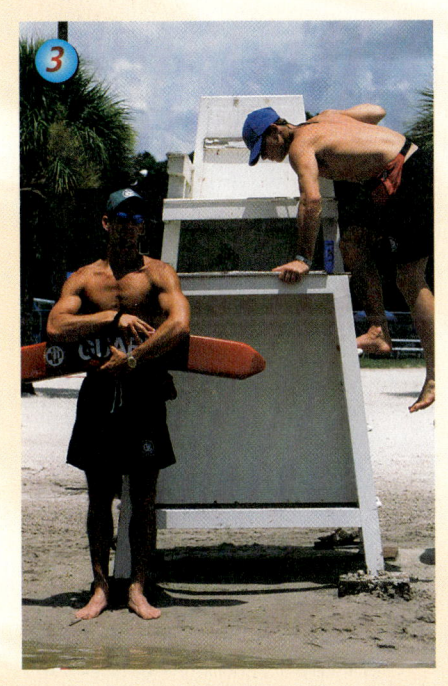

3. Incoming lifeguard watches zone while outgoing lifeguard exits the chair.

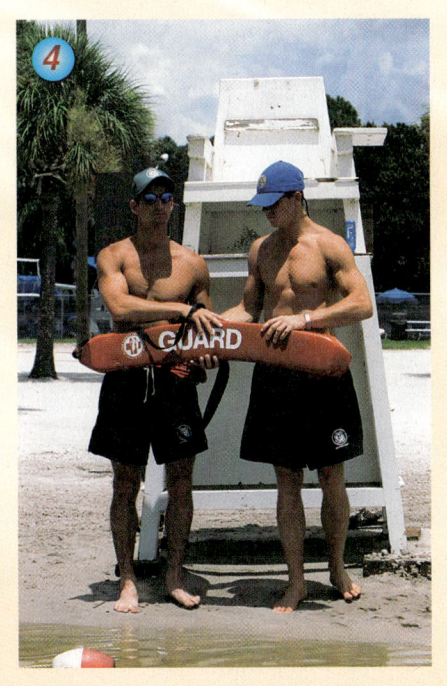

4. Equipment is transferred back to outgoing lifeguard.

continued on following page

Incoming Lifeguard Has No Rescue Tube
Figure 2.12 (continued)

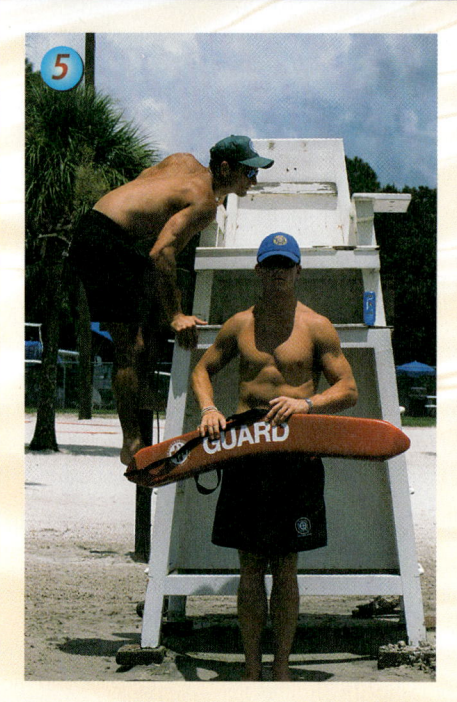

5. Incoming lifeguard enters stand while outgoing lifeguard watches zone.

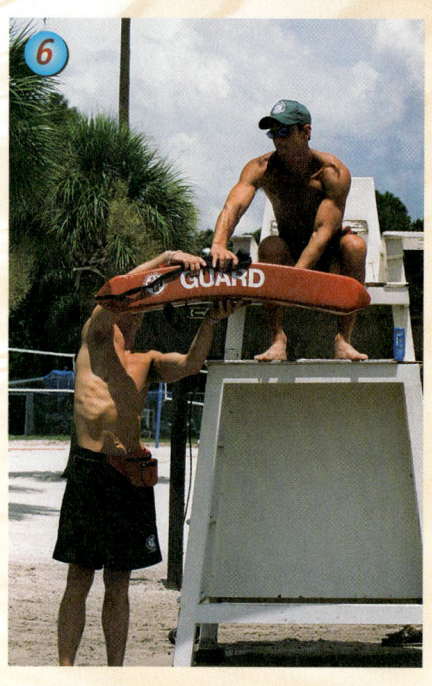

6. Equipment is transferred back to incoming lifeguard in stand.

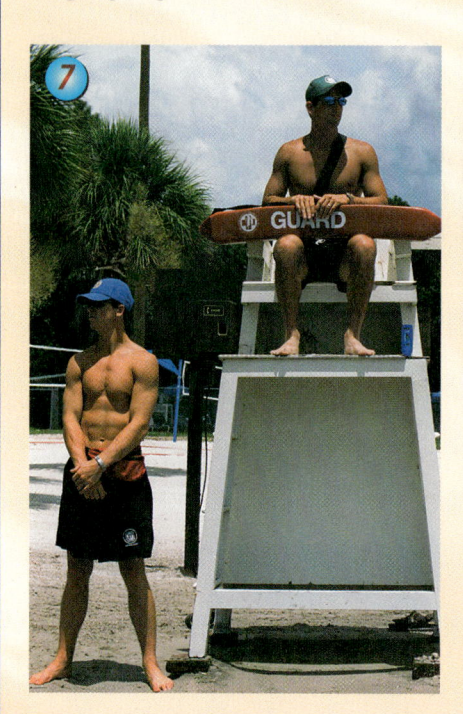

7. Outgoing lifeguard scans zone. Both lifeguards agree that the bottom is clear.

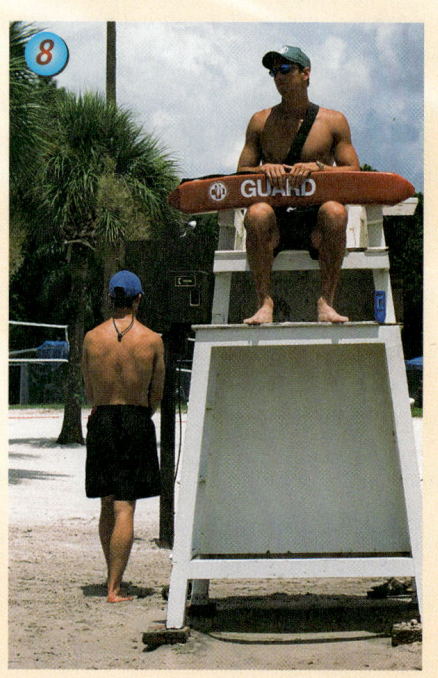

8. Outgoing lifeguard leaves only after information is shared and incoming lifeguard is ready, assuming responsibility of the zone. Rotation is complete.

CHAPTER 2 • AWARENESS AND RECOGNITION   23

Both Lifeguards Have Rescue Tubes - Figure 2.13

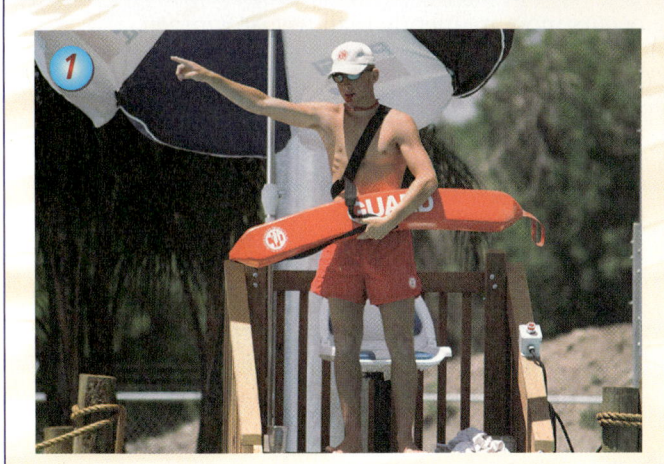

1. Lifeguard in stand prior to rotation.

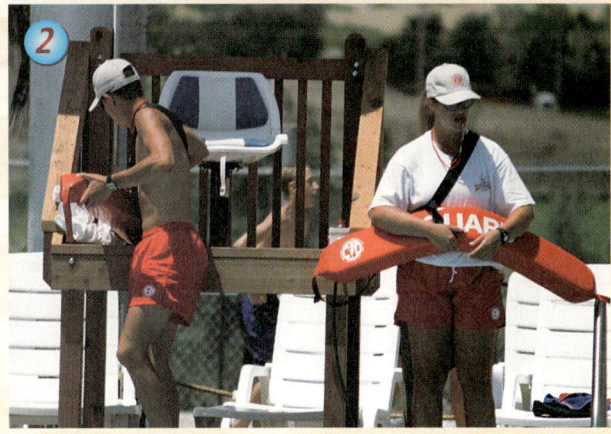

2. Incoming lifeguard scans bottom, stands at side of chair, begins scanning, and assumes responsibility for zone.

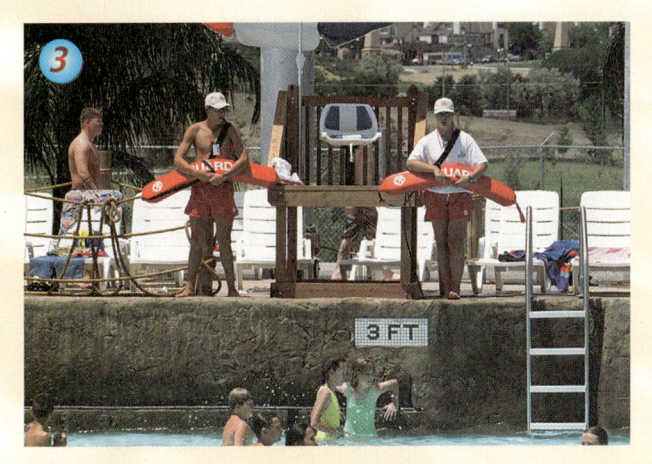

3. Outgoing lifeguard watches zone.

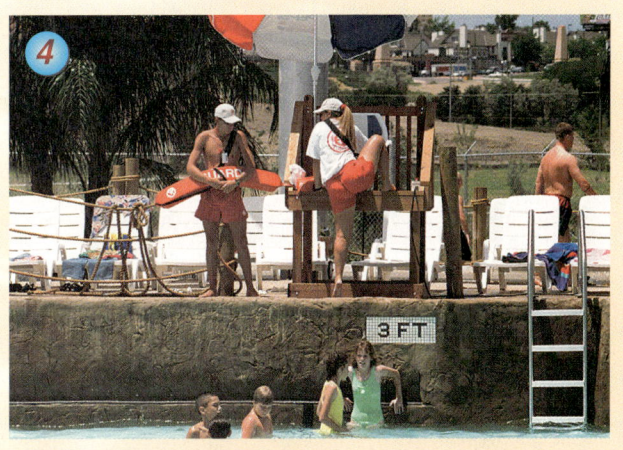

4. Incoming lifeguard enters stand.

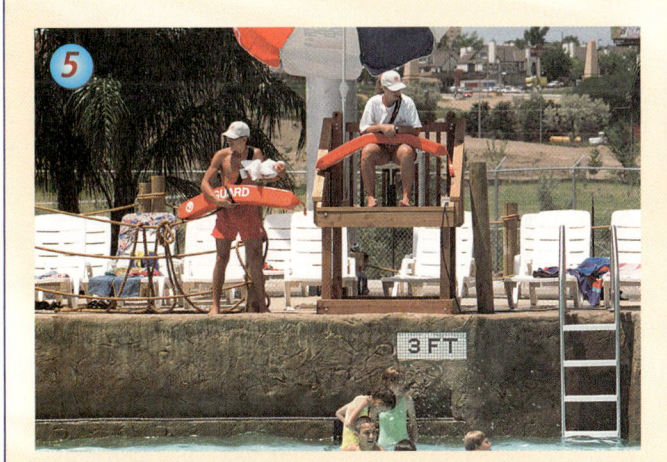

5. Incoming lifeguard assumes responsibility for zone. Information is exchanged and outgoing lifeguard scans zone. Both lifeguards agree that the bottom is clear.

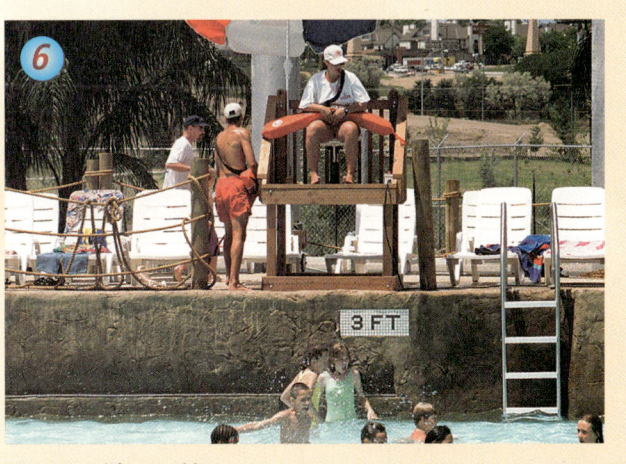

6. Outgoing lifeguard leaves.

REVIEW QUESTIONS

1. Dry drowning occurs more frequently than wet drowning.

2. Name four types of guests who would be considered high risk.

   a. _____

   b. _____

   c. _____

   d. _____

3. Most rescues occur at what time of day? _____

4. (T) (F) A guest on the bottom will be easy to see.

5. (T) (F) Guests can be conscious on the bottom and still need to be rescued.

6. (T) (F) Scanning patterns for a zone should not be changed.

7. (T) (F) When rotating, it is important to look professional and maintain the 10/20 Protection Rule.

8. The 10/20 Protection Rule allows you _____ seconds to see and recognize an aquatic emergency, and _____ seconds to preform a rescue and begin management of the situation.

9. (T) (F) You should only scan the area of your facility where guests are present.

10. Name three locations of an aquatic facility that have greater numbers of rescues.

    a. _____

    b. _____

    c. _____

CHAPTER 2 • AWARENESS AND RECOGNITION   25

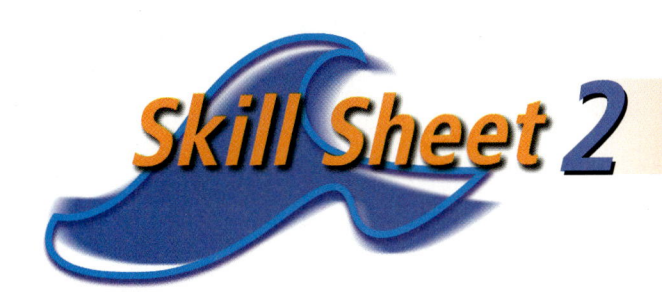

Skill Sheet 2

SCANNING AND ROTATION

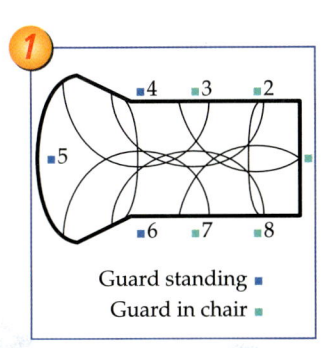

1 Know your zone.

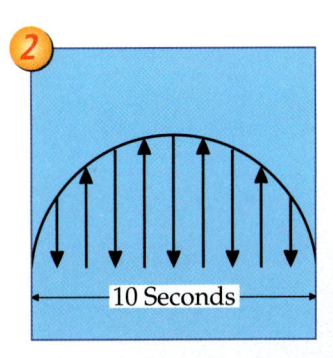

2 Scan zone every 10 seconds.

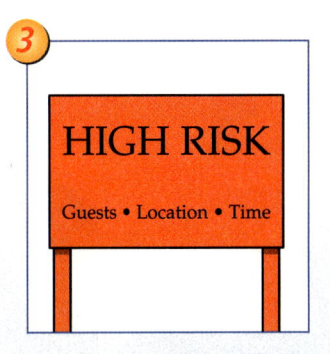

3 Watch for high risk guests, locations, and times.

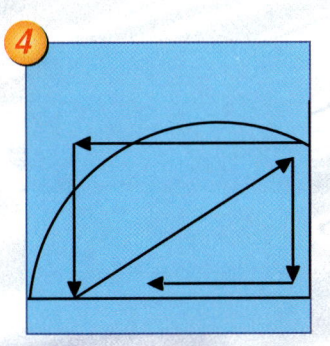

4 Have a scanning pattern.

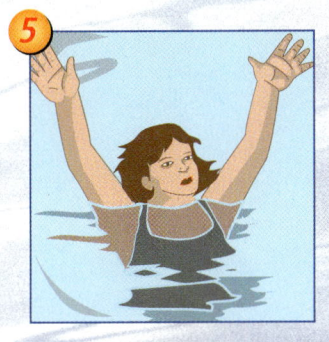

5 Know what to look for.

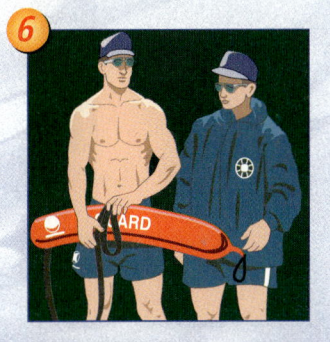

6 Rotate professionally.

KEY POINTS:

- Never compromise diligence.
- Complete rotations while maintaining the 10/20 Protection Rule.
- Change scanning patterns occasionally.
- Scan your zone from the bottom up before and after your rotation.

CRITICAL THINKING:

1. What are some situations that would change your scanning?
2. How does the 10/20 Protection Rule affect what you do?
3. What circumstances might make it more difficult for you to remain diligent? How can you control them?
4. What can you do to keep your attention level up no matter what the circumstances?

Reaction

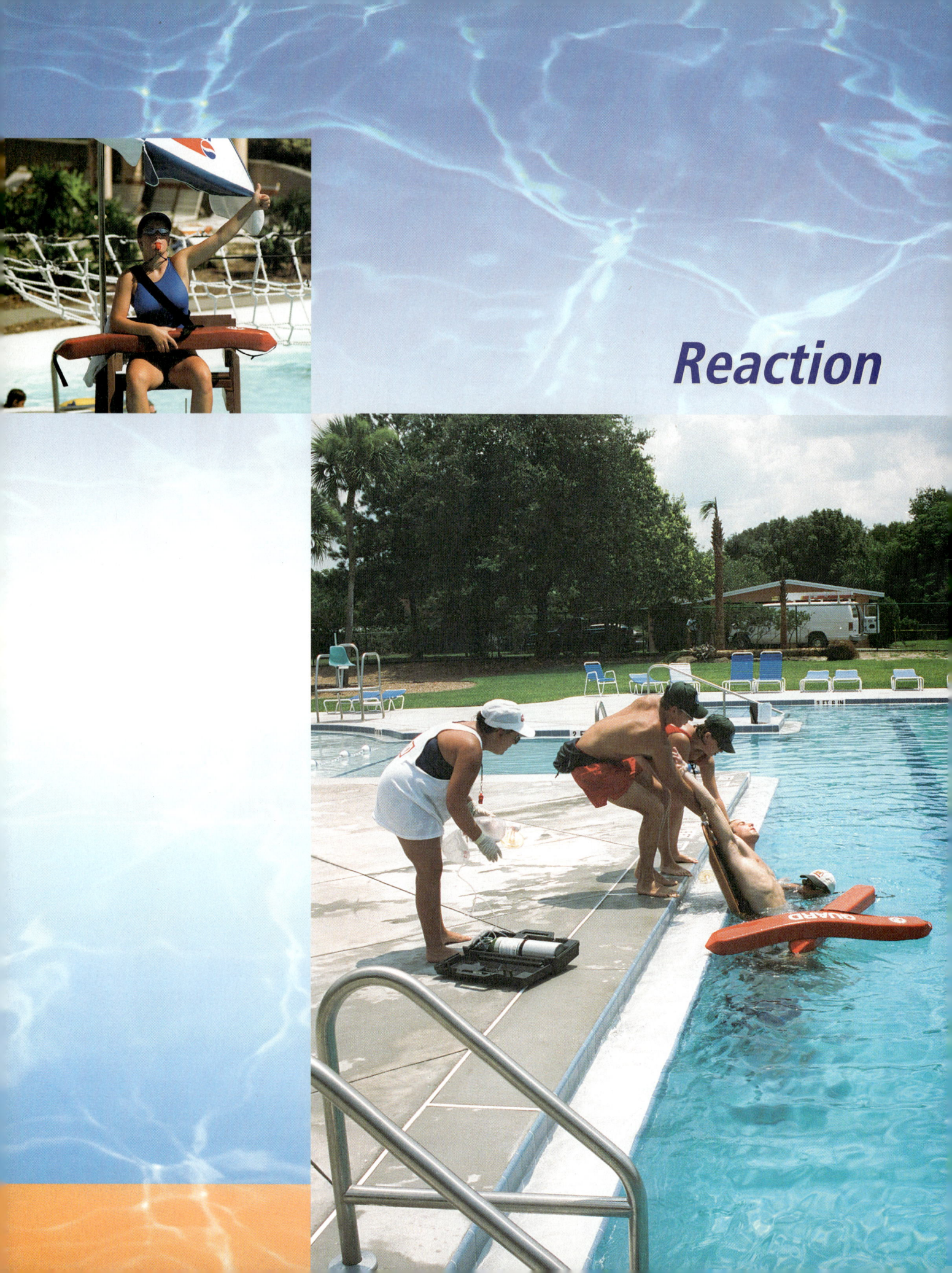

chapter 3

OBJECTIVES

After reading this chapter and completing the related course work, you should be able to:

1. Explain the purpose of an Emergency Action System.
2. Demonstrate methods of lifeguard communication.
3. Describe the concept of team lifeguarding.
4. Identify the differences between an assist and a rescue.
5. Recognize the importance of nonbody-contact rescues and the use of the rescue tube.

THREE

In every emergency situation, people become confused and excited. They react, often without thinking. In doing so, they put themselves and others at even greater risk than the situation warrants. It isn't something people do on purpose, it just happens because there is no plan of action.

EMERGENCY ACTION SYSTEM

As a **professional lifeguard**, you cannot become confused or excited during an emergency. You must be in control of your actions and know what must be done. You cannot expose any of your guests, or yourself, to greater risk. You must follow a plan of action. Your job is to minimize risk and prevent any further injury. The way you do that is to follow your facility's *Emergency Action System (EAS)*. This is a chain of events that will help you and your fellow lifeguards manage the situation in the best manner possible.

Your facility will have a written plan for using the EAS, and it will be designed specifically for your location. You need to read, discuss, and **practice** the plan. The EAS covers all types of emergencies. Samples of the Emergency Action System for both an Active Guest in Distress and a Passive Guest are detailed in Appendix A.

Each EAS outlines what should happen during an emergency. It will start with the recognition of the emergency and go through the lifeguard's reaction, rescue, and care provided to the guest. The plan will include all additional facility personnel that become involved in the emergency. And, if necessary, it will follow the guest through the transfer of care to the Emergency Medical Personnel. The plan will also include gathering information about the emergency, such as witness statements and accident reports. All critiques and follow-up meetings will also be included in the plan.

The number of steps in an Emergency Action System will depend on the size of the facility and the number of staff available. Every facility will operate differently. No matter how large or small the EAS may be, the most important part of the total plan is the *lifeguard*. If the lifeguard fails to recognize the emergency or fails to activate the plan, none of it matters. Someone may be injured or may die.

You, the *professional lifeguard*, must recognize the emergency and activate the plan. You activate the Emergency Action System by blowing your whistle. This alerts other lifeguards that you are responding to an emergency and that you may need assistance. Even if you do not need help with the actual rescue, the guests in the water in your zone still need to be supervised.

> As a professional lifeguard, you cannot become confused or excited during an emergency.

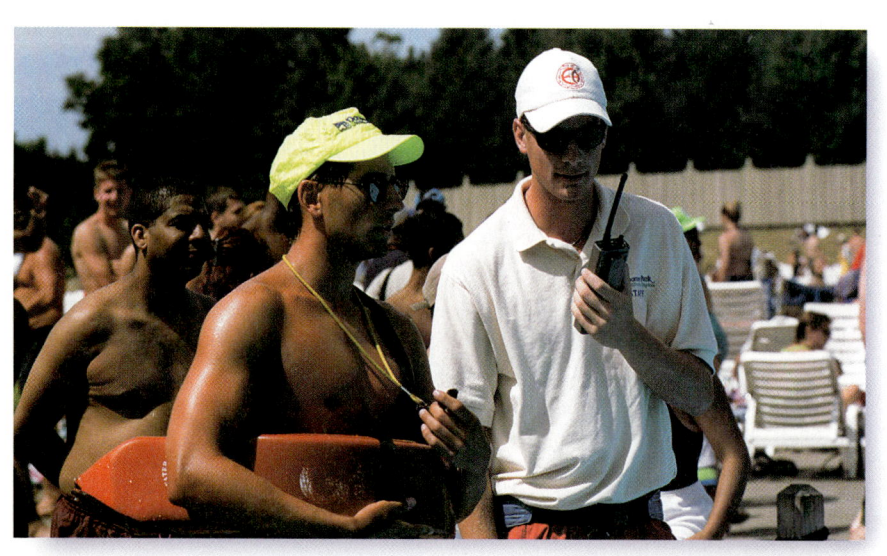

FIG 3.1 Understand your EAS plan so you can communicate your need for assistance effectively with your fellow lifeguards.

Basic Principles of the Emergency Action System

Lifeguard to Your Left Covers Both Zones

The EAS must be set up to insure that your zone is still covered while you are assisting a guest, and that another lifeguard will back you up if you need assistance.

When you leave the stand during an emergency, the lifeguard **to your left** will usually assume responsibility for your zone, and if you need assistance, this lifeguard will also be your back-up. This also means that you are the back-up for the lifeguard to your right.

When you hear a whistle signaling an emergency, you should immediately check the lifeguard to your right. If that lifeguard has left the stand to assist a guest, you now have to expand your scanning pattern to cover his or her zone. You continue to scan both zones. Watch and be ready to assist that lifeguard if she signals for help.

There may be situations where you are in a stand and there is no lifeguard stand to your left. An example of this would be on the wall of a wave pool.

There are two methods of dealing with this situation:

1. The lifeguard to your right covers your zone and is your back-up.
2. Depending on the size of the facility, the lifeguard across the pool will cover your zone and be your back-up.

The specific procedure will be determined by your facility management.

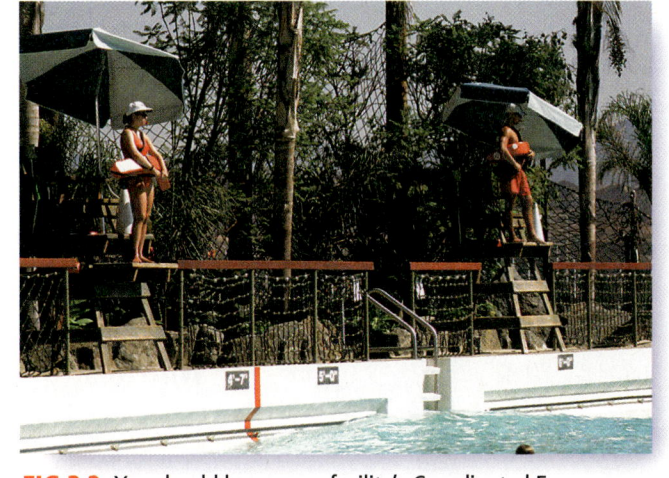

FIG 3.2 You should know your facility's Coordinated Emergency Action System.

Two or More Lifeguards Involved—Stop the Activity

When two or more lifeguards are required to leave their stations for a rescue, the "Guard to Your Left" rule may not work. The zones may be too large for the remaining lifeguards to cover. If this is the situation, the activity must be stopped. Once the emergency has passed and the lifeguards have returned to their stands, the activity can be reopened.

If there are enough lifeguards to safely cover all zones, the activity may remain open. The EAS should provide for other lifeguards who may be on break, to cover the zones of the lifeguards involved in the rescue.

In facilities with only one or two lifeguards, the EAS must involve other staff who can clear the water and control the crowd. They may also be trained to assist with the rescue once the guest is on the pool deck.

COMMUNICATIONS

In an aquatic facility, communication can be difficult because of crowd noise, weather, acoustics, or distance. You must be able to communicate with guests to enforce rules. You must also be able to communicate with other lifeguards and supervisors.

Whistles and hand signals are good ways to communicate. Many facilities also use telephones, two-way radios, megaphones, or other communication devices.

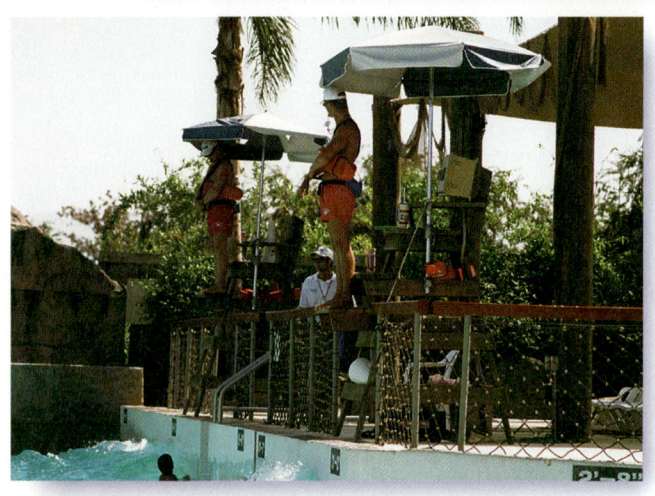

FIG 3.3 Lifeguard hears whistle and looks to his right.

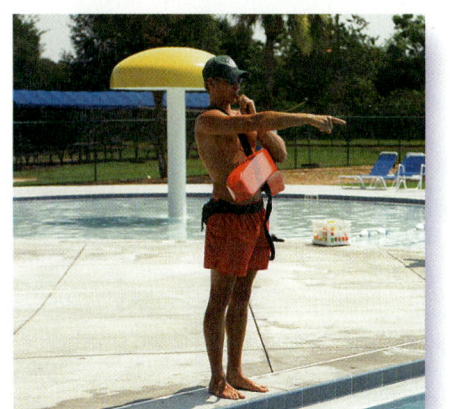

FIG 3.4 Whistle initiates Emergency Action System.

When you are in a stand, there are several situations during which you need to communicate:

- When you need to get the attention of a guest.
- When you want to get the attention of another lifeguard or a supervisor.
- When you have to leave your stand to assist a guest and someone has to watch your zone. This is not an emergency.
- When there is an emergency. You must leave your stand, someone has to cover your zone, and additional personnel are needed.
- When there is a major emergency. This may be a life-threatening situation, two or more lifeguards are involved, or the activity must be closed immediately.

The following examples of communication allow you to control your area and be able to notify other lifeguards or supervisors in different situations. Your facility may use these common signals or develop its own communication system. You need to know **and practice** the communication signals used in your facility.

Whistles

Your whistle will be your most frequently used piece of equipment. You will be required to have a whistle with you at all times when you are on duty.

Your whistle should be in good working order, with a shrill tone that cuts through crowd noise. When you have to use your whistle, you should **blow it loudly and firmly**. You should have regular "whistle-blowing practice." This teaches you to blow it properly, and it also teaches you to **recognize its sound** over crowd noise and other distractions.

Whistle Signals

One Short Blast: To get the attention of a guest. After you get the guest's attention, it is best to use hand signals and speak clearly if you need to give further instructions. A megaphone helps when you have to talk to a guest in a crowded facility.

Two Short Blasts: To get the attention of another lifeguard or supervisor. As you blow your whistle, raise your hand or tap the top of your head. This lets the other lifeguards or your supervisor know who has whistled and what you want.

One Long Blast: To activate the Emergency Action System. This indicates that you are going to do a rescue. This means that you are leaving your stand, someone has to cover your zone, and additional personnel may be needed. Wherever you are working, you should point to where you are going, and hit the emergency stop button (E-stop). The lifeguard to your left covers your zone (in addition to his own). In a wave pool or slide, this lifeguard is also responsible for making sure that the waves or dispatch of riders has been stopped.

A head lifeguard or supervisor should respond to all emergencies whenever possible or practical. A rescue report may be required or the guest may need additional assistance.

Two Long Blasts: To indicate a major emergency. This may be a life-threatening situation in which several lifeguards or facility personnel are involved or needed. The activity may need to be closed immediately and guests cleared from the area. Other lifeguards who are not involved in your rescue attempts are responsible for securing the pool before providing additional support to the emergency.

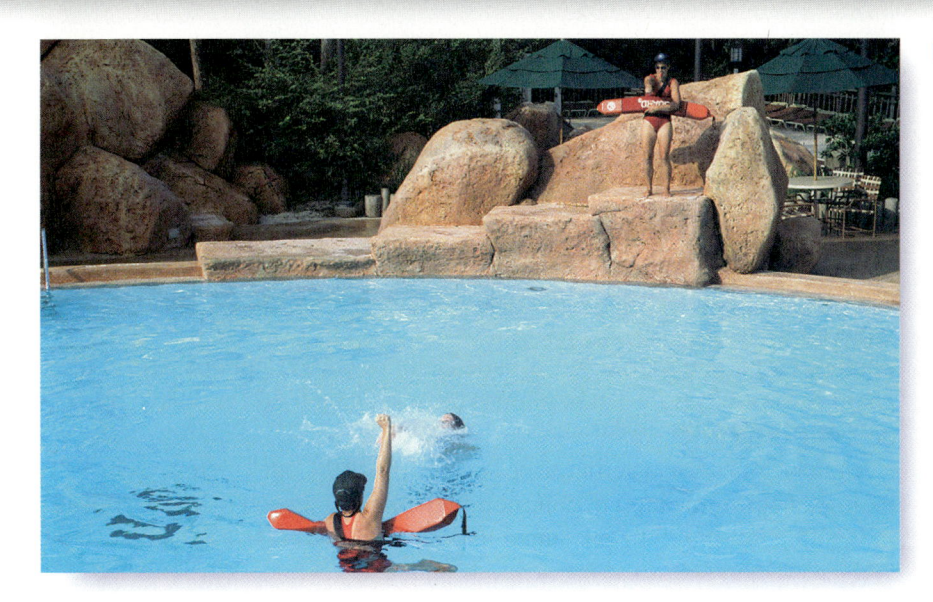

FIG 3.5 Lifeguard signaling for help.

Hand Signals

Hand signals are primarily used with whistles to help communicate. When possible, you should hold the hand signal for 5 seconds to make sure it is noticed.

Pointing. Point to give direction. Pointing can be used with a whistle blast to indicate to guests what you would like them to do. This is also helpful when you would like to point out a certain guest to another lifeguard or supervisor.

Raised Clenched Fist. This means that you need help. If you are on the deck, at the side of the pool, or still in your stand, this may be used with whistle blasts. If you are in the water, you may not be able to use your whistle. (Remember, the lifeguard to your left should already be covering your zone and watching to see if you need help.)

Crossed Arms above the Head. Use this signal to stop dispatch. This is generally used on slides, tube rides, or other water attractions. It can be used with whistle blasts to indicate a rescue in progress. It is also used by the catch pool lifeguard to signal to the lifeguard on dispatch that it is necessary to retrieve a lost article (sunglasses, etc.) from the activity area or catch pool.

Thumbs Up. This indicates it is all right to resume the activity. It is usually accompanied by whistle blasts.

Tapping the Top of Your Head. This signal means "Watch My Area." It indicates that you need another lifeguard to cover your area for a brief time. It is usually accompanied with whistle blasts. The lifeguard you are signaling should acknowledge the signal, and become responsible for covering your area.

Other Communication Devices

In addition to whistles and hand signals, there are other communication devices used at aquatic facilities.

Megaphones. These are used to project your voice toward another person. These are especially useful in large or crowded facilities.

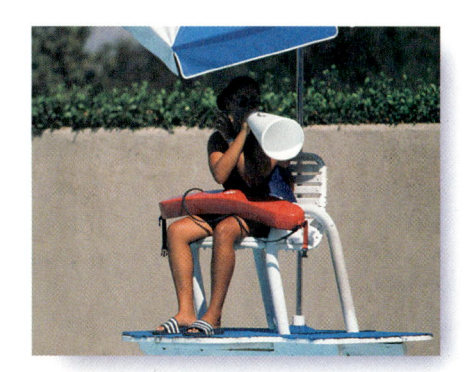

FIG 3.6 Use of a megaphone as a communication device.

Lifeguard telephones must only be used for official business or emergencies.

Telephones. Telephones must be available for emergencies. The telephone numbers for emergency services must be posted near the telephone and be clearly visible. It is also recommended that the telephone number for the Poison Control Center be clearly posted. If cordless phones are used, a standard wall phone should also be available as a back-up in case of malfunction of the cordless phone. If a pay phone is the only means of communication, the appropriate change must be kept in a location known only to employees. Hidden coins should be checked daily and replaced if missing. Emergency numbers should be displayed at such phones. Large waterparks and aquatic facilities have telephones to aid lifeguard communication. These phones must only be used for official business or emergencies.

Some facilities use a verbal code such as the "10 Code" system to aid in quick communication of common information. If such a system is used in your facility, it will be explained in your EAS.

2-Way Radios. These are used primarily between supervisors and for medical staff.

Public Address Systems. These are used for announcements, music, and other information of a general nature. If needed, emergency information can be communicated to your entire facility very quickly.

TEAM LIFEGUARDING

No matter what size aquatic facility you work in, or the number of lifeguards on duty at any time, as a professional lifeguard, you are a member of an emergency response team. Once you activate the EAS, your signal is meant to draw together other lifeguard and support personnel. This is your team. They may cover your zone or provide other forms of assistance.

Be aware that whatever the situation, there will always be someone to back you up. Even in one-lifeguard facilities, additional personnel, such as locker room attendants or cashiers, can provide the necessary assistance.

All team members must know their responsibilities during an emergency. The ultimate goal is to prevent drowning. The more each staff member can be part of the team process, the more effective the EAS will be.

All team members must know their responsibilities during an emergency. The ultimate goal is to prevent drownings. The more each staff member can be part of the team process, the more effective the EAS will be.

RESCUES vs. ASSISTS

An *assist* occurs when you help a guest, either from the deck or in the water, and you are still able to maintain zone coverage within the 10/20 Protection Rule. An example is using a pole for an extension assist.

A *rescue* occurs when you must leave your stand to help a guest and cannot maintain the 10/20 Protection Rule within your zone. It applies to any situation for which the EAS is activated.

Anytime you enter the water to rescue a guest, you endanger your life and/or risk personal injury.

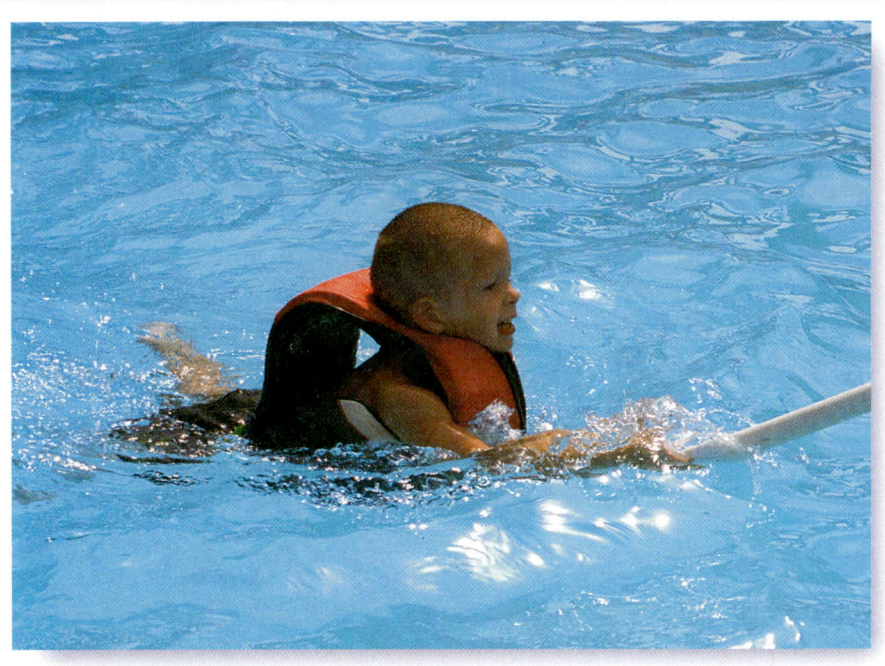

FIG 3.7 Use of a pole for an Extension Assist.

RESCUE TUBES

Rescue tubes are used to help minimize personal danger when you are performing a rescue. The rescue tube has been proven to be the safest and most effective rescue device available. All lifeguards must have a rescue tube at their lifeguard station. There will be some lifeguard stations where the tube will not be used as part of your direct responsibilities, such as doing dispatch at the top of a slide.

The flotation quality of the average rescue tube can support up to five people in the water. This greatly reduces the danger and risk to both the guest and the lifeguard during a rescue. Traditional body contact rescues are dangerous for both the guest (victim) and the lifeguard. That is why nonbody-contact rescues with the rescue tube are advocated. This does not mean that the fitness of the lifeguard during a rescue is not important when using equipment-based rescue techniques. Ellis & Associates stress that regular exercise is necessary to maintain fitness. Personal conditioning and skill-specific training should be part of all inservice training programs.

Experience has shown that equipment-based rescues provide additional flotation during a rescue. This reduces the energy you need to move the guest to safety. You can also use the rescue tube for self-protection. By keeping the rescue tube between you and the guest, it reduces the chance of the guest grabbing you during a rescue. Even if the guest does grab you, the rescue tube will assist in keeping both of your heads above water. In addition, should the guest need resuscitation, you can initiate resuscitative efforts in the water.

The rescue techniques presented in this manual and covered in this course are designed specifically for effective lifeguarding with a rescue tube.

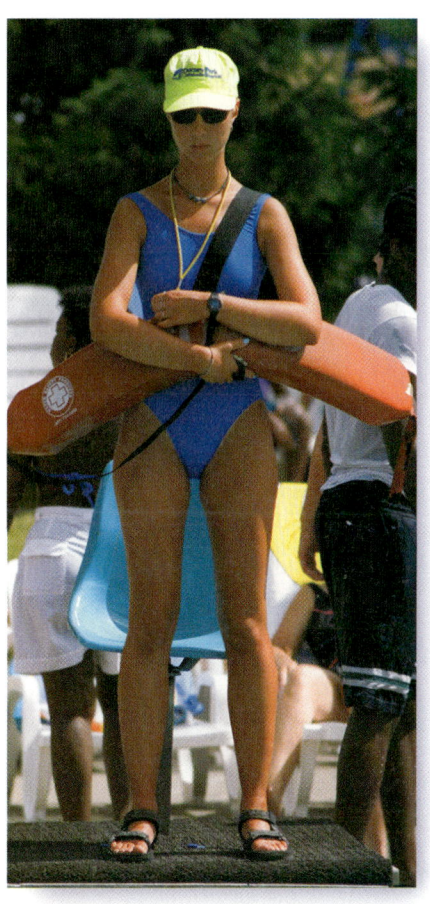

FIG 3.8 Hold your rescue tube in a manner that allows you to respond quickly to an emergency.

Wearing and Holding the Rescue Tube on the Stand

How you wear or hold the rescue tube while you are on duty depends on the responsibilities of your position and the needs or regulations of the facility. For example, a lifeguard at a wave pool must wear a rescue tube at all times, but a lifeguard dispatching guests at the top of a slide may not be required to wear a rescue tube. Other positions may have the rescue tube placed within arms' reach, where it is immediately available. You must look professional and have your rescue tube immediately available for use. The shoulder strap of the tube should fit diagonally across your chest when you are wearing the tube. The following are some examples of proper wearing of the rescue tube when you are on duty.

- You may hold the rescue tube in front of you.
- You may hold it at your side while you are standing.
- You may sit in a chair with the tube across your lap.

In all of these positions, you must *secure the line* so that it does not get caught on anything when you move around or enter the water in an emergency.

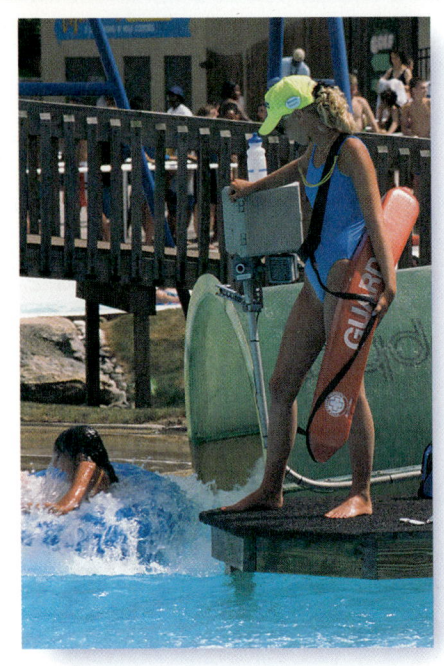

FIG 3.9 You may hold the rescue tube at your side while you are standing.

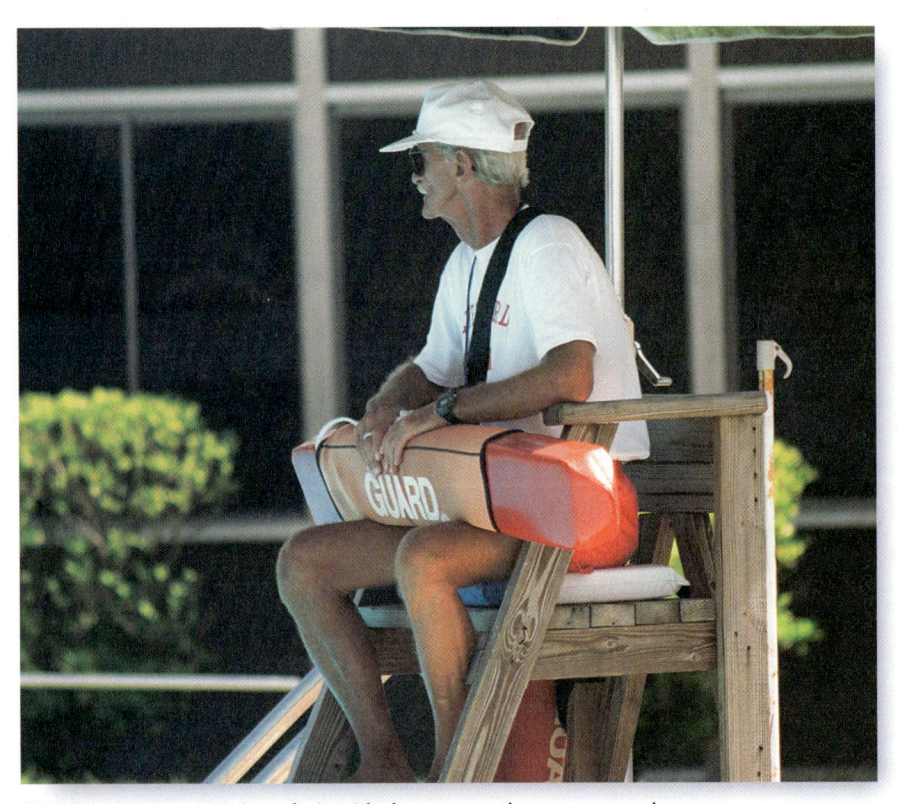

FIG 3.10 You may sit in a chair with the rescue tube across your lap.

REVIEW QUESTIONS

1. The Emergency Action System is activated by _____.

2. While a lifeguard is making a rescue, who covers his or her zone?

3. Match the communication signal with its use:

   _____ One short whistle   a. Major emergency

   _____ Raised Fist   b. Give direction

   _____ Two long whistles   c. Gain swimmer attention

   _____ Crossed arms   d. Watch my area

   _____ Tapping head   e. Resume activity

   _____ One long whistle   f. Rescue in progress

   _____ Pointing   g. Lifeguard needs help

   _____ Thumbs up   h. Stop dispatch

4. What information should be posted next to the telephone?

   a. _____

   b. _____

   c. _____

5. What is the difference between an assist and a rescue?

6. When making an assist or rescue, it is important to reassure the guest by _____ to him or her.

7. (T) (F) The rescue tube is an optional piece of equipment for lifeguards at wave pools.

Skill Sheet 3

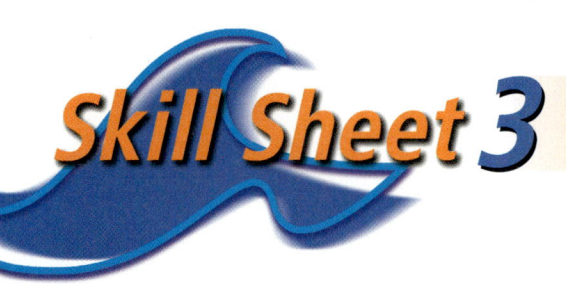

COMMUNICATIONS

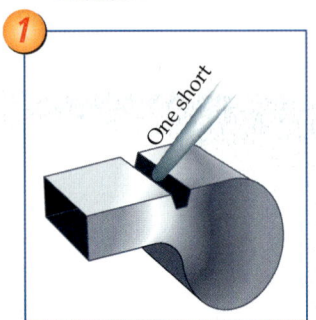

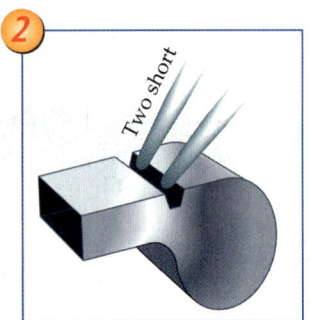

1 One short — Guest's attention.

2 Two short — Guard's attention.

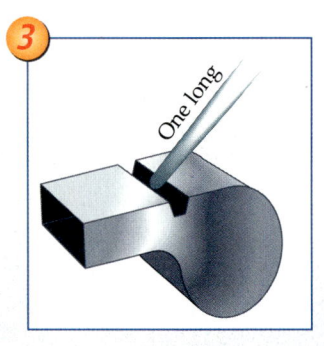

3 One long — Activate EAS.

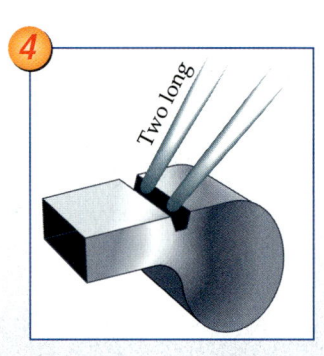

4 Two long — Major emergency.

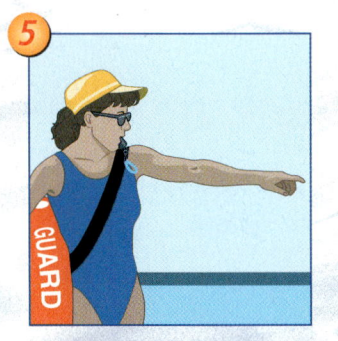

5 Give direction.

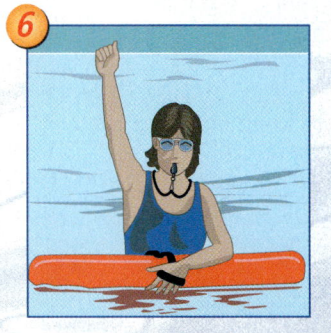

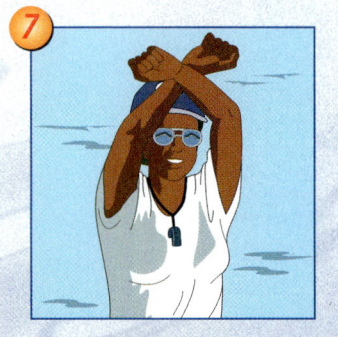

6 Help.

7 Stop dispatch.

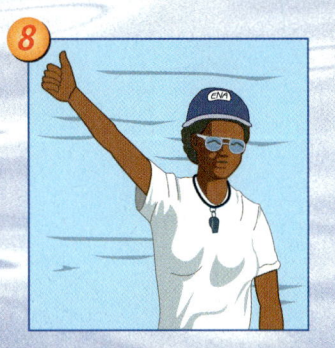

8 Resume activity.

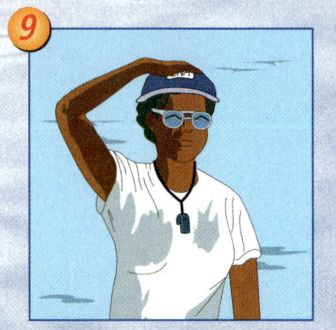

9 Watch zone.

KEY POINTS:

- Blow whistle loudly and firmly.
- Combine whistle and hand signals.
- Avoid unnecessary communication; blow your whistle only when necessary.

CRITICAL THINKING:

1. What do you do if the guard to your right is making a rescue and raises a clenched fist?
2. When does an activity have to be cleared of remaining swimmers?
3. What is the difference between an assist and a rescue?
4. Why should a stand-mounted phone be used for emergency or business use only?

part 2
TWO

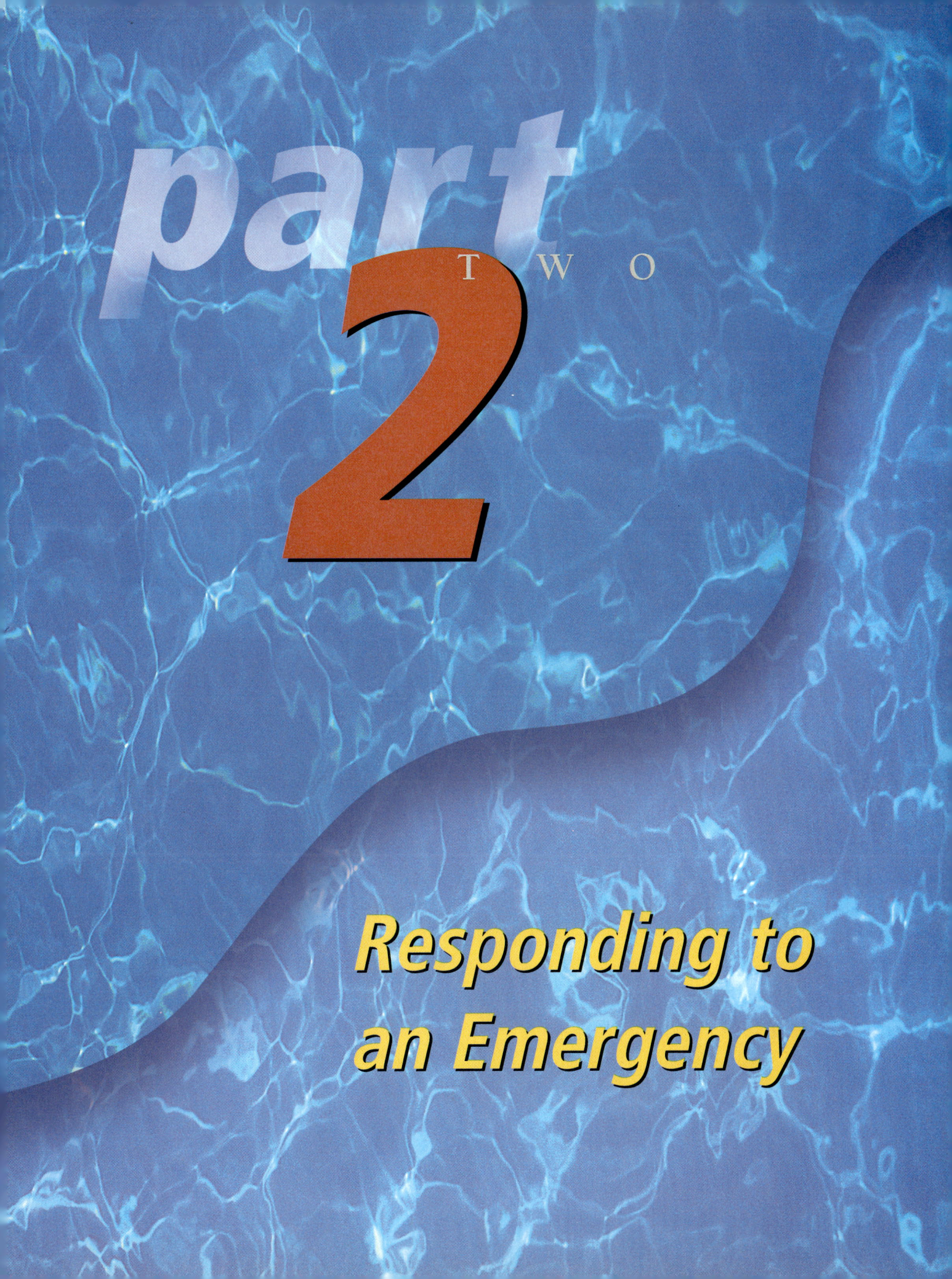

Responding to an Emergency

Guest on the Surface —Breathing

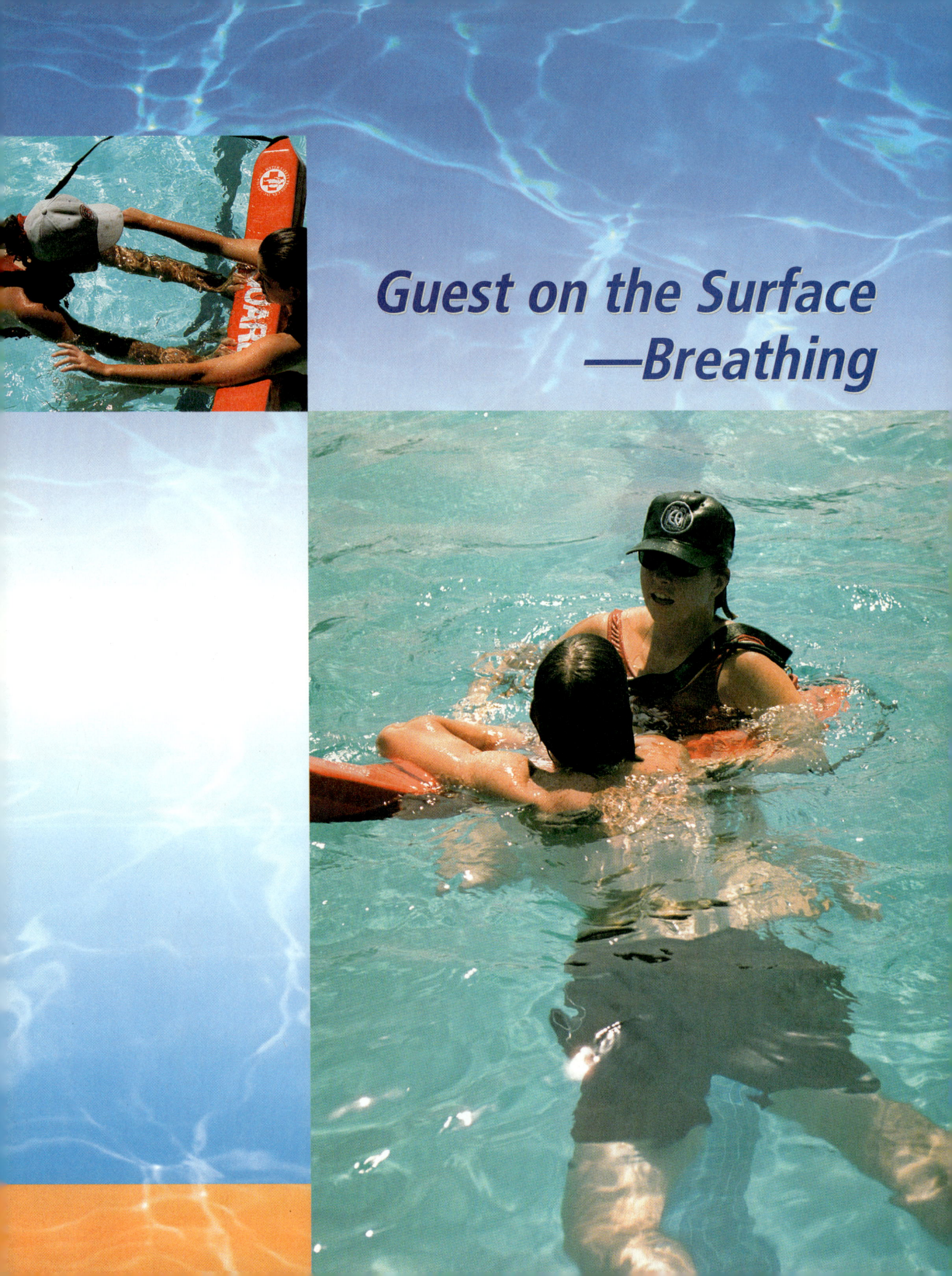

chapter 4

OBJECTIVES

After reading this chapter and completing the related course work, you should be able to:

1. Identify the differences in managing distressed swimmer and near-drowning rescues.

2. Demonstrate a compact jump entry and an approach stroke.

3. Demonstrate a front drive.

4. Demonstrate a rear huggie.

5. Demonstrate a two-lifeguard rescue.

In previous chapters, you learned to recognize guests in the water who need assistance. You have learned the difference between an assist and a rescue. This chapter will expand your knowledge by introducing you to the skills required to properly handle these situations.

Any repetition of information in this chapter is meant to reinforce the importance of diligence required by you as a professional lifeguard.

Executing an Assist

When executing an assist, you should:

- Reassure the guest. Talk to the guest while doing the assist. You may be able to talk some guests to safety.

- Support the guest. Remember that guests are generally able to assist themselves once they have hold of an extension device.

- Caution the guest. The guest's safety is your main concern. You may point out more appropriate areas of your facility for the guest's ability level, or suggest the use of a lifejacket. If you do suggest using a lifejacket, remember that some people may be uncomfortable in a lifejacket at first. The buoyancy around the chest may make it difficult for them to stand or regain their footing. You may need to continue to assist these guests until they become comfortable in lifejackets.

ASSISTS

Providing assistance to guests who need help can often be done without compromising your ability to maintain the 10/20 Protection Rule. As previously stated, an *assist* occurs when you help a guest, either from the deck or in the water, and you are still able to maintain zone coverage within the 10/20 Protection Rule. It is not necessary to activate your Emergency Action System or complete a rescue report for an assist.

Guests may need an assist if they lose their footing, are slightly disoriented, have difficulty exiting the pool or standing up, or have a physical disability. You can assist these guests to safety by extending a body part, pole, or rescue tube.

These types of assists are called reaching, or **extension assists**. They can be safely performed while standing or kneeling on the pool deck. If you are in the water (such as in a catch pool), you can also assist the guest by supporting him. Remember to keep your rescue tube between you and the guest you are assisting.

EXTENSION ASSISTS

Body Part

To use a part of your body for an extension assist, you should:

1. Keep your body down low and your weight away from the water.
2. Grasp the guest's wrist or arm, rather than letting the guest grasp you.
3. Assist the guest to the deck, if necessary. Do **not** lift the guest by pulling on the arms. Grasp underneath the armpits to avoid shoulder injury.
4. Assist the guest out of the water, if he or she wishes to get out of the pool.

Pole Extension

To use a pole for an extension assist, you should:

1. Keep your body weight as low as possible and lean back away from the water.
2. Extend the pole out slightly beyond and to the side of the guest.
3. Slowly bring the pole toward the side of the guest. Encourage the guest to reach for and grasp the pole. A distressed non-swimmer may have the eyes closed, or hair and water may be blocking vision. Touch the extension device against the guest's arm or shoulder.

CHAPTER 4 • GUEST ON SURFACE–BREATHING   41

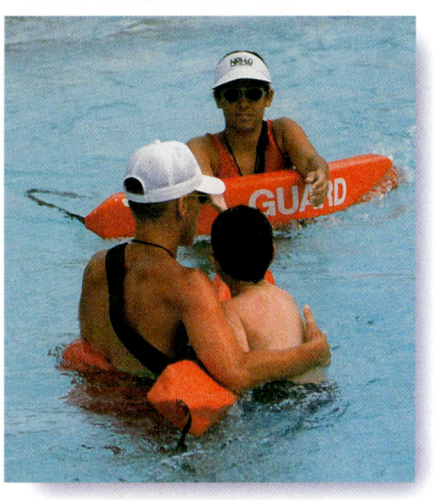

FIG 4.1 Extension assist of a high risk guest.

FIG 4.2 In-water assist.

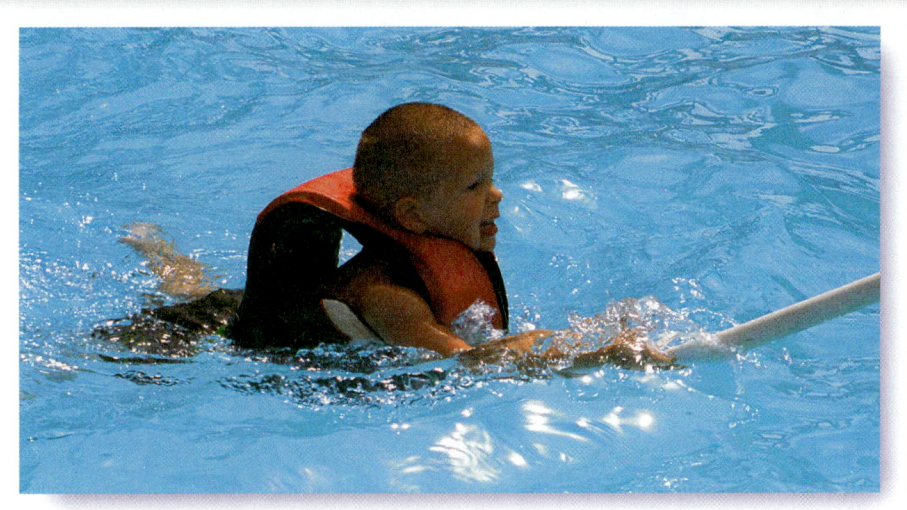

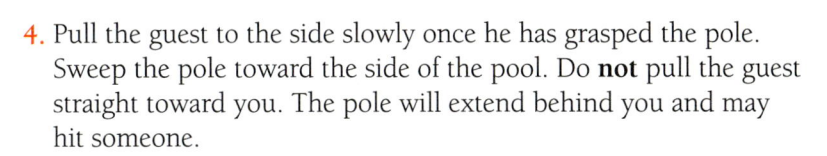

4. Pull the guest to the side slowly once he has grasped the pole. Sweep the pole toward the side of the pool. Do **not** pull the guest straight toward you. The pole will extend behind you and may hit someone.

5. Be cautious about other guests who may be swimming in the water or walking around you.

Rescue Tube or Other Extension Device

To use a rescue tube or other extension device for an extension assist, you should:

1. Place the equipment in the guest's hands. The guest may be unable to see the equipment, even if it is within her reach.

2. Be careful not to hit the guest with the equipment.

3. Bring the guest to the side of the pool once he or she has a firm grasp on the equipment. Assist the guest out of the water, if necessary.

Assists may be done in either shallow or deep water. As a professional lifeguard, you must make the judgment of whether or not you can maintain the 10/20 Protection Rule while assisting the guest. If not, you must activate your Emergency Action System and execute a *rescue*.

RESCUES

A *Rescue* occurs when you must leave your stand to assist a guest and cannot maintain the 10/20 Protection Rule within your zone. You must activate your Emergency Action System by blowing your whistle and using the proper signal, such as pointing to an area of concern, before you enter the water. A rescue report must also be completed after the rescue has been accomplished. For documentation and reporting purposes, rescues will be classified in two ways, depending on the severity of the incident:

- Distressed Swimmer Rescue
- Near Drowning Rescue

A *Distressed Swimmer Rescue* involves a guest who exhibits behavior indicating the inability to remain on, or return to the surface of the water. The situation may result in death by drowning if the swimmer is not aided by a lifeguard. In all such cases, the professional lifeguard must recognize and react to the situation before it becomes life threatening.

A *Near Drowning Rescue* involves a guest who is rendered unconscious during an immersion incident, rescued by a lifeguard, and successfully revived by the initiation of appropriate resuscitative efforts.

ENTRY AND APPROACH

There are three primary objectives when entering the water and approaching a guest in trouble:

1. To safely enter the water from a height.
2. To maintain control of the rescue tube.
3. To approach the guest in a safe manner that will allow you to evaluate and control the situation.

Once you recognize that a guest is in distress, as a professional lifeguard, you must do several things simultaneously:

1. Activate the Emergency Action System. Use the appropriate signal and blow your whistle loudly.
2. Point in the direction of the guest you are going to rescue. This alerts other lifeguards to the area where you will be during the rescue.
3. Push the Emergency Stop (E-Stop) button if there is one at your lifeguard station. This stops the next wave from being generated in a wave pool. In other locations, it may notify a base station that a rescue is in progress and you need assistance.
4. Enter the water in a safe manner and approach the guest.

The **compact jump entry** is used to enter the water to perform a rescue. When performing the compact jump entry:

1. Keep your eyes on the guest while preparing to jump.
2. Secure the excess line on your rescue tube so that it will not hook onto something when you jump. You can hold the line in your hand or secure it in any manner that keeps it out of the way. Remember that after you enter the water, the line must be able to be extended to its full length. Be careful about tying any kind of knots in the line, as they may not release when they are wet or drying.
3. Bring the rescue tube up high across your chest. Reach over the tube with both arms and press it against your body to lock it in place. You can press the tube against your body with your elbows.
4. Jump from the lifeguard chair or pool deck. Keep your legs together and your feet flat. You want to hit the water with the soles of your feet. If you hit the bottom of the pool with your toes pointed, you could injure yourself.

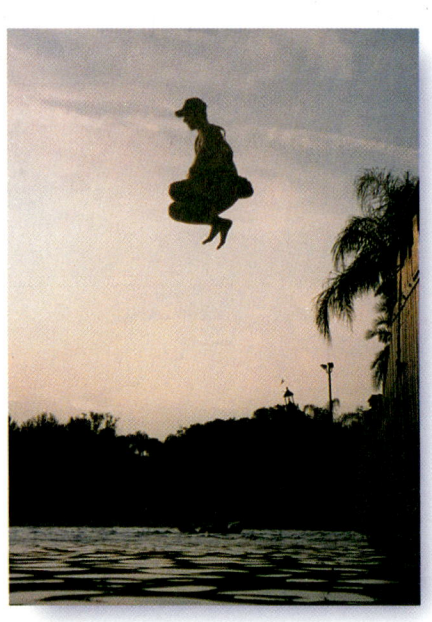

FIG 4.3 The compact jump entry is used to enter the water to do a rescue.

5. As you leave the chair or deck, bend your knees. This should not be a tight tuck position. Just bend your knees as if you were sitting in a chair. Be prepared to hit the bottom with flat feet. Your legs will absorb the shock.

6. You may go underneath the water briefly. The buoyancy of the rescue tube will bring you back to the surface quickly.

After entering the water with a compact jump entry, you must reach the distressed guest as quickly as possible. Some lifeguards prefer to use a breaststroke as an *approach stroke*, when swimming toward a guest, others prefer to use a crawl stroke. You should use whatever combination of arm and leg movements allow you to make the fastest forward progress toward the guest.

As you approach the guest, you should:

1. Keep your eyes on the guest at all times.

2. Keep the rescue tube in front of your chest, between you and the guest at all times. This puts you in the safest position to do the rescue and reduces the chance of other guests grabbing the rescue tube.

The only exception to this would be if there is an area of your facility in which you would compromise the 10/20 Protection Rule when using the rescue tube during your initial approach to the guest. In this situation, it may be faster if you allow the rescue tube to trail behind you as you swim. An example would be if you had to swim through a current or out from a waterfront area. In these cases, Ellis & Associates grants a variance, which allows you to pull the tube behind you during the approach stroke. Then, when you are approximately 3 body lengths (15 to 20 feet) from the distressed guest, you could pull the rescue tube across in front of you into the approach stroke position.

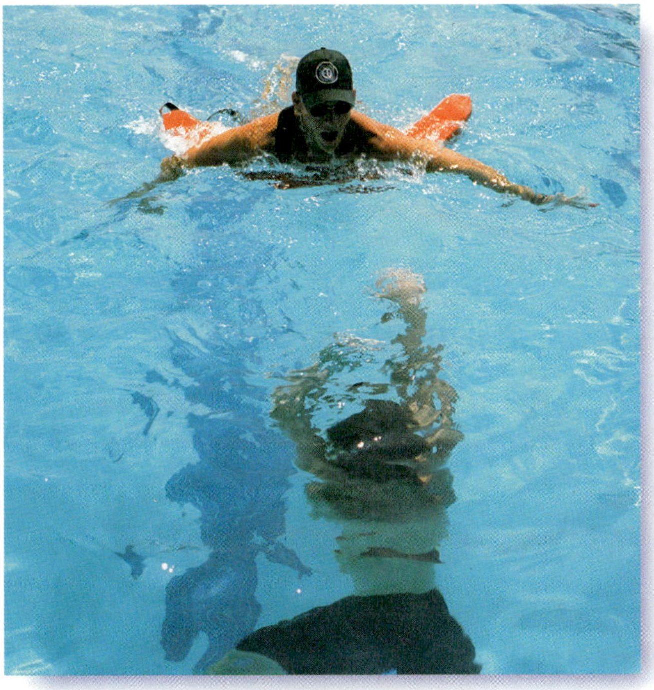

FIG 4.4a Approach stroke, breast.

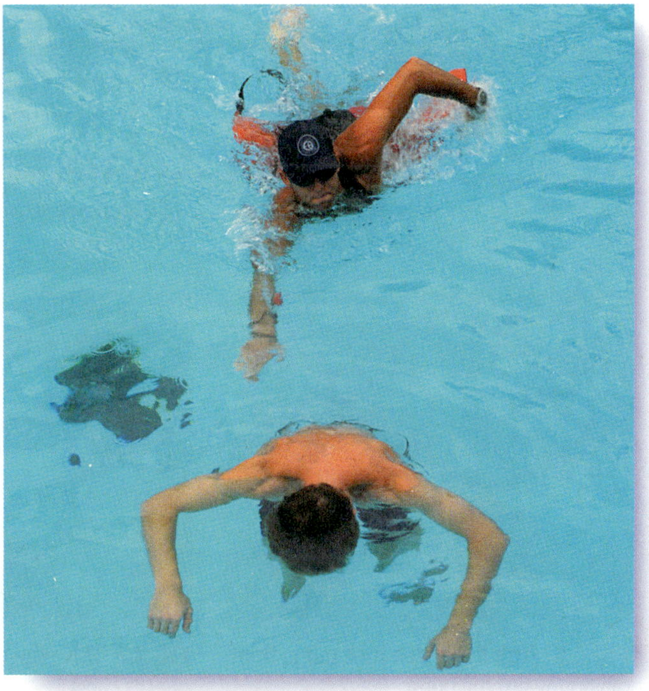

FIG 4.4b Approach stroke, front crawl.

FRONT DRIVE

The objectives of the front drive are to:

1. Provide support to a guest in the water by placing the rescue tube under his arms and against his chest.

2. Maintain control of the rescue tube and the guest as you move to safety.

When the distressed guest is on the surface, breathing, and facing you, you will execute a *front drive*. This can be done in either deep or shallow water.

To execute the front drive:

1. Whistle, point to the guest, hit the E-Stop (if there is one), do a compact jump entry, and approach stroke toward the distressed guest.

2. When you are about one body length from the guest, pull the rescue tube from under your arms and push it out in front of you with both hands. Keep your arms straight with your elbows locked. Keep the tube pushed out in front of you as far as possible.

3. As you get near the guest, forcefully kick to push the tube slightly under water to get it below the guest's arms. Push the tube into the chest of the guest, "driving" the guest backward. Keep your arms straight with your elbows locked. This will help to prevent the guest from reaching across the tube and grabbing your head. If she does reach for you, you can move your head underwater or to the side to avoid being grabbed.

4. Keep kicking and driving. Maintain your momentum and move the guest backward. Tell the guest you are a lifeguard and that you are there to help. Encourage the guest to hold on to the tube. Try to stay on your stomach with your hips up toward the surface of the water.

5. Move toward an exit point or the side of the pool. Keep your arms straight and your elbows locked. Continue to talk to the guest to reassure her.

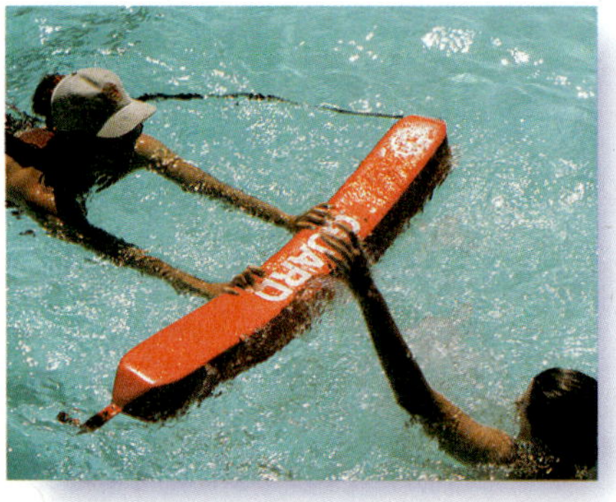

FIG 4.5 Push the rescue tube out in front of you toward the guest.

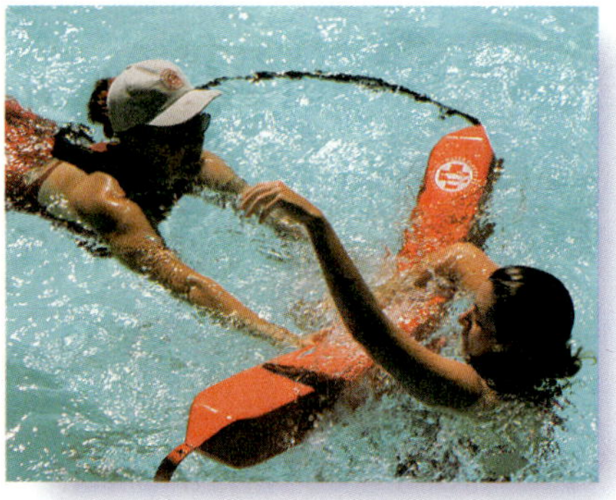

FIG 4.6 Drive the rescue tube into the guest's chest.

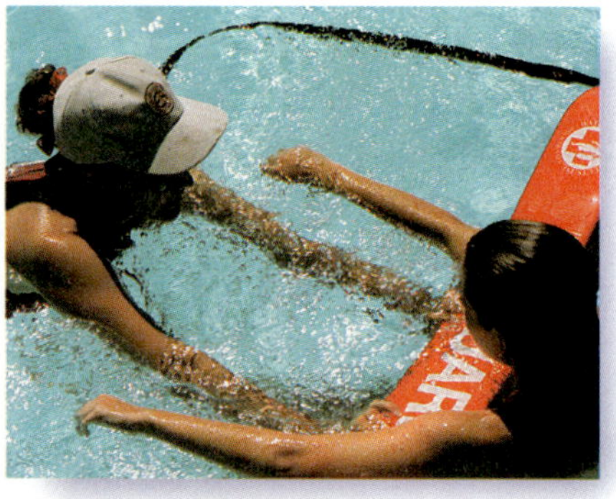

FIG 4.7 Keep driving.

6. Assist the guest from the water and make sure that he or she is all right before you leave. Your Emergency Action System should explain exactly what procedure you should follow at this time. Fill out the rescue report.

If the guest should grab you during a front drive rescue, there are several things you can do to prevent injury to yourself while still executing an effective rescue:

1. **Use a front huggie position.** Keep the rescue tube between you and the guest. If your head is still above water after the guest grabs you, continue to move toward an exit or the side of the pool. Reach under the guest's arms and "hug." It is very important to keep your head and body a little to the side of the guest so he cannot hurt you if his head moves quickly toward you.

2. **Use a flip-over.** Keep the rescue tube between you and the guest. If you are being forced underwater, execute a flip-over to position yourself on top of the guest. This puts the guest on his back. Keep kicking and moving forward. As the guest attempts to climb onto you to get higher out of the water, you can actually use his efforts to help leverage the flip-over. Try not to allow yourself to be forced into a vertical position or onto your back.

3. **Use a push-away.** If you cannot control the situation because of the way the guest has grabbed you, or you are choking, or you have lost your rescue tube, it is safer if you separate from the guest and execute another rescue procedure To execute a push-away, get some air, tuck your chin, and submerge. Push yourself away from the guest, recover your rescue tube, and position it between you and the guest. Either approach the guest again or signal for help from a second lifeguard.

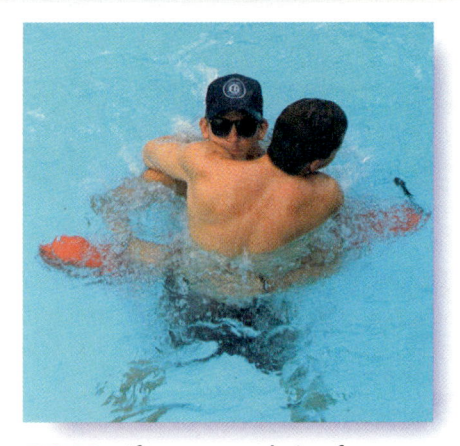

FIG 4.8a If you are caught in a front huggie, keep the rescue tube between you and the guest.

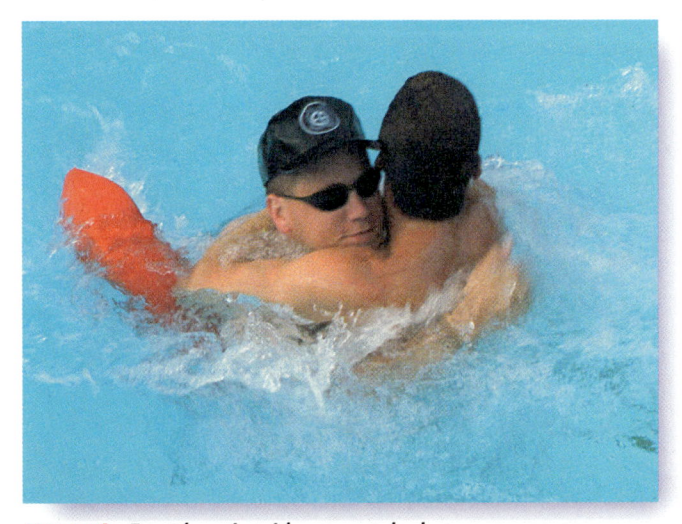

FIG 4.8b Front huggie with rescue tube between rescuer and guest.

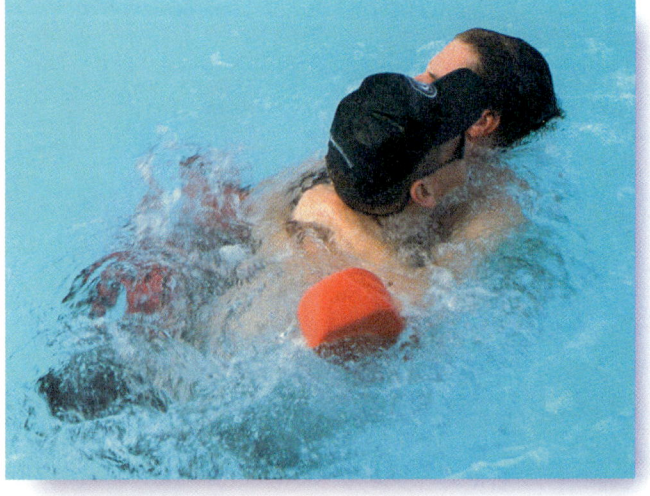

FIG 4.8c Executing the flip-over technique.

REAR HUGGIE

The objectives of the rear huggie are to:

1. Provide support to a guest in the water by reaching across the rescue tube with both hands and grasping the guest from behind.
2. Maintain control of the rescue tube and the guest as you move to safety.

When the distressed guest is on the surface, breathing, and facing away from you, you will execute a *rear huggie*. This can be done in either deep or shallow water.

To execute the rear huggie:

1. Whistle, point to the guest, hit the E-Stop (if there is one), do a compact jump entry, and approach stroke to a position directly behind the distressed guest.
2. Keep the rescue tube in the approach stroke position, right up against your chest and under your arms.
3. Watch the distressed guest's movements, and, as quickly as possible, extend your arms under the guest's armpits and wrap your hands around her shoulders. Or, you may wrap your arms around the guest's chest. Either of these techniques can be done even if the guest is slightly underwater.
4. Keep your body a little to the side of the guest. Turn your head to the side to avoid injury if the guest should snap her head backward toward you.
5. Immediately begin to talk to the guest to reassure her.
6. Keep the rescue tube between you and the guest.
7. Move toward an exit point or the side of the pool. Maintain a firm hold on the guest.
8. Assist the guest from the water and make sure that she is all right before you leave. Your Emergency Action Plan should explain exactly what procedure you should follow at this time. Fill out the rescue report.

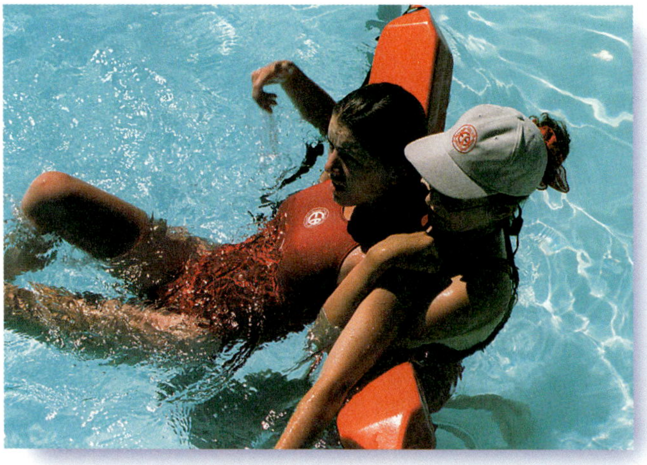

FIG 4.9 Rear huggie, shoulders. Remember to protect your face.

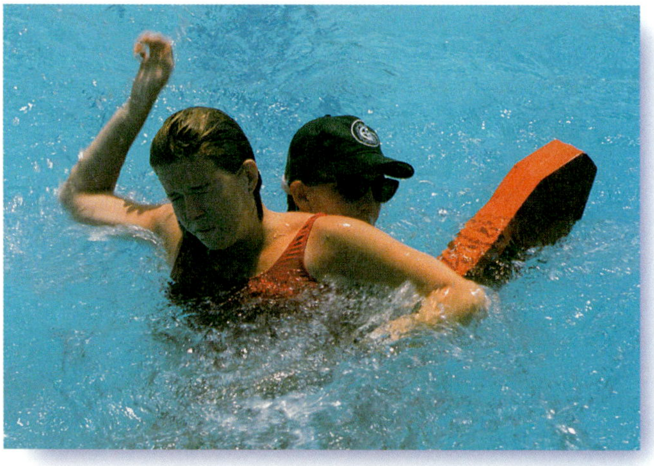

FIG 4.10 Rear huggie, chest. Remember to protect your face.

CHAPTER 4 • GUEST ON SURFACE–BREATHING   47

TWO-LIFEGUARD RESCUE

The objectives of the two-lifeguard rescue are to:

1. Provide support to a guest in the water by simultaneously placing two rescue tubes against the guest, one against his chest and the other against his back.
2. Maintain control of the rescue tubes and the guest as the two of you move the guest to safety.

When a distressed guest is on the surface, breathing, and too active for one lifeguard to handle safely, you will execute a *two-lifeguard rescue*.

There may be times when a guest is too active for you to handle safely alone. This can happen especially if the guest is under the influence of alcohol or drugs. The two-lifeguard rescue combines the front drive and the rear huggie. Even the most difficult guests can be handled safely with this technique.

If you feel you need assistance while making a rescue, to execute the two-lifeguard rescue:

1. Raise your fist above your head. Continue to attempt the rescue of the guest. Reassure the guest.
2. Keep the rescue tube between you and the guest. Keep your hips up and your body horizontal.
3. At this point, your back-up lifeguard (in the station to the left of yours) blows his whistle.
4. The remaining lifeguards clear the pool while covering the open zone. There are some facilities, such as large wave pools, where this is not practical. This is covered in your facility's Emergency Action System.
5. Your back-up lifeguard does a compact jump entry and approach strokes to a position on the opposite side of the guest. This positions the guest between the two lifeguards. You should still be attempting to assist the guest.
6. At this point, the lifeguards prepare to make contact with the guest. Communication between the lifeguards is very important. Each lifeguard must know when the other will move to make contact with the distressed guest.
7. At the signal to move (this signal must be one that the lifeguards know and have practiced as part of their in-service training program), the lifeguard behind the distressed guest will execute the rear huggie. The lifeguard in front of the guest will execute the front drive.
8. The lifeguard doing the rear huggie has to present a "target" for the lifeguard in front of the guest to place his rescue tube against. To do this, as he pushes his arms under the guest's armpits, the rear lifeguard brings his forearms up, with the palms of his hands facing the front lifeguard.

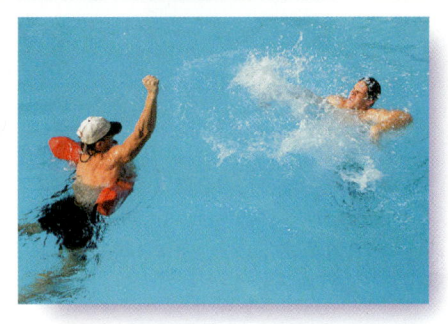

FIG 4.11 Lifeguard rescue signal for help.

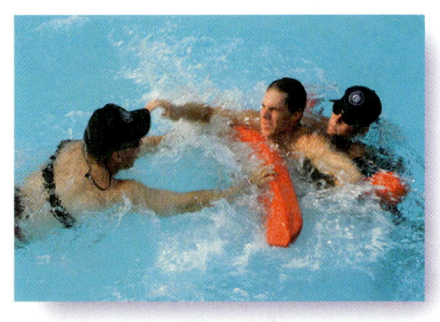

FIG 4.12 Two-lifeguard rescue. The front lifeguard executes a front drive while the rear lifeguard performs a rear huggie.

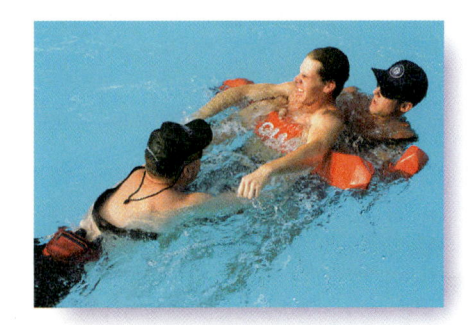

FIG 4.13 In a two-lifeguard rescue, the rear lifeguard pulls the resuce tube against the guest's chest, and the front lifeguard helps drive toward safety.

9. As the rear lifeguard presents the "target," the front lifeguard drives into the distressed guest. He places his rescue tube against the arms of the rear lifeguard.

10. As he feels the front lifeguard's rescue tube make contact with his forearms, the rear lifeguard should reach over the rescue tube to secure it and pull it against the chest of the guest. This "sandwiches" the guest between the two rescue tubes and lifeguards.

11. The front drive and the rear huggie should be executed as close to the same time as possible. Communication is important so that both lifeguards execute their skill simultaneously.

12. The front lifeguard watches the guest and the rear lifeguard starts to move toward an exit area or the side of the pool.

13. Both lifeguards should continue to reassure the guest while they are moving through the water.

14. Assist the guest from the water and make sure that he or she is all right before you leave. Your Emergency Action System should explain exactly what procedure you should follow at this time. Fill out the rescue report.

REVIEW QUESTIONS

1. (T) (F) The difference between a distressed swimmer assist and a near-drowning rescue is that in a near-drowning, the guest is unconscious.

2. (T) (F) The compact jump entry is performed with the legs apart.

3. (T) (F) In order for a front drive to be the most successful, you must keep your arms straight and keep driving and kicking.

4. (T) (F) Active guests in distress must always be approached from the front.

5. (T) (F) Communication between lifeguards in a two-lifeguard rescue is not important.

6. Why is it important to always try to grab underneath the armpit, as soon as possible, when you are assisting a guest?

CHAPTER 4 • GUEST ON SURFACE—BREATHING   49

Skill Sheet 4

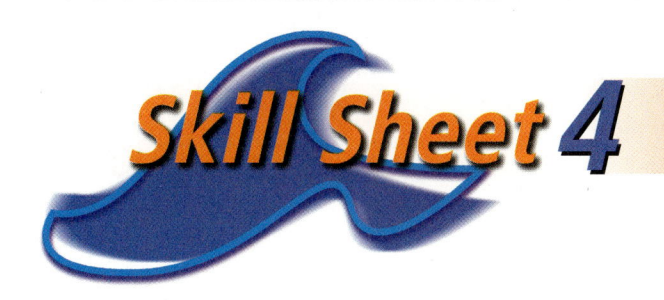

THE FRONT DRIVE

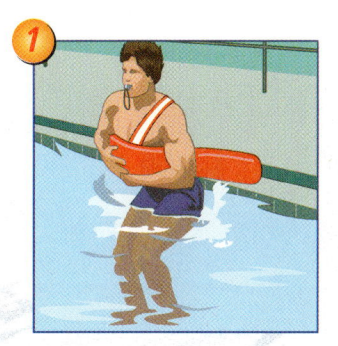

1. Whistle; compact jump with feet flat.

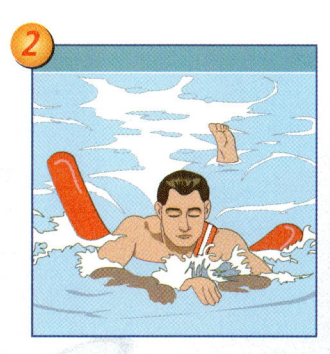

2. Approach stroke; kick and pull.

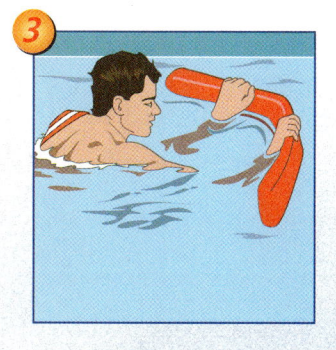

3. Extend rescue tube; lock elbows.

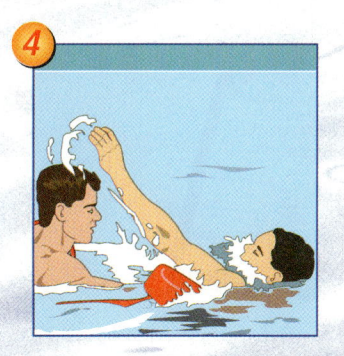

4. Drive rescue tube; keep kicking.

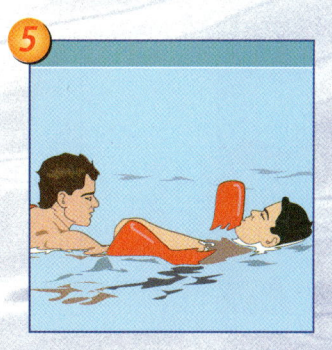

5. Keep driving; talk.

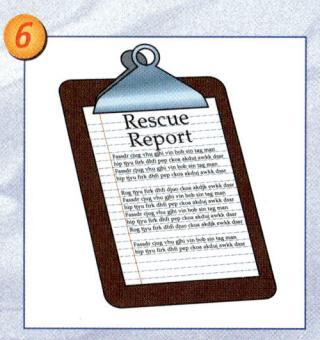

6. Secure guest at side; complete rescue report.

KEY POINTS:

- Keep kicking—hips up!
- Push tube slightly underwater before driving.
- Get tube under guest's arms.
- Keep talking; have guest hold onto tube.
- Keep tube between yourself and the guest.

CRITICAL THINKING:

1. What are some of the things you can do if a guest grabs you while you are executing a front drive?

2. Why should you talk to the guest? What should you say?

3. What type of distressed guest is the front drive rescue designed for?

PART 2 • RESPONDING TO AN EMERGENCY

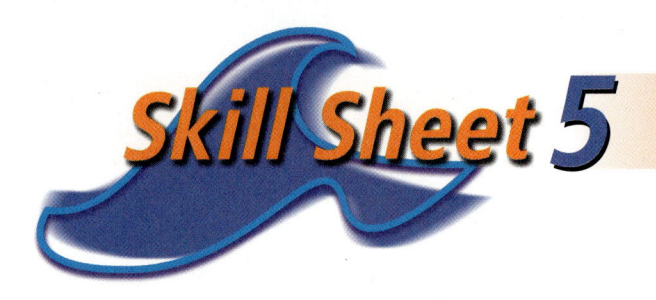

Skill Sheet 5

REAR HUGGIE

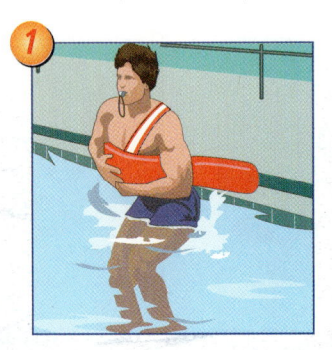

1. Whistle; compact jump with feet flat.

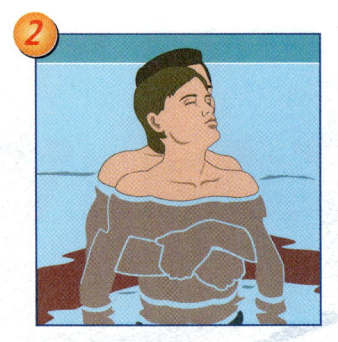

2. Hug under armpits, around body.

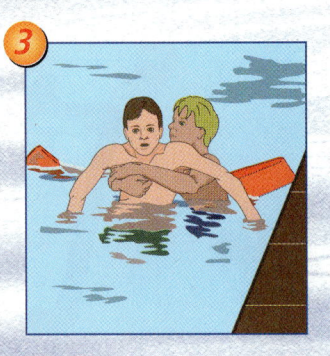

3. Talk; proceed to side.

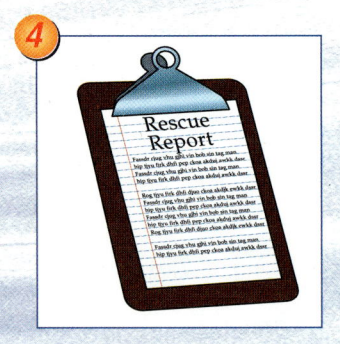

4. Secure and remove; complete rescue report.

KEY POINTS:

- Keep your body off-center and your head down.
- Kick–keep moving after contact.
- Keep tube next to your body, under your armpits.

CRITICAL THINKING:

1. What would you do if the guest struggles?
2. What if the guest is too big for you to wrap your arms around him or her?

CHAPTER 4 • GUEST ON SURFACE–BREATHING   51

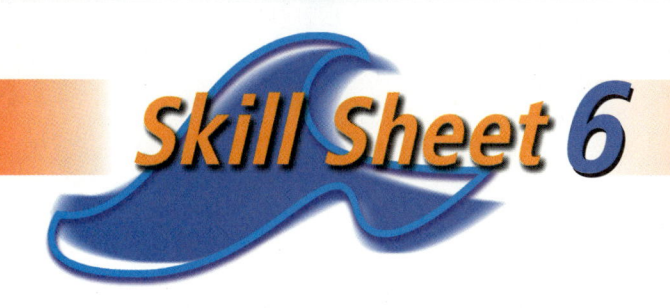

Skill Sheet 6

TWO-LIFEGUARD RESCUE

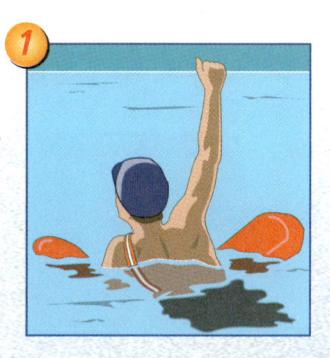

1. Signal for help; keep trying to drive.

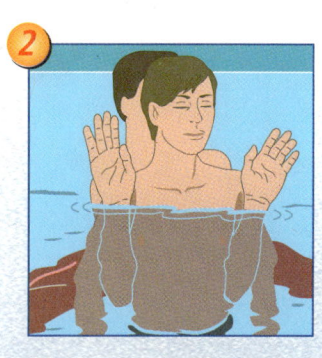

2. Lifeguard behind does rear huggie—"target."

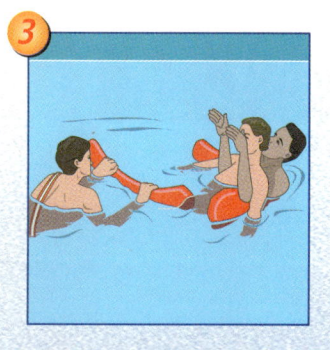

3. Lifeguard in front performs front drive.

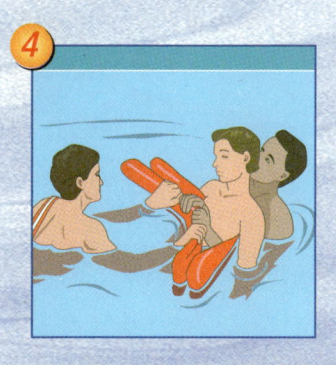

4. Rear lifeguard locks hands over front tube.

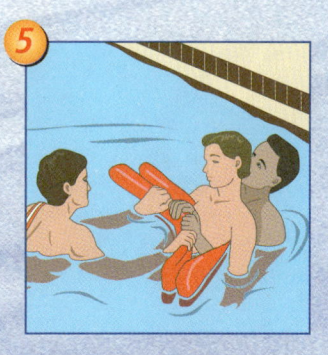

5. Talk to guest; progress to side.

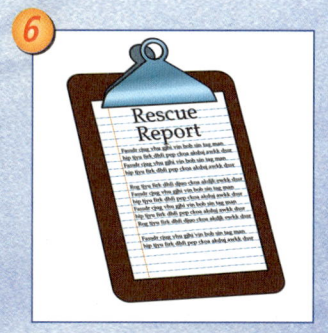

6. Secure and remove guest; complete rescue report.

KEY POINTS:

- Keep hips up.
- Communicate.
- Rear huggie and front drive at the same time if possible.
- Watch your head–keep it down.
- Practice being first and second rescuer.

CRITICAL THINKING:

1. What would you do if the guest became unconscious after the rescue was complete?
2. What is necessary for effective teamwork?
3. What situations might cause a guest to be out of control and make a two-guard rescue necessary?

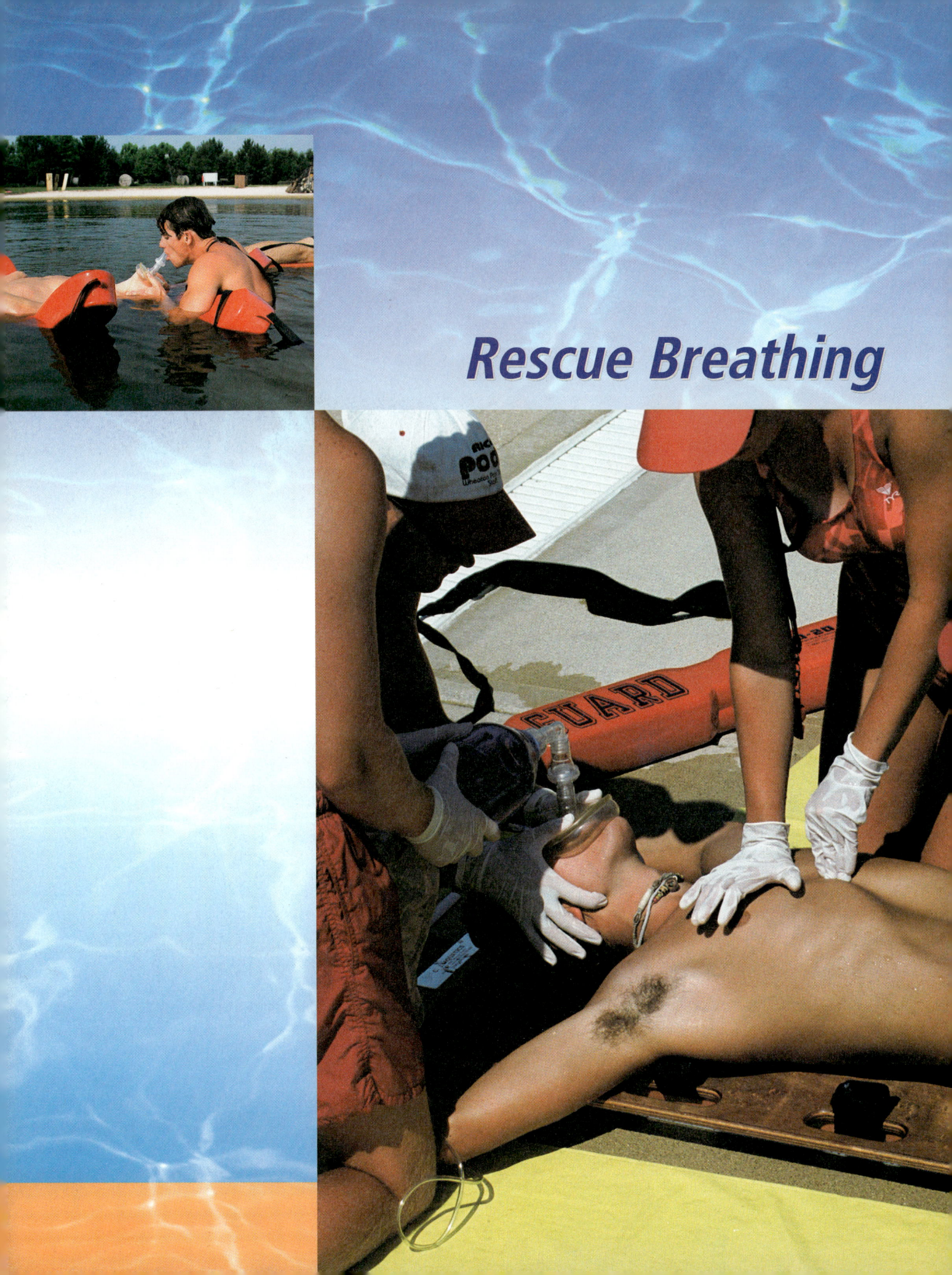

Rescue Breathing

chapter 5

OBJECTIVES

After reading this chapter and completing the related course work, you should be able to:

1. Demonstrate how to open an airway.

2. Demonstrate how to perform rescue breathing using a resuscitation mask.

3. Demonstrate how to perform two-lifeguard rescue breathing using a Bag-Valve-Mask (BVM).

4. Demonstrate how to clear an airway using a manual suction device.

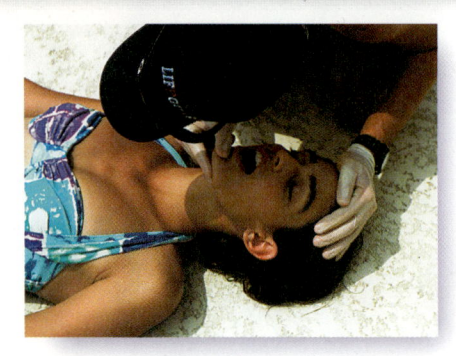

FIG 5.1 Head-tilt/chin-lift.

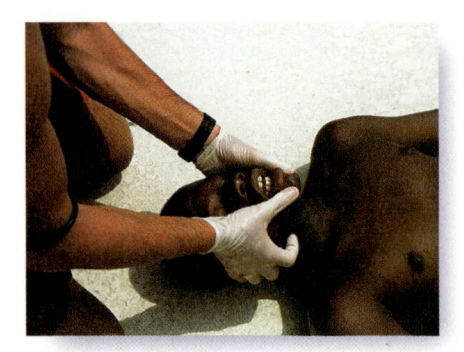

FIG 5.2 Jaw-thrust.

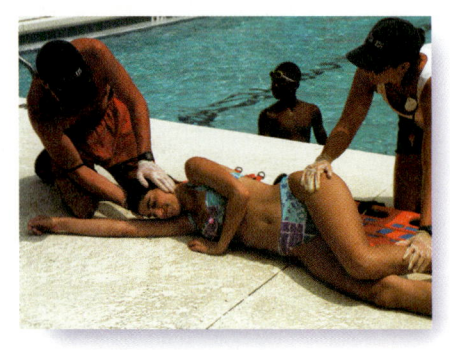

FIG 5.3 Recovery position.

*E*llis & Associates believes that the core of a successful resuscitation training program is its staff's ability to transfer a complete understanding of basic airway management skills to its students. Of the many skills you will learn in your resuscitation training program, airway management will likely be the most difficult to master.

BASIC AIRWAY MANAGEMENT

Of the various problems you may encounter in obstructed airway situations with unconscious guests, the most common is managing the anatomical obstruction of the tongue. When a person loses consciousness, he loses skeletal muscle tone, including those muscles connected to the tongue. The tongue relaxes enough in most cases to block the exchange of air through the airway, especially when the person is positioned on his back.

The basic procedure for relieving tongue obstructions and the core of basic airway management is the manual positioning of the guest's head. Tilting the guest's head back and/or lifting his jaw will move his tongue away from the back of his throat. Standard airway techniques such as the head-tilt/chin-lift and the jaw-thrust are based on these concepts.

It has been established that the combination of hyperextension and forward jaw displacement is much more effective in opening an obstructed airway than the use of either technique by itself. You should only modify this technique if you suspect a spinal injury, in which case you should not attempt to hyperextend the head initially. In suspected spinal injury cases, jaw displacement alone may open an obstructed airway.

There are two procedures for displacing a person's jaw: the head-tilt/chin-lift and the jaw-thrust:

1. You can accomplish the head-tilt/chin-lift by hooking two of your fingers underneath the bony part of the guest's jaw, and lifting his chin upward. At the same time, place one hand on the guest's forehead and tilt his head back, being careful not to shut his mouth completely nor to compress the soft tissue under his jaw—because either action may obstruct his airway.

2. You can accomplish the jaw-thrust by pushing the guest's jaw forward from just below his ear. To do this, hook your index or middle finger behind the angle of the guest's jaw, putting counter pressure against his cheekbones.

The jaw-thrust procedure is a more efficient method of airway management than the head-tilt/chin lift procedure because you do not have the potential of compressing the soft tissue under the guest's jaw, nor do you have a tendency to close the guest's mouth. The jaw-thrust is also the most effective procedure for you to follow as a lifeguard, because you may not have the option available of using an airway device.

Another valuable procedure for you to use if a guest is breathing but unconscious is to place her on her side in the *Recovery Position*. The recovery position uses gravity to assist in moving the guest's tongue off the back of the throat, and allows for the passive drainage of fluids from the mouth.

ENHANCED AIRWAY MANAGEMENT

To provide you with an improved approach to managing airways, we will discuss the use of three supporting devices that you can use as tools to "enhance" your overall management of a resuscitation incident. These devices are simple to use (with practice), and you can learn to use them correctly in a short period of time, but you should not consider them a replacement for your basic ability to physically manage an airway.

The Enhanced Airway Management devices are the:

1. Resuscitation Mask
2. Bag-Valve-Mask
3. Hand Suction

THE RESUSCITATION MASK

A resuscitation mask allows you to ventilate a nonbreathing person by covering his mouth and nose with a clear plastic mask, and blowing through an opening in the top of the device. A one-way valve can be attached to this opening to stop the guest's exhaled breath from passing toward you, and to eliminate direct mouth-to-mouth contact between you and the guest. This method is consistent with OSHA guidelines to lower your risk of exposure to infectious diseases. Another benefit of using a resuscitation mask is that when you connect it to an oxygen delivery source, you have the ability to increase the percentage of oxygen you are delivering to the guest.

One of the main advantages in using a resuscitation mask is that it allows you to move from the victim's side to over his head. If you are positioned above his head, you can use the jaw-thrust technique with head-tilt to establish an open airway.

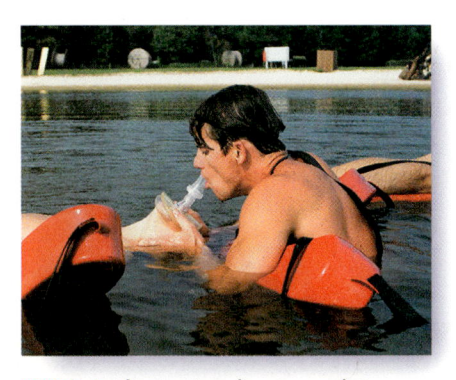

FIG 5.4 Eliminating direct mouth to mouth contact between you and the guest is one of the main advantages in using a resuscitation mask.

Follow these guidelines when you are using a resuscitation mask:

1. Inspect the mask before you use it. If you have a one-way valve available, correctly connect it to the mask. Examine the cuff's inflation to make certain that it is adequate before you place it on the guest's face.

2. Position yourself comfortably above the guest's head.

3. Properly place the mask on the guest's face. Some masks will cover both the mouth and the nose, while others may only have a single opening to place over their mouth.

4. Some masks may require different positioning for an adult or child. Practice frequently with the mask(s) available at your facility.

5. Place your palms completely on the mask, over the guest's cheekbones. Point your thumbs toward the guest's feet and as close to the neck of the mask as possible. Place your index fingers behind the angles of the guest's jaw on both sides of his head, near the base of his ears.

6. To open the airway, lift the guest's jaw and tilt his head back.

Determine the volume of the breath you should give the guest by watching his chest for an obvious rise.

7. To ventilate the guest, take a deep breath. The purpose of this breath is to provide the control you will need to give a slow and steady ventilation. Do not consider this deep breath to be the volume of the breath you will give. Determine the volume of the breath you should give the guest by watching his chest for an obvious rise.
8. Seal your mouth around the airway valve port of the mask, and breathe. The goal of ventilating a guest is to create a slow and steady rise of his chest while preventing gastric distention.
9. Allow the guest to fully exhale after each ventilation you give. This exhalation will prevent the build-up of pressure in his airway and gastric distention. A relief port in the one-way valve will direct the guest's exhaled breath away from your face.

Complications of Using a Resuscitation Mask

The most common problem that arises for rescuers using a resuscitation mask is the difficulty or inability of maintaining an open airway while ventilating the guest. If you are completely focused on sealing the mask and not on establishing an open airway, you will place downward pressure on the mask without any head-tilt or jaw displacement measures.

Other problems that arise for rescuers using a resuscitation mask involve the improper placement of their hands. If the heels of your hands are low, or they are not on the mask at all, you will have difficulty thrusting the guest's jaw. You will also have difficulty if you allow your fingers to creep around the guest's jaw angle, because this finger placement will simply close his mouth. Placing your index fingers behind the angle of the guest's jaw will prevent his mouth from closing, and will also place your (stronger) index fingers in a position to thrust the jaw.

THE BAG-VALVE-MASK (BVM)

A bag-valve-mask (BVM) is a device that allows you to ventilate a non-breathing guest without having to breathe through a resuscitation mask. You can accomplish ventilations by compressing a self-refilling bag and forcing air through a one-way valve.

The use of the BVM may allow you to feel more comfortable in providing ventilations, because it does not require you to be face to face with the guest, as you are when you use a resuscitation mask.

The biggest advantage of using the BVM is its ability to provide almost 100 percent oxygen delivery to the guest when it is attached to supplemental oxygen. In comparison, even the use of supplemental oxygen with the resuscitation mask only approaches 50 percent oxygen delivery.

The ability to achieve an almost 100 percent oxygen delivery concentration with a BVM is dependent upon having an oxygen reservoir system. These systems use a secondary plastic reservoir that supplies oxygen to the primary bag.

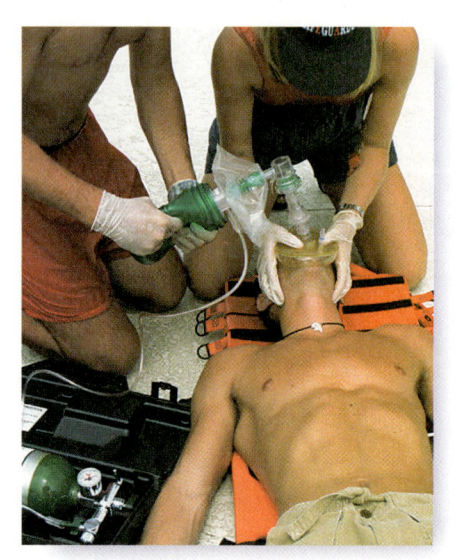

FIG 5.5 Using the bag-valve-resuscitation mask.

An adequate BVM should include the following features:
- A self-refilling bag
- A non-jam valve system allowing a minimum oxygen inlet flow of 15 lpm (liters per minute)
- Standard 15mm/22mm fittings
- A reservoir system for delivering high concentrations of oxygen
- A non-rebreathing valve
- The ability to perform under various environmental conditions
- Correct size masks must be used on both children and adults

Using a BVM

To understand the operation of a BVM, begin with the reservoir bag. When filled completely with 100 percent oxygen from an oxygen source, one-way movement of the oxygen is started. When the rescuer compresses the primary bag, air is forced from the main bag toward the guest. A one-way valve between the mask and the primary bag prevents the bag from refilling through the mask. Some primary bags fill completely from the reservoir bag through another one-way valve. Others may fill directly from an oxygen source. When the primary bag is compressed again, this valve will close and the reservoir bag will refill from the oxygen source. According to BLS guidelines, a minimum oxygen flow rate of at least 15 lpm is required to keep the reservoir bag refilled when ventilating.

As with the resuscitation mask, it is important for you to focus on your central purpose. Using a BVM without maintaining an open airway provides no benefit.

Two rescuers are required to correctly use the BVM. One rescuer maintains an open airway and mask seal, while the second rescuer squeezes the bag. Although there are techniques that allow a single person to use the device, research has shown that the two-rescuer approach is more effective in obtaining the desired ventilation results.

In order to establish a single approach for using the BVM, use an adult-size bag for all victims over one year of age. You can avoid causing gastric distension in younger victims by slowly squeezing the bag until you note a chest rise.

To reduce the length of time that it takes to set up a BVM for use, you should store the device so that it is ready to use again. You or your supervisor should establish a system of periodic inspections to verify "rescue ready" storage.

Follow these guidelines for using the BVM:
1. Perform ventilation with a resuscitation mask while the BVM is being prepared for use.
2. Verify that all BVM parts are present, including a mask, the self-refilling bag, a reservoir system, and an oxygen-connecting tube.
3. With the connecting tube, connect the BVM to an oxygen source that is capable of delivering a 15 lpm flow.
4. Begin the oxygen flow and allow the reservoir bag to fill completely.

critical POINT
Using a BVM without maintaining an open airway provides no benefit.

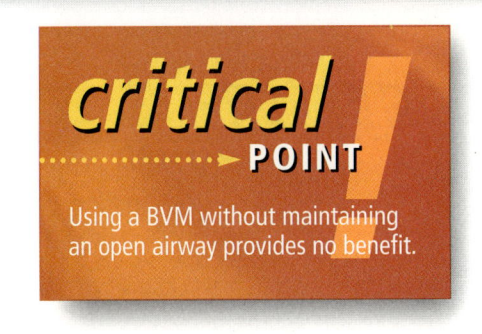

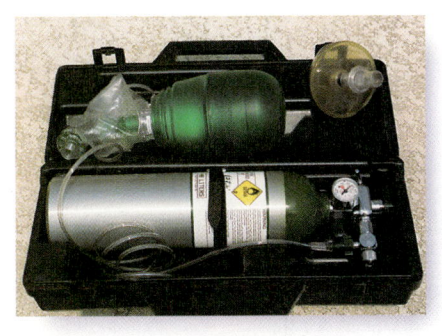

FIG 5.6 A BVM and supplemental oxygen system can provide nearly 100% oxygen to a guest.

critical POINT

The best way to protect yourself from legal liability is to be attentive, conscientious, efficient, and skilled. Airway management skills need to be practiced frequently.

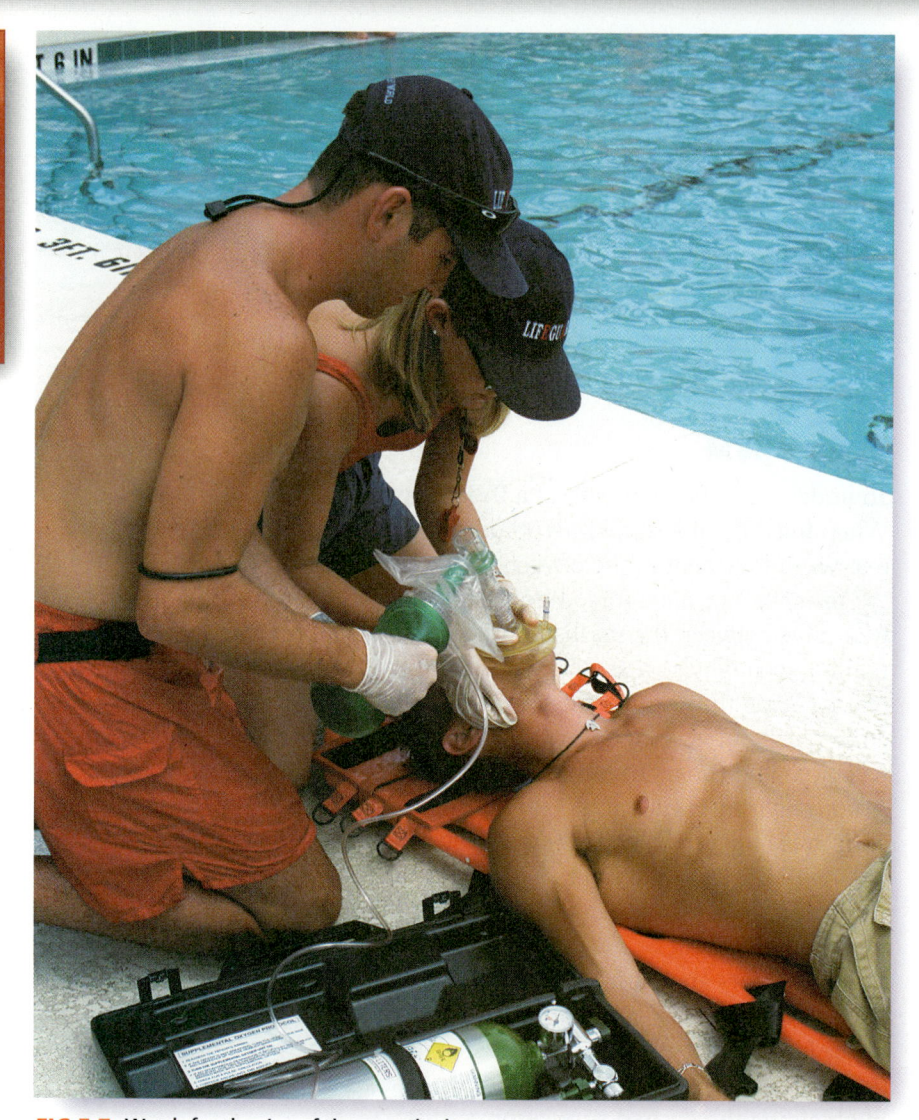

FIG 5.7 Watch for the rise of the guest's chest.

The first rescuer's position will be above the guest's head. This rescuer is responsible for managing the airway and is in control of the mask. Perform the jaw-thrust technique with head-tilt while applying the resuscitation mask to the guest.

The second rescuer's position will be at the guest's side, near his head. This rescuer is responsible for compressing the bag. The rescuer should use two hands, slightly offset, to gain optimal compression of the bag. Integrate the use of the BVM smoothly into the resuscitation process as quickly as possible. Place the mask on the guest's face and open the airway correctly.

Once the first rescuer has placed the BVM correctly and opened the guest's airway, the second rescuer should begin compressing the bag. Both rescuers should look for an obvious chest rise with each breath provided.

Whenever you suspect a neck injury, modify your technique by using the jaw-thrust maneuver without tilting his head. If you are unable to establish an airway this way, tilt the guest's head back slightly.

If, for any reason, using the BVM does not result in adequate ventilations, immediately return to ventilating the guest with a resuscitation mask. Never delay ventilations while correcting problems with a BVM.

Complications of the BVM

If you do not see an obvious chest rise during ventilation, the resuscitation is inadequate. You must attempt to correct this problem immediately.

The most common problem associated with using a BVM is the inability to provide enough oxygen volume. This problem is typically caused by the rescuer's inexperience in maintaining an airtight mask seal to the victim's face.

The standard bag volume is about 1600 ml of space. Even when a rescuer compresses it with both hands, an average volume of just over 1000 ml is displaced. Considering that the adult requires a minimum of 800 ml per ventilation, this leaves a very narrow error margin. The two-rescuer approach to using the BVM is designed to minimize the loss of a seal during resuscitation.

A lack of chest rise could be the result of an inadequate airway. Always keep in mind that the underlying importance of the manual positioning of the airway is to remove the guest's tongue away from the rear of his throat.

Monitor the reservoir bag for total collapse. If the reservoir bag is empty, the BVM can only provide the same oxygen percentage that is found in room air. A collapsed reservoir bag can be caused by:

- An oxygen flow rate of less than 15 lpm (Check the oxygen source for any problems).
- An empty oxygen tank (Continue to use the BVM with room air. Consider using another tank if one is available).
- An improperly attached connecting tube.
- A damaged reservoir bag or BVM (Switch back to a resuscitation mask. Replace the BVM if one is available).
- A too rapid ventilation rate (Slow down to BLS guidelines).
- A too slow ventilation rate.

MANUAL SUCTION DEVICE

Overview

The purpose of a manual (hand-operated) suction device is to assist you in removing fluids from the guest's mouth during resuscitation.

One of the most difficult situations you can encounter during resuscitation is when a victim vomits. Studies have shown that vomiting occurs in most drowning situations in which CPR is performed. Always treat vomiting as an immediate and serious threat to a guest's airway.

The largest risk a guest runs if he vomits is that he may aspirate the material into his lungs. Other problems from vomiting can range from the immediate blockage of the small airways in the lungs to the development of serious lung infections.

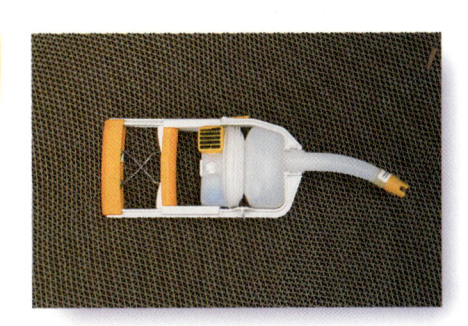

FIG 5.8 Manual suction device.

Always treat vomiting as an immediate and serious threat to a guest's airway.

You should always consider the fluid in the vomit to be an immediate concern. Log-rolling a guest to the recovery position can help keep fluid from entering the lungs.

Unfortunately, solid matter usually accompanies the fluid, and you will need to clear debris from the guest's mouth. A quick finger sweep of the mouth can usually remove most of the vomit.

In some cases, the volume and consistency of the vomit may present a hurdle for you to clear if you are performing basic airway care. During these instances, the additional use of a suction device can dramatically improve the condition of the guest's airway.

Follow these guidelines for using a manual suction device:

- Provide basic airway care such as log-rolling and finger sweeps of the mouth until the suction device is available.
- An unused cartridge should be pre-installed into the suction device. If one is not, one should be inserted.
- The protective cap should be removed from tip of the suction catheter.
- Spread the guest's teeth using the cross-finger technique.
- With your other hand, insert the catheter into the guest's mouth, toward the back of his throat. Insert the catheter only to the base of the guest's tongue.
- Squeeze the suction handle and hold until suction stops.
- Repeat the handle squeeze as necessary.
- Suction no longer than 10 seconds. Return to resuscitation as soon as possible.
- Cartridges are intended to be disposable, and should be disposed of as biohazard waste. After using the device, keep the tip pointing up to prevent the cartridge from leaking.
- Do not attempt to clean or re-use cartridges.

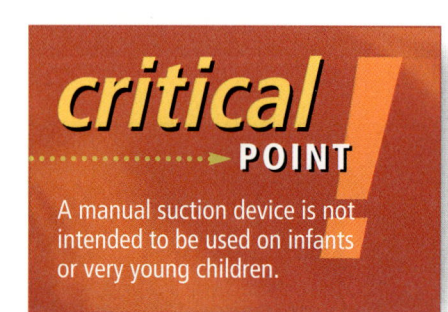

Additional Points to Consider

Leave the stroke adjustment of the suction device in position for maximum pressure. Be especially careful if you are using the suction device on children. *The device IS NOT intended to be used on infants or very young children.* Let the size of the guest's mouth be a guide as to when to use the device. Suction only the guest's mouth cavity.

critical POINT

A manual suction device is not intended to be used on infants or very young children.

Complications of the Suction Device

Clogging of the intake filter may occur when a particle is too large to fit through the catheter tip. You can tell when this happens because you will feel increased resistance as you squeeze the handle. Remove the particle from the victim's mouth by keeping the handle squeezed. Remove the particle from the catheter tip by brushing it against another object.

If the cartridge fills to capacity, excess fluid will spill out through the exhaust port, and sometimes the exhaust port will clog with large solid particles. If this happens, the handle will squeeze, but will not return to its original position. In this case, you can flip the exhaust port cover open and remove the filter to clear the clog.

If the suction handle does not squeeze from the start, check to be sure that the catheter tip was removed prior to use.

REVIEW QUESTIONS

1. Two commonly used techniques for clearing an obstructed airway are the head-tilt/chin-lift and the jaw-thrust. What is a third possible manuever you can use to clear an obstructed airway?

2. Which procedure is the more efficient method of airway management for a guest without a suspected spinal injury?
   a. the jaw-thrust
   b. the head-tilt/chin-lift

3. Use of which part of a resuscitation mask lowers your risk of exposure to infectious diseases?

4. How should you determine the volume of breath you give to a guest?

5. Name two complications that can occur when you are using a resuscitation mask.

   a. _____

   b. _____

6. How many rescuers are needed to most effectively use a Bag-Valve-Mask?

7. What is the largest danger a vomiting guest has?

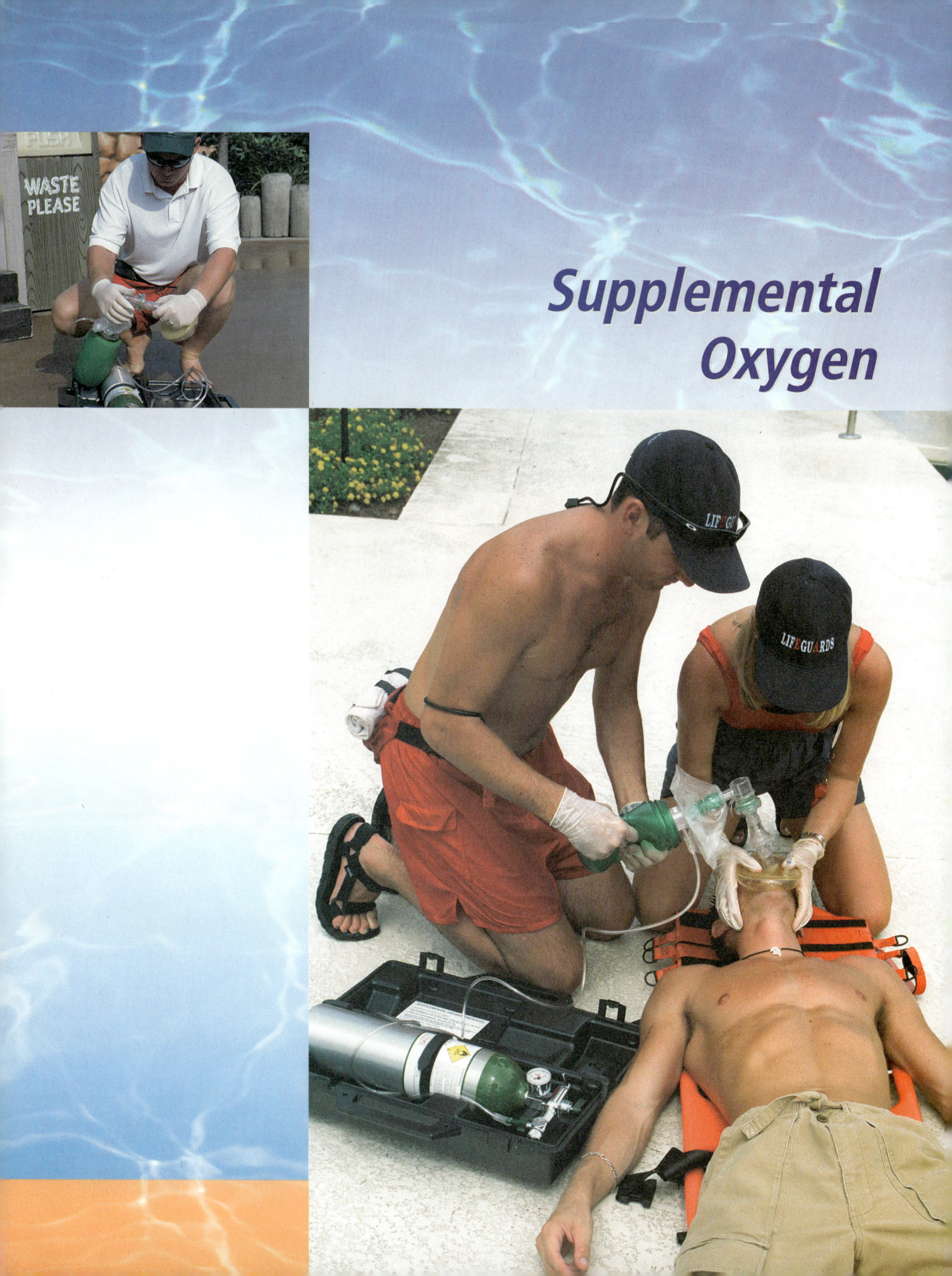

Supplemental Oxygen

chapter 6

OBJECTIVES

After reading this chapter and completing the related course work, you should be able to:

1. Summarize your role as a lifeguard first responder in an aquatic emergency.

2. Describe the importance of activating the EAS/EMS immediately.

3. Explain the benefits of using supplemental oxygen during resuscitation efforts.

4. Demonstrate how to use an automated oxygen delivery system to assist resuscitation efforts.

5. Explain the safety precautions necessary when using an oxygen delivery system.

6. Explain the difference between an automated and non-automated oxygen delivery system.

7. Demonstrate how to activate and deactivate an automated oxygen delivery system.

8. Explain the basic care and maintenance of oxygen delivery systems.

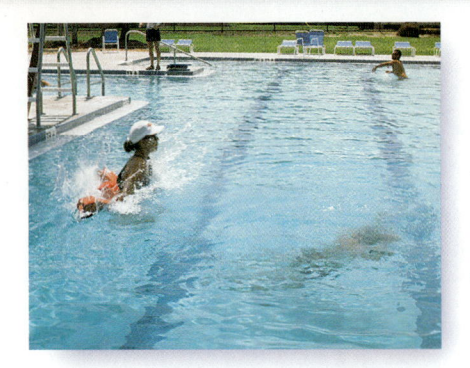

FIG 6.1 Understand the importance of vigilance and response.

Throughout the last quarter of the century, the skillful application of rescue breathing and cardiopulmonary resuscitation (CPR) have emerged as the mainstay of first-line emergency care in near-drowning incidents. Long supported by scientific evidence, both of these procedures have accrued an impressive statistical record of lifesaving and are now an expected part of any aquatic emergency action system, beginning at the lifeguard level.

Scientific literature and practical experience have recently identified the tremendous value of the early application of oxygen (O_2) to resuscitation efforts.

An additional noteworthy development has been the increasing familiarity of lifeguards and other aquatic personnel with the use of compressed gas systems (i.e., scuba diving) and resuscitation masks, both of which are the basic equipment components of supplemental oxygen delivery systems. These advances set the stage for the use of supplemental oxygen to support resuscitation efforts by lifeguards.

As a lifeguard, it is your role to anticipate, recognize, and manage an aquatic emergency. When you manage a life-threatening situation, you are responsible for activating the EAS/EMS and managing the guest's ABC's until more advanced EMS personnel arrive. Within these parameters, your training in airway management, CPR, bleeding control, and infectious disease protection is critical.

The addition of supplemental oxygen support in drowning and near-drowning situations will improve the standard of care you give a distressed guest until EMS personnel arrive. This can be accomplished without adding a burden that would be outside the scope of your duties as an Ellis & Associates lifeguard.

By participating in this training program and having the availability of supplemental oxygen support for resuscitation efforts, you are clearly setting the stage for creating a new level of expected management of aquatic emergencies.

THE LIFEGUARD FIRST RESPONDER AND SUPPLEMENTAL OXYGEN

Your primary responsibilities as a lifeguard are to anticipate, recognize, and manage aquatic emergencies. One of your lifeguarding roles is to be the first responder in aquatic emergencies. These emergency management responsibilities include:

- Promptly rescuing and removing distressed guests from the water.
- Performing a primary survey assessing the guest's condition.
- Checking ABC's (A-Airway, B-Breathing, C-Circulation).
- Activating your facility's EAS, or the local EMS.
- Providing emergency care until trained EMS personnel arrive.

Time is a critical factor when an aquatic emergency occurs that involves a guest who is not breathing, considering the heart's and brain's need of oxygen during resuscitation efforts. The medical benefits of adding supplemental oxygen to resuscitation efforts have been clearly substantiated. With the availability of fairly inexpensive, easily deployed oxygen delivery systems, lifeguards and others involved in a facility emergency action plan can successfully deliver supplemental oxygen to distressed guests.

As a lifeguard trained in the Supplemental Oxygen Support (SOS) program, you will use supplemental oxygen with resuscitation efforts and other medical emergencies when EMS has been called. The only exception to this will be if you are following the orders of a medical professional.

Your equipment will be designed specifically to meet the needs of a nonbreathing guest during an aquatic emergency. The simple design of the equipment reduces or eliminates possible distractions. This will allow you to quickly and efficiently perform your primary duty of basic life support, while simultaneously providing supplemental oxygen in what is often a tense emotional environment.

THE HUMAN BODY AND THE NEED FOR OXYGEN

Oxygen is a colorless, odorless, and tasteless gas. All living cells in the human body depend on oxygen as the fuel that keeps the body systems functioning. Although each body system has a specialized function, the systems rely on each other to maintain a state of normal, balanced function.

Some systems, such as the nervous and circulatory systems, require a high, continuous supply of oxygen and will begin to die in minutes if this requirement is not met. The central nervous system including the brain, alone requires almost 20 percent of the total oxygen transported continuously by the cardiovascular system.

The cardiovascular and respiratory systems work together and are closely interlinked in their function to provide oxygen and nutrients and eliminate waste for the entire body. Because these two systems provide such critical functions, anything that happens to them can quickly affect every cell in the body. It is necessary for you to have a basic understanding of the functions of the cardiovascular and respiratory systems to appreciate the need for oxygen.

The Cardiovascular System

The cardiovascular system consists of the heart, blood vessels, and blood. This system provides the body with a pump and a closed system of tubing through which approximately 1 gallon of blood (adult) continuously circulates. In this way the red blood cells pick-up oxygen in the lungs and deliver it to every living cell, and remove wastes to be disposed of by the lungs and kidneys.

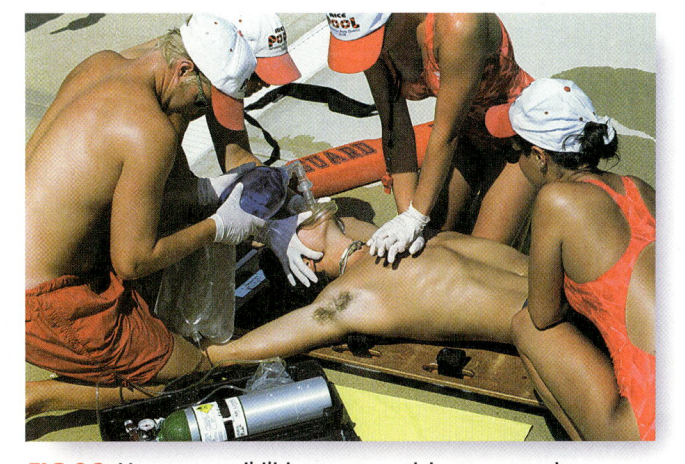

FIG 6.2 Your responsibilities are to anticipate, recognize, and manage aquatic emergenicies.

The heart is an electrically activated, four-chambered muscular pump that contracts rhythmically to move blood through the arteries and veins. Circulation of blood takes place in the following way:

1. Oxygenated blood from the lungs enters the left side of the heart and is forced out to the large aorta artery, which supplies this oxygen-rich blood to all parts of the body.
2. Simultaneously, deoxygenated blood returning from the tissues fills the right side of the heart, and is forced out through the two pulmonary arteries (right and left) to the lungs. The lungs then remove the waste gases and reoxygenate the blood to complete the cycle.

The Respiratory System

Most parts of the respiratory system, such as the mouth and nose openings, trachea, bronchi and bronchioles are simply air transfer passageways, often referred to as "dead air space." No actual transfer of gases into the bloodstream takes place at these sites.

The actual site for contact between the breathing gases and the blood is the terminal portion of the lungs called the alveoli. The alveoli are air sacs surrounded by pulmonary capillaries through which oxygen and carbon dioxide are exchanged.

Respiration, or breathing, is controlled by the brain. The body is able to automatically monitor the oxygen and carbon dioxide levels in the blood. When the oxygen level gets low and the carbon dioxide level is high, the breathing reflex is automatically stimulated and the body takes in more oxygen. This process takes place continuously and does not require any conscious effort because it is controlled by the autonomic nervous system. If the autonomic nervous system or the spinal cord that carries the nervous system impulses are damaged, the brain will not tell the body to perform vital life functions such as breathing and blood circulation.

DROWNING EMERGENCIES

In every aquatic emergency resulting in respiratory or cardiac arrest, time is critical. In near-drownings where the distressed guest has stopped breathing, there may be enough oxygen in her lungs and bloodstream to support life for 4 to 6 minutes. After the guest stops breathing, his heart may continue to beat for several minutes, circulating the existing oxygen to the brain and vital organs.

Once a person's heart stops or begins to beat inefficiently due to the interruption of its oxygen supply, any remaining oxygen in the bloodstream cannot be circulated. Without emergency basic life support in the form of CPR, brain death will begin. The actual amount of time until brain death begins depends on factors such as the victim's age, physical fitness, state of health, and even the temperature of the water. In most instances, however, irreversible brain damage occurs in 4 to 6 minutes after breathing and circulation have stopped.

During submersion, oxygen is not supplied to the brain, nervous system, and heart—which demand a continuous supply. Not only is the body not able to take in any oxygen, but the oxygen transfer sites at the alveoli are also damaged or poorly functioning.

CHAPTER 6 • SUPPLEMENTAL OXYGEN

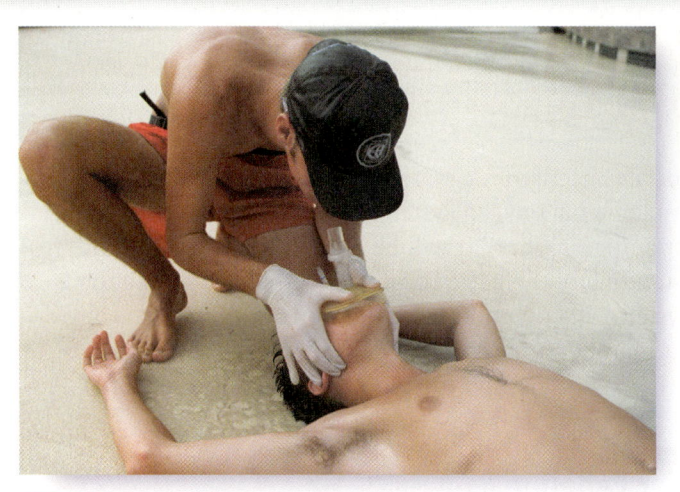

FIG 6.3 Time is critical in every aquatic emergency.

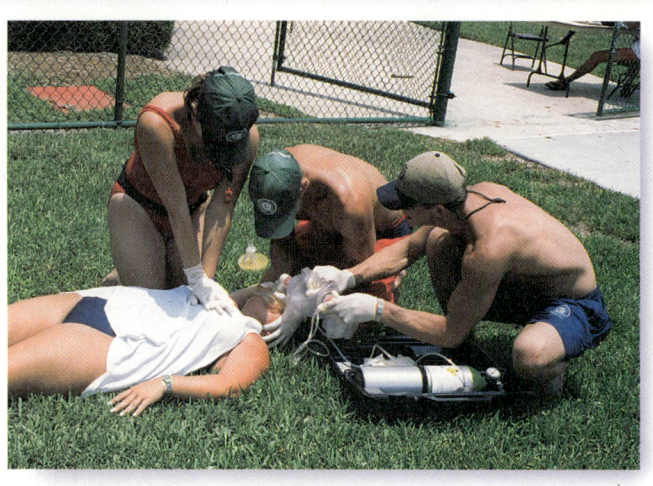

FIG 6.4 To counter-act the effects of drowning, begin efforts to restore the guest's ABCs as quickly as possible.

There are two types of drowning: "wet" and "dry." Wet drownings account for 80 percent of drowning incidents, and the specific cardiopulmonary response to wet drowning depends upon the type of water the victim aspirates (breathes in). Salt water will cause different changes and complications for the victim than fresh water. However, these changes and complications pose no practical significance to you as a lifeguard.

Dry drownings occur when a person's larynx is irritated by water droplets that enter the mouth and/or nose. The larynx constricts in an involuntary spasm to block fluid from entering the lungs. Unfortunately, this spasm of the larynx also keeps air from entering the lungs, and suffocation occurs. Once a person's body begins to suffer the effects of drowning, regardless of how the incident occurred, you can best manage the situation by restoring the guest's Airway (A), Breathing (B), Circulation (C), and increasing the oxygen delivery to the guest.

Rescue breathing or CPR provide approximately 16 percent oxygen to the nonbreathing guest. This percentage is the amount of oxygen that is not used by the body of the rescuer and is expelled every time a person breathes out. By increasing the percentage of oxygen that is available to the lungs to 50 to 100 percent, the partially functioning transfer sites can more effectively improve the delivery of oxygen. Therefore, providing supplemental oxygen support with CPR during basic life support efforts can improve oxygenation of the brain and heart, and prevent the death of these critical organs. In addition, the early delivery of supplemental oxygen can also enhance the advanced life support efforts of EMS personnel when they arrive.

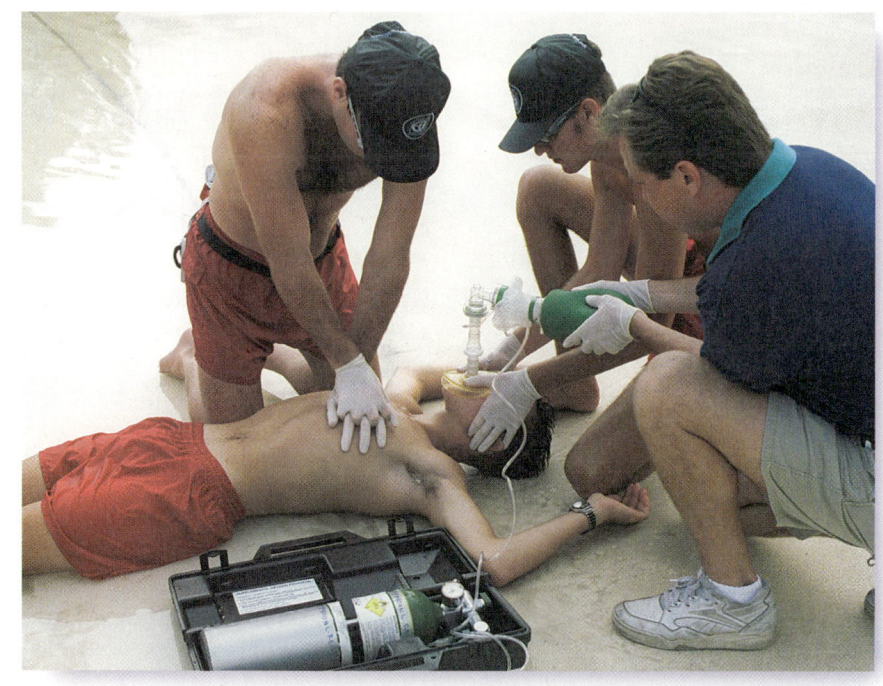

FIG 6.5 You can increase the precentage of oxygen to the guest by using a supplemental oxygen support (SOS) system.

COMPONENTS OF A SUPPLEMENTAL OXYGEN SUPPORT (SOS) SYSTEM

As an Ellis & Associates licensed lifeguard, you will be provided with a specific supplemental oxygen system (SOS) that meets the standards of our training program. It will be helpful, however, for you to have an understanding of the basic components that make up a total oxygen support system, whether automated or nonautomated. It is also necessary for you to have an understanding of the safety considerations when handling oxygen systems, and the guidelines for basic care and maintenance.

Oxygen Cylinder Labeling

Some states regulate the use or purchase of oxygen. The regulations vary from state to state, and usually apply to the purchase of oxygen for use in nonemergency situations. For example, some individuals have medical conditions that require a physician to prescribe oxygen as a treatment. It is the responsibility of the facility management where you work to provide oxygen systems, training, and protocols that will meet any local, state, or federal regulations.

Oxygen Cylinders

Medical oxygen utilized during resuscitation efforts will be contained in a seamless steel or aluminum alloy cylinder filled to a working pressure of approximately 2000+ psi (pounds per square inch). The size of the cylinder is identified by code letters. The most common sizes are D, E, or M cylinders and are rated to hold 359 to 3029 liters of oxygen at 2000 psi at 70 degrees Fahrenheit. The larger the cylinder, the more oxygen it can hold. The amount of time that the oxygen will last when the cylinder is open depends not only on how much is in the cylinder, but also on how fast it is allowed to flow.

Oxygen cylinders in the United States have a distinctive green coloration and a highly visible yellow diamond marking indicating "OXIDIZER." The product label will indicate "HIGH PRESSURE COMPRESSED OXYGEN GAS" with appropriate warnings concerning administration and proper handling of the cylinder. U.S. federal law requires that most common refillable oxygen cylinders be hydrostatically tested every five years. Hydrostatic testing checks the ability of the cylinder to withstand the pressure of holding the compressed oxygen, and makes sure the cylinder is in good condition. Your oxygen supplier will be able to give you information on how to have your cylinder tested.

Oxygen Cylinder Valves

Oxygen cylinder valves allow high pressure gas in the tank to be delivered by a pressure regulator. The valve has three holes that allow the mating of an oxygen pressure regulator. A rubber valve seat gasket or "O" ring must be present on the top prong in order to create a leak-proof connection between the cylinder valve and the regulator.

Oxygen cylinder valves also contain safety relief devices (rupture/safety disks) that are designed to safely release gas from an overpressurized tank.

The following cylinder valve safety precautions include:
- Valves and safety relief devices should only be removed and replaced by trained personnel using complete replacement assemblies supplied by the valve manufacturer.
- Safety discs should not be altered.

Pressure Regulator

To administer oxygen at a safe working pressure, and to control the speed of the flow of oxygen out of the cylinder, a regulator must be placed on the cylinder valve. The pressure regulators used on smaller oxygen cylinders have metal prongs that engage matching holes on the cylinder valve. The "O" ring must be in place to make a leakproof seal between the valve and regulator as oxygen is being delivered.

The regulator is equipped with a pressure gauge that indicates how much oxygen pressure is in the cylinder. By checking the gauge, you can see how full the tank is, and estimate the amount of time oxygen can be delivered if you know how long the tank should last when it is full. The regulator also houses a flowmeter, which controls the amount of oxygen delivered in liters per minute (lpm).

Flowmeters are able to deliver oxygen at 1 to 25 liters per minute. A continuous oxygen flow rate of 15 lpm is recommended for resuscitation efforts for nonbreathing guests.

A continuous oxygen flow rate of 15 lpm is recommended for resuscitation efforts for nonbreathing guests.

Resuscitation Masks

There are many models of resuscitation masks on the market. You have already learned the importance of proper mask placement and enhanced airway management skills with the resuscitation mask.

Most masks either have an oxygen inlet built in, or can be fitted with an adapter to allow easy attachment to an oxygen system. A one-way valve should also be attached to the mask to prevent exhaled air or bodily fluids from the guest from returning to your mouth.

The resuscitation mask is attached to the flowmeter outlet by clear, plastic tubing. A headstrap might also be included to help you maintain an effective seal between the mask and the guest's face.

Equipment Design for the SOS Program

The equipment design specifications for the delivery systems to be used by lifeguards trained in the SOS program were carefully chosen to:

- Meet the specific needs of aquatic emergencies, with a continuous flow rate of 15 lpm.
- Maintain simplicity in use and in training.
- Have superior reliability.
- Maintain the highest safety standards for the aquatic environment.

There are many types of rescue and resuscitation devices on the market that are designed to be used in nonbreathing/CPR emergencies. All of these devices require regular practice and frequent use to maintain a high level of skill in using them. Other devices provide options that are unnecessary for the level of care that you will be providing until EMS arrives.

If your facility chooses to use an oxygen delivery system that is different from the equipment used in this training course, you must receive additional training from your facility in the use of their equipment.

CARE AND MAINTENANCE OF OXYGEN SYSTEMS

Oxygen delivery systems require little maintenance. However, to ensure safe use and optimum performance, several guidelines should be followed:

- Keep the system out of the reach of children.
- Do not expose the cylinder to temperatures above 130 degrees Fahrenheit.
- Do not puncture, drop, or allow the cylinder to rust.
- Do not use any type of grease or oils (even Vaseline or suntan oil) on any device that will be attached to the cylinder.
- Oxygen supports combustion (speeds burning). Do not use oxygen near a fire or open flame.
- Release internal pressure before disposing of an oxygen cylinder, and do not incinerate.
- Never remove the valve of an oxygen cylinder.
- Have the cylinders refilled by a professional medical oxygen supplier. If you have had your oxygen cylinder for more than five years, U.S. federal law requires that it be hydrostatically tested before it can be refilled. Engraved markings on the cylinder will indicate the last date of testing.
- Keep the cylinder secure in a carry case. If you must remove the cylinder from its protective case, take care not to drop it. If you set the cylinder down, position it so that it will not be knocked over or bumped into, or roll away.
- After use in training, the resuscitation mask may be cleaned and disinfected. While still attached to the oxygen cylinder, one-way valves will have to be either disinfected or replaced. The mask and tubing should always be replaced after use in actual rescue breathing or CPR applications.

Oxygen systems should be checked and logged on a regular basis. The check should examine:

- The amount of oxygen in the cylinder. Check the pressure gauge or the time remaining gauge. Refill or replace with a fully charged cylinder if there is less than 15 minutes of oxygen remaining.
- The masks and hoses. Check to see that they are attached to the resuscitation mask and the cylinder. Check that they are clean, in proper condition, and properly stored for your system.
- Check the O-ring, regulator, on–off handle, and pressure gauge of non-automated systems to make sure all parts are present and in the proper working order. Additional O-rings should be kept on hand in case one is damaged or missing.
- External tank for valve damage. If any is found, do not use the equipment until it has been hydrostatically tested.

The oxygen delivery system must be thoroughly maintained on an annual schedule. It is important to maintain accurate records about your oxygen system. You should include the date of purchase, purchase receipts, receipts for any refills or hydrostatic tests, and all operating manuals or instructions from the manufacturer.

SUPPLEMENTAL OXYGEN DELIVERY

Since time is a critical factor in resuscitation emergencies, oxygen delivery equipment should be either totally automatic or assembled and checked for functioning at the beginning of each workday as a facility opening procedure. This will allow you to respond more efficiently to aquatic emergencies without equipment distractions. Depending upon the equipment you have, the system may or may not be left assembled at the end of each day. Refer to the manufacturer's instructions for your system.

The use of supplemental oxygen should be integrated into your emergency action plan. This can be as simple as designating a member of the lifeguard team, or even a bystander, to bring the oxygen system to the rescuer. It is critical that you simulate rescue scenarios and practice with the equipment that will be used at your facility so that you become familiar with the manufacturer's instructions for use.

Common Questions about Emergency Medical Oxygen

- **Can oxygen ever be harmful?**
  Oxygen is never harmful during resuscitation efforts. It always increases the likelihood of a better outcome for the guest.

- **Will supplemental oxygen substitute for rescue breathing?**
  No. In the nonbreathing guest, application of oxygen without rescue breathing will ensure the death of the victim. *It must be coupled with rescue breathing though a resuscitation mask.*

- **Is oxygen indicated after the guest revives?**
  Yes! Oxygen should be continued until EMS personnel can determine further need. Keeping oxygen on the guest may prevent him from relapsing into cardiac or respiratory arrest.

- **When should oxygen be started?**
  Immediately. However, if there is a delay retrieving the oxygen unit, you should use mouth-to-mouth rescue breathing during the delay.

- **If I am not sure whether the guest is breathing, should I perform rescue breathing or should I put the oxygen mask on the guest and wait and see?**
  If it is unclear whether the guest is breathing, start rescue breathing. By responding in this manner, you will not harm the person if he or she is breathing. However, DO NOT put on the oxygen mask and just wait and see if the guest is breathing.

- **If the near-drowning guest appears to be having difficulty breathing, should I apply supplemental oxygen?**
  Yes. If the guest is having difficulty breathing, applying supplemental oxygen is important.

The use of supplemental oxygen should be integrated into your emergency action plan.

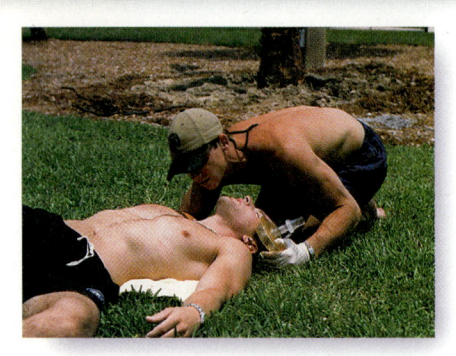

FIG 6.6 Assess the status of the guest's breathing and pulse.

- **Does medical oxygen require a physician's prescription?**

  Oxygen is classified as a drug when it is given in concentrations beyond what is normally found in the air and when it is used for medical treatment. The U.S. Food and Drug Administration (FDA) requires a prescription for medical oxygen, but has exempted this requirement since 1972 in emergency applications. According to federal guidelines, in order to qualify for that exemption and be regarded as an over-the-counter (OTC) device (non-prescription), the oxygen delivery systems must provide a flow rate of at least 6 lpm for a minimum time of 15 minutes.

- **Who can use an emergency medical oxygen system?**

  Anyone properly instructed in its use.

- **What are the legal requirements for maintaining an emergency medical oxygen delivery system?**

  U.S. federal regulations (under DOT) regarding refillable cylinders require hydrostatic testing of the cylinder every five years if the cylinder is refilled. Disposable cylinders do not have this requirement, but may not under any circumstances be refilled.

  Common sense requirements should include checking the contents and integrity of components periodically, performing function checks with documentation, and following any service/maintenance recommendations of the manufacturer.

REVIEW QUESTIONS

1. (T) (F) Gas exchange in the lungs occurs in the brochi.

2. (T) (F) The value of aiding resuscitation procedures by applying supplemental oxygen has not been clearly established.

3. (T) (F) The delivery systems recommended for lifeguard use employ a portable oxygen cylinder with a continuous flow regulator providing oxygen at a rate of up to 15 lpm.

4. (T) (F) The oxygen delivery system should be checked for function, and observations logged at the beginning of each day.

5. (T) (F) In a drowning or near-drowning situation, supplemental oxygen should be supplied to the resuscitation process as soon as possible.

CHAPTER 6 • SUPPLEMENTAL OXYGEN

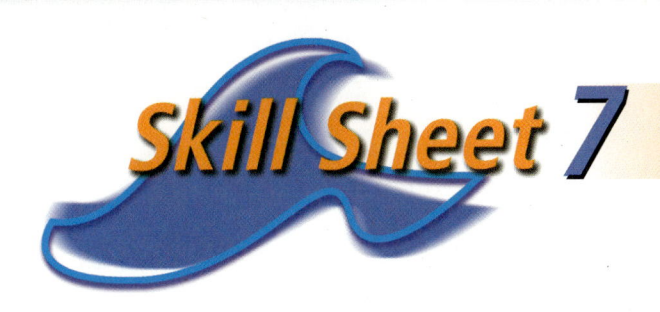

Skill Sheet 7

SUPPLEMENTAL OXYGEN DELIVERY

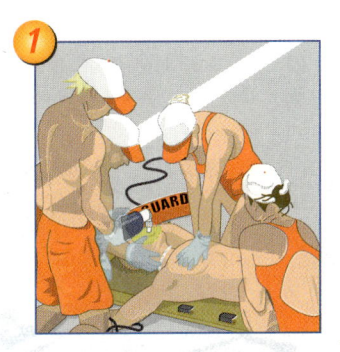

1. Assess the guest's ABCs and need for supplemental oxygen.

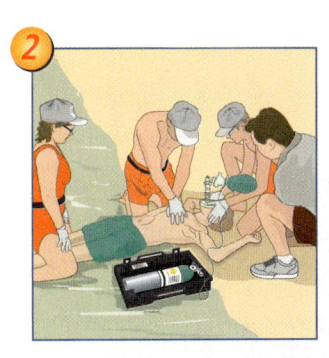

2. Provide supplemental oxygen.

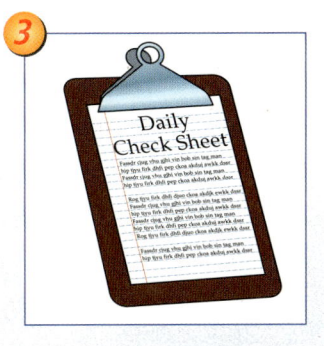

3. Provide proper care maintenance of oxygen system.

KEY POINTS:

- Check equipment daily.
- Do not delay basic care while waiting for supplemental oxygen.
- Supplemental oxygen delivery can increase the chance of survival in a respiratory or cardiac emergency.

CRITICAL THINKING:

1. How would you supply supplemental oxygen to a nonbreathing guest if you were alone?
2. When should an oxygen cylinder be replaced?

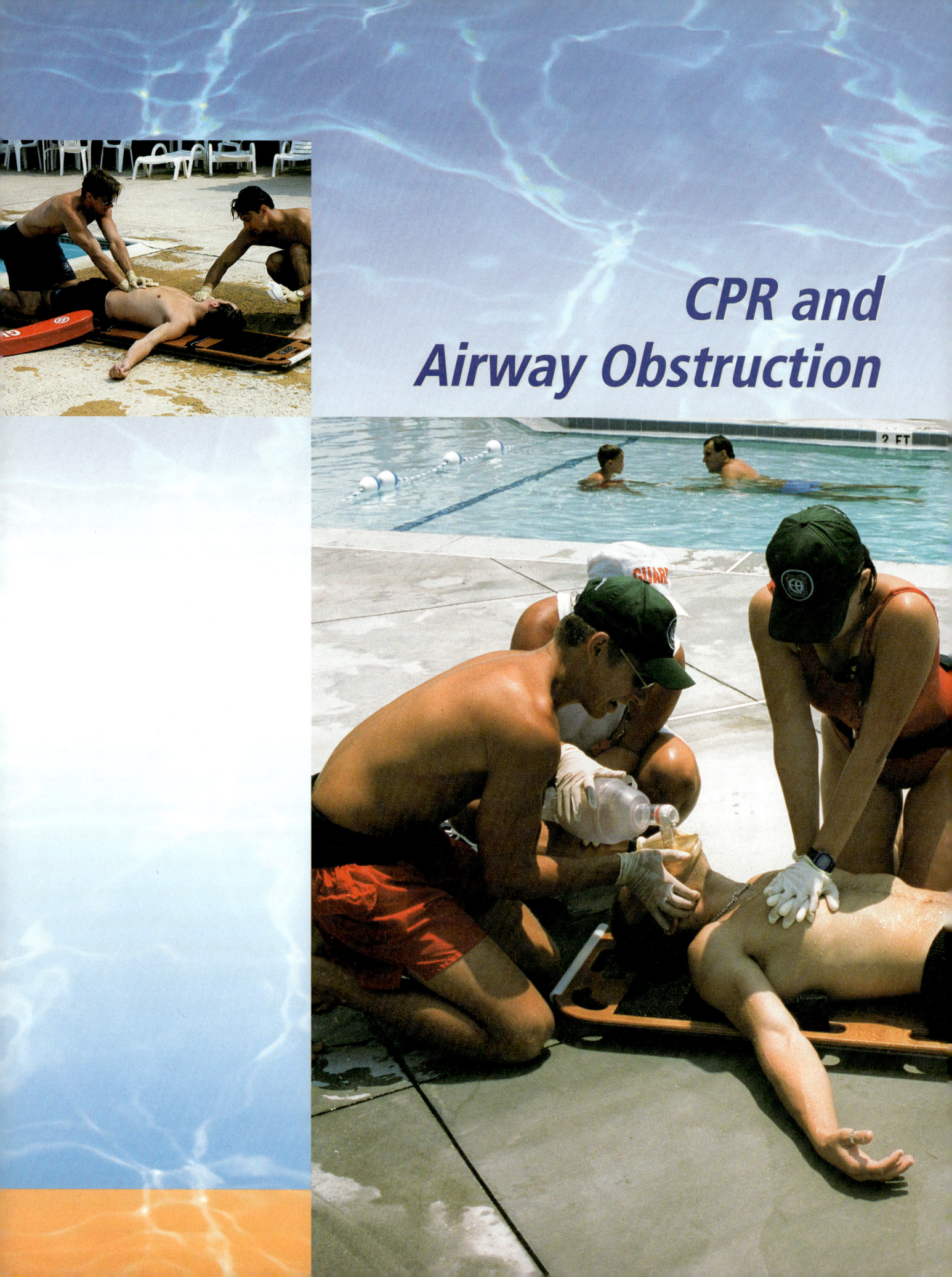

CPR and Airway Obstruction

chapter 7

OBJECTIVES

After reading this chapter and completing the related course work, you should be able to:

1. Conduct an initial assessment (primary survey).
2. Describe when to perform CPR.
3. Demonstrate proper chest compression techniques for adult, child, and infant.
4. Demonstrate how to remove a foreign body airway obstruction from an adult, child, or infant who is conscious or unconscious.
5. Demonstrate how to perform two-lifeguard CPR.

S E V E N

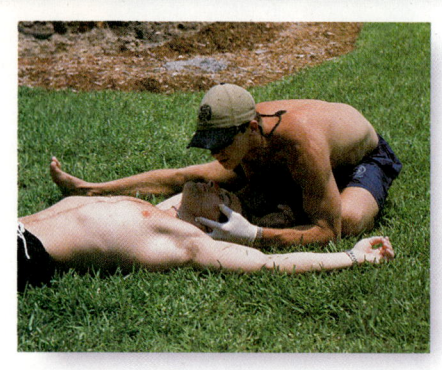

FIG 7.1 Practice your ABC assessment skills frequently to maintain your test-ready skill level.

Lifeguards have saved countless lives over the years using a basic resuscitation technique called Cardiopulmonary Resuscitation, or CPR. Components of this lifesaving technique include assessing consciousness, activating the EAS/EMS, opening the airway, assessing the status of the guest's breathing, performing rescue breathing (artificial ventilations), checking for a pulse, and performing chest compressions. You learned how to assess a guest for breathing, and perform rescue breathing in earlier chapters. In this chapter you will learn how to perform chest compressions on a nonbreathing and pulseless person.

CPR definitions and skills related to the adult guest are presented first, with techniques for children second, and infants last. Within each of these different sections, information on foreign body airway obstruction management will be covered at the same time.

While CPR skills are not difficult to learn, they can be difficult to remember months after you complete your training. For this reason, it is important to practice these skills frequently, so that you can recall them easily during an actual emergency event.

THE PURPOSE OF CPR

"Cardio" refers to the heart, and "pulmonary" refers to the lungs. Thus, cardiopulmonary resuscitation (CPR) represents a set of assessment techniques and skills designed to temporarily assist heart and lung function. CPR is only a temporary solution to a significant problem; it keeps oxygen-rich blood circulating to the brain until EMS personnel can provide advanced cardiac life support.

CPR AND DISEASE TRANSMISSION

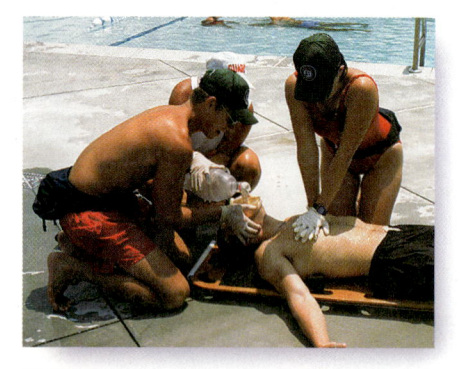

FIG 7.2 Know the ratios for compressions to breaths for adult, child and infant CPR.

In all medical emergencies, you should use appropriate barriers for personal protection before you make physical contact with the guest. The use of personal protective equipment from the beginning of an incident, including hand, eye, and airway protection, is particularly important when you are managing guests who require CPR, because during resuscitation efforts, guests frequently vomit with little or no warning signs, exposing you to various bodily fluids that could contain infectious bloodborne diseases.

ADULT CPR

The first step in adult CPR is to complete a scene survey to ensure your safety. If you conclude that a scene is unsafe, wait for professional help to arrive before you enter it. Do not become a victim yourself by forgetting to assess the safety of every scene. Once the scene is safe, and you have taken precautions against disease transmission, perform your initial assessment of the guest.

CHAPTER 7 • CPR AND AIRWAY OBSTRUCTION

FIG 7.3 Shake and shout.

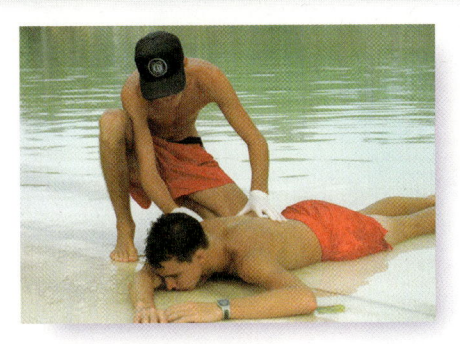

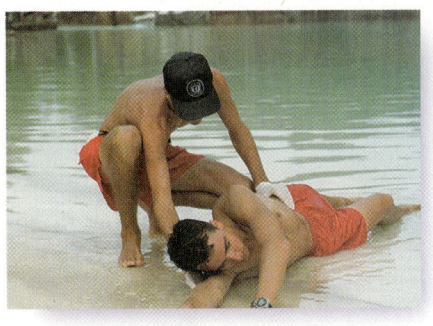

FIG 7.4 Roll injured guest as a unit

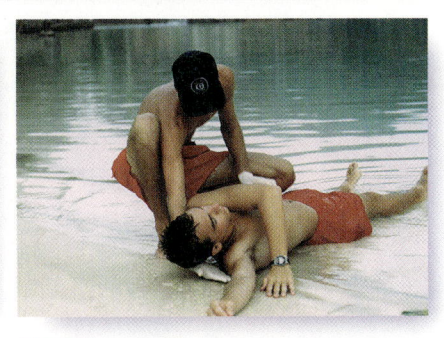

FIG 7.5 Roll injured guest onto back, protecting head.

The steps for CPR are:

1. Determine the guest's level of consciousness (shake and shout, "Are you O.K.? ")
2. If the guest does not respond, he is likely unconscious. In this case, immediately activate the EAS/EMS. If the guest is lying on his stomach, gently roll him onto his back. If you suspect that the guest is suffering from a head or neck injury, request assistance and carefully logroll the guest onto his back. Attempt to maintain a straight line between the guest's nose and navel. If you are in a two-rescuer situation, the rescuer holding the guest's head calls for the roll.
3. Open the guest's airway using the head-tilt/chin-lift method, or the jaw-thrust method if you suspect a head or neck injury.
4. Determine the status of the guest's breathing by *looking* at the guest's chest for movement. *Listen* for air passing through the guest's nose and mouth, and *feel* for exhaled air against your cheek.
5. If the guest is breathing, he will have a pulse. If you do not suspect any head, neck, or back injury, place the guest on his side in the recovery position, and continue to monitor the his ABC's. Have a manual suction device available. If you lose the guest's pulse or if he stops breathing on his own, lay him on his back and begin the next step.

critical POINT

Do not become a victim yourself by forgetting to assess the safety of every scene.

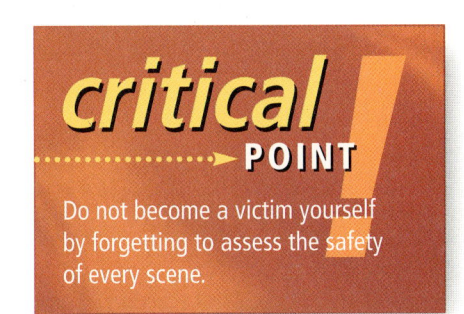

FIG 7.6 Open airway.

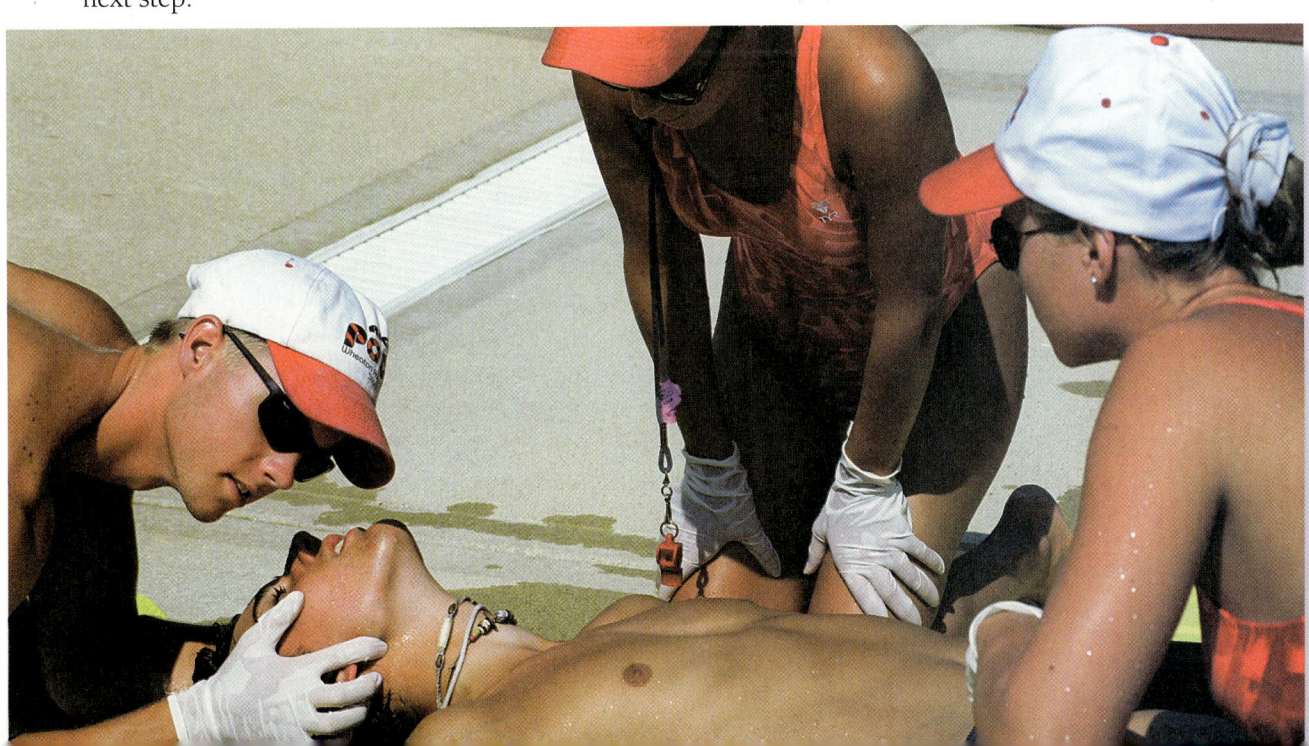

FIG 7.7 Recovery position.

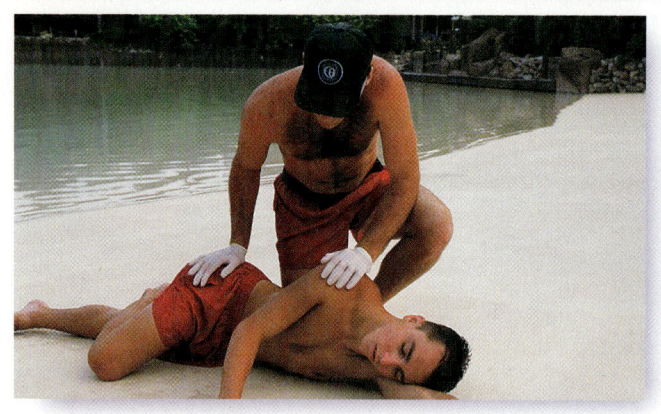

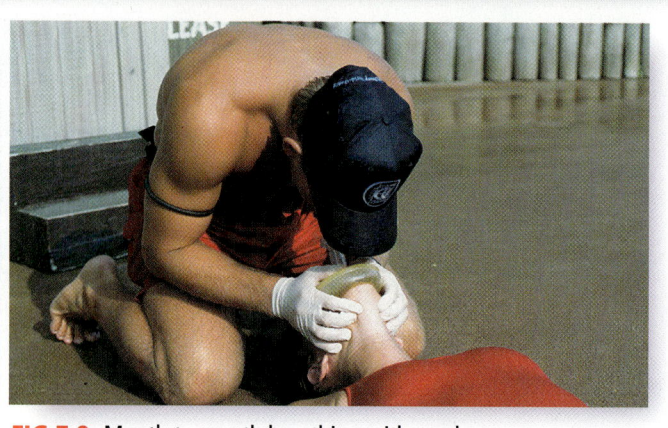

FIG 7.8 Mouth to mouth breathing with mask.

6. If the guest is not breathing, place a resuscitation mask over his mouth and nose and administer 2 slow breaths. Each breath should take 1.5 to 2.0 seconds to deliver. Watch the rise and fall of the guest's chest during each breath.

   If you are trained in the use of the Bag-Valve-Mask (BVM) device, and have one available, attach it to oxygen and provide ventilations. Otherwise, attach the oxygen to the resuscitation mask.

7. If your initial attempt at rescue breathing is unsuccessful, reposition the guest's airway and attempt a second ventilation. If your second attempt is also unsuccessful, immediately begin the appropriate foreign body airway obstruction (choking) removal techniques, which will be described later in this chapter.

8. Once you have successfully provided the guest with two slow breaths, assess his circulation.

9. The pulse in an adult is found at either of the two carotid arteries in the neck. Using two or three fingers, locate the Adam's apple, and slide your fingers into the groove at the side of the neck closest to you. Feel for a pulse for 5 to 10 seconds.

10. If the guest has a pulse, but is not breathing spontaneously, begin rescue breathing and re-check his pulse each minute

11. If the guest is pulseless, begin CPR.

Chest Compressions

To correctly perform chest compressions, you must find the appropriate landmarks so that you can correctly position your hands. If you place your hands incorrectly, you can cause the following injuries to your guest: collapsed lungs, lacerated abdominal organs, and internal bleeding.

To find the correct chest compression landmarks:

1. Remove any thick clothing that is covering the guest's chest. Kneel beside the guest's chest and run two fingers up along her rib cage until you feel the xiphoid process, a triangle-like bone at the lower end of the sternum.

2. Slide your two fingers up toward the guest's head, two finger-widths above the xiphoid bone. Keep those two fingers in place.

3. Place the heel of your free hand directly beside (toward the head) your two fingers.

4. Remove your two fingers and place this free hand on top of your other hand, which is in the center of the guest's chest, and interlock your fingers.
5. Lock your elbows, place your shoulders directly over your hands and compress the guest's chest 1.5 to 2 inches. Perform 15 compression about every 10 seconds. This will equal a rate of 80-100 compressions a minute. Compressing the heart in this manner only provides the patient with 25 percent of the blood flow normally produced by a healthy beating heart.

Do not be alarmed if a few of the guest's ribs fracture while you are performing compressions. However, exercise caution and try not to be overly aggressive with your compression depth. If possible, have someone help you determine the right depth of compressions.

Your best indicator of effective chest compressions is the generation of an artificial pulse in the carotid arteries.

Coordinating Chest Compressions and Rescue Breathing (Ventilations)

A ratio is the comparison of two or more numbers. The ratio of compressions-to-ventilations in adult CPR is 15 compressions for every two ventilations, or 15:2. Every time you complete 15 compressions and 2 ventilations, this a **cycle**. For an adult guest, during one minute of resuscitation, you should be able to complete 4 cycles.

At the end of 4 complete cycles, or if the guest shows signs of improved consciousness (moaning, moving, etc.), you should immediately stop compressions and check the guest's pulse for 5 to 10 seconds.

If you find a pulse, check the quality of the guest's breathing by using the head-tilt/chin-lift or jaw-thrust methods to open their airway, and look, listen, and feel for breaths. If the guest is not spontaneously breathing, continue rescue breathing techniques and monitor his pulse. If you do not find a pulse, continue chest compressions and rescue breathing cycles. Recheck the guest's pulse after every few minutes.

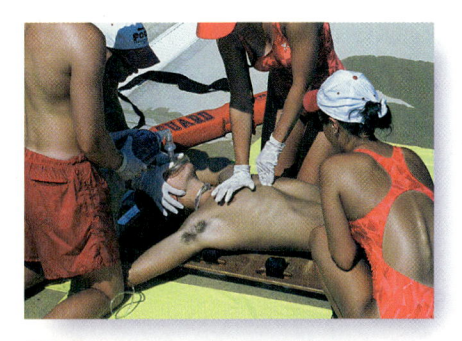

FIG 7.9 Compressions position.

Common CPR performance problems

There are several common problems with CPR performance, including:
- Incorrect hand position.
- Incorrect depth of compressions.
- Failure to maintain an adequate mask seal.
- Bending arms or "jabbing" during compressions.
- Using too much force when ventilating.
- High flow oxygen not attached or flowing.
- Failure to maintain correct open airway position.
- Failure to activate the EAS/EMS early.
- Failure to recognize either pulselessness or breathlessness.

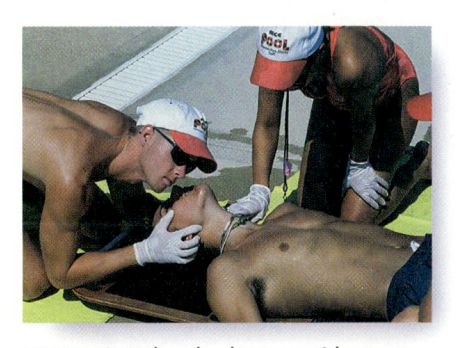

FIG 7.10 Pulse check at carotid artery.

Two-Lifeguard CPR

In many emergency situations, more than one lifeguard will be involved. Two lifeguard CPR can help reduce your fatigue and improve your efficiency. The tasks of providing chest compressions and rescue breathing are physically demanding. Do not hesitate to ask for relief when you are performing CPR.

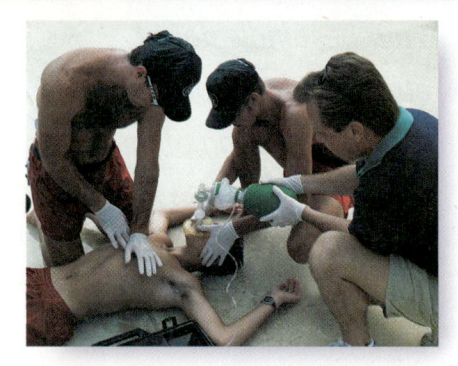

FIG 7.11 Performing two-lifeguard CPR is less tiring and more effective than one-lifeguard CPR.

Only a few minor modifications are required during two-lifeguard CPR. The major differences in the CPR steps involve the ratio of compressions to ventilations and the number of cycles completed before reassessing the patient's pulse.

For two-lifeguard CPR, the compression-to-ventilation ratio changes from 15:2 to 5:1. With this new ratio, about 12 cycles should be completed prior to reassessing the guest's pulse. In the typical resuscitation event, one person performs chest compressions, while the other person performs ventilations using a resuscitation mask. If either of the rescuers becomes exhausted, he or she should ask for a change of tasks at the end of the next cycle. Commonly, a shift in positions occurs at the end of one minute and while the guest's carotid pulse is being assessed.

FOREIGN BODY AIRWAY OBSTRUCTION (FBAO) MANAGEMENT

Occasionally, a complete airway obstruction may cause unconsciousness and respiratory or cardiac arrest. The most common cause of upper airway obstruction in the unconscious adult is the tongue. When a person becomes unconscious, muscle control is lost, and consequently, the tongue (a muscle) falls back against the upper airway, blocking it. Upper airway obstruction can also occur from almost any object that someone can place in their mouth. In adults, alcohol consumption is a contributing factor in airway obstruction cases.

Partial Foreign-Body Airway Obstruction

There are two categories of FBAO: partial and complete. A partial airway obstruction allows limited air movement past the vocal cords, and usually stimulates the gag reflex. In this case, the guest will be coughing or gagging, making a forceful attempt to dislodge the object. She may appear anxious and frightened, and will sometimes be clutching her throat in the Universal Distress Sign of Choking.

Partial foreign body airway obstruction treatment

Follow these steps to treat a guest with a partial foreign body airway obstruction:

1. Assess the amount of air exchange occurring. Can the guest talk? Does her gagging and coughing appear to be dislodging the object?

2. Reassure the guest and coach her as she attempts to naturally dislodge the object.

3. Monitor the guest's condition until either the object is removed or the obstruction becomes complete. If partial obstruction persists, activate the EAS/EMS.

4. Do not attempt to forcefully dislodge the object with back blows or other similar techniques. Using these sorts of techniques can cause the obstruction to lodge deeper in the airway, and cause a complete airway obstruction.

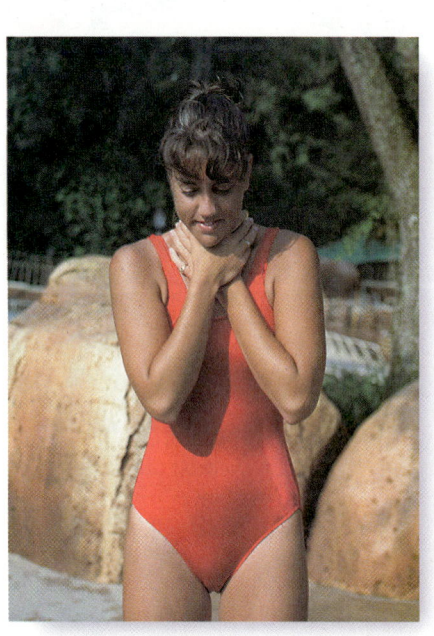

FIG 7.12 Universal sign of distress: clasping the throat.

Complete Foreign Body Airway Obstruction

A complete foreign body airway obstruction is just what is sounds like; little or no air is able to enter or leave the guest's airway. This is a life-threatening emergency! The guest will be unable to breathe, cough, or talk. Her skin color will quickly become cyanotic (blue), especially around her lips and fingers. Because the guest will be unable to talk or communicate, she will usually use the Universal Distress Sign of Choking.

Complete foreign body airway obstruction treatment for a conscious adult

Follow these steps for a conscious adult with a complete airway obstruction:

1. Ask the guest "Are you choking?"
2. If she is unable to respond, tell her you are going to help relieve the object using the Heimlich Maneuver.
3. Quickly stand behind the guest and wrap your arms around her waist. Support and stabilize yourself to hold her full weight if she suddenly loses consciousness. Remember that she cannot talk and will not be able to prepare you for her fall.
4. Place the thumb side of one fisted hand against the guest's abdomen, just above her navel. Grasp your fisted hand with your other hand.
5. Perform abdominal thrusts to dislodge the object. Abdominal thrusts are quick, upward motions that push the abdomen inward and upward against the diaphragm. The thrusts are designed to produce an artificial cough that forces air back up the patient's airway.
6. Continue providing these thrusts until the object is removed or the guest loses consciousness.
7. If the guest becomes unconscious, assist her to the floor, protecting her head and neck from injury. Make sure you have activated the EAS/EMS!

Complete foreign body airway obstruction treatment for an unconscious adult

Follow these steps for an unconscious adult with a complete airway obstruction:

1. Activate the EAS/EMS.
2. Perform an initial assessment.
3. For a nonbreathing guest, begin rescue breathing. If ventilation is difficult or you feel resistance, reposition the guest's head and attempt to ventilate again. If your second ventilation attempt is unsuccessful, the guest's airway is likely obstructed.

    Straddle the guest with your knees aside her knees. Find the navel and xiphoid process. Place your hands just above the navel, and well below the xiphoid process.

> **critical POINT**
> A complete foreign body airway obstruction is a life threatening emergency!

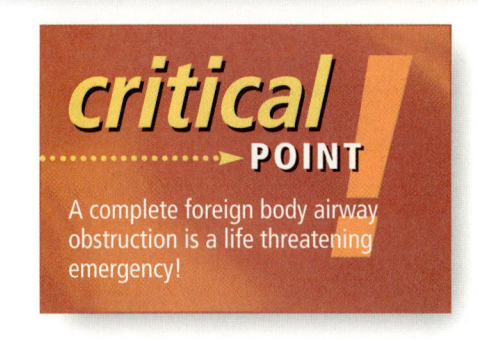

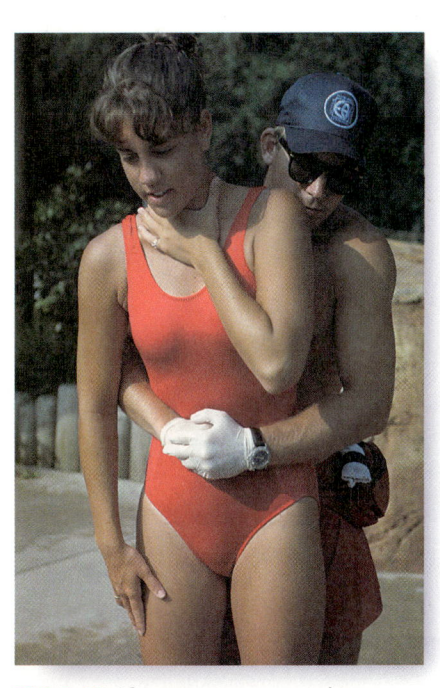

FIG 7.13 If you see a guest making the Universal Distress Sign of Choking, act immediately!

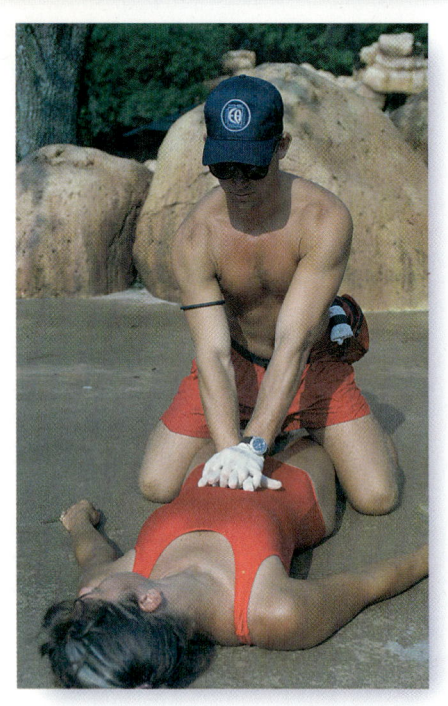

FIG 7.14 Body and hand position for an unconscious adult with a foreign body airway obstruction.

4. Perform up to 5 abdominal thrusts.
5. Open the guest's mouth by grasping his tongue and lower jaw, and lifting. Insert your other hand's index finger along the inside of the guest's cheek, to the back of her mouth. Using a hooking action, attempt to remove the object if you find it.
6. Attempt to perform ventilation, repositioning the airway if it is necessary.

If the guest's airway remains obstructed, repeat thrusts, finger sweep, and ventilations until the object is dislodged or EAS/EMS arrives.

Foreign body airway obstruction management in the pregnant or obese person

The foreign body airway obstruction sequences remain the same for pregnant or obese persons. However, the hand position is moved upwards to the same location as chest compressions in CPR. Remember that you are trying to create an artificial cough. You are not squeezing the chest in a "bear hug" style. With pregnant guests, be particularly careful that you do not press directly over the woman's abdomen.

CHILD CPR AND FOREIGN BODY AIRWAY OBSTRUCTION

Because of the large number of children that participate in aquatic activities, lifeguards must be familiar with the skills needed to perform CPR on a child. You should treat guests between the ages of one and eight years as children. This is only a guideline, and adjustments must be made for individual children.

Nearly all the CPR and FBAO techniques used for the adult guest are also performed on children, with only minor changes. The differences between adult and child CPR and FBAO techniques are:

- If you are acting alone, activate the EAS/EMS after 1 minute of CPR. If bystandards are available, have one of them activate the EAS/EMS system immediately.
- Reduce the amount of air you breathe into a child, appropriate to the child's size (i.e., half a breath or smaller breath). If you are using a BVM, be sure to use the correct size bag and mask.
- Take 1.0 to 1.5 seconds to complete ventilations.
- Any resuscitation mask you use must provide a good face seal.
- Reduce chest compression depth to 1.0 to 1.5 inches.
- Perform chest compressions using only the heel of one hand.
- The chest compression-to-ventilation ratio is 5 compressions to 1 breath, or 5:1 (20 cycles in approximately 1 minute).
- The chest compression rate should equal 100 per minute.
- Perform rescue breathing at a rate of 1 breath every 3 seconds, or 1:3 (20 times a minute).

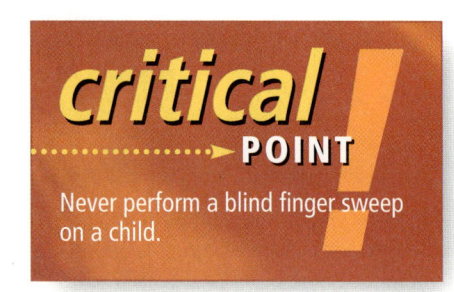

critical POINT
Never perform a blind finger sweep on a child.

- Perform abdominal thrusts with less force, and if necessary, only one hand.
- You must see the object before you attempt to sweep it from the child's mouth. Do not perform blind finger sweeps.

INFANT CPR

Infant cardiopulmonary resuscitation is performed on guests who are between birth and one year of age. The initial CPR assessment for infants is altered slightly in comparison to children and adults. Some significant changes include:

- If you are acting alone, you must activate the EAS/EMS after 1 minute of CPR on an unresponsive infant. If bystanders are available, have one of them activate the EAS/EMS immediately. If the infant does not require CPR, activate EAS/EMS immediately or simultaneously with other life-saving intervention efforts.
- If you are acting alone, pick up the infant and move quickly to the nearest telephone. Continue performing CPR while contacting the EAS/EMS.
- When assessing an infant's airway, do not hyperextend the neck as this can block his airway.
- Assess the infant's breathing by looking, listening, and feeling. Pay particular attention to the rise and fall of his abdomen, as many infants are "belly breathers."
- Perform rescue breathing at a rate of 1 breath every 3 seconds, or a ratio of 1:3 (20 times a minute). Cover the infant's mouth and nose with your mouth or the correct face mask. Reduce ventilation volume to small "cheek puffs."
- Perform a pulse check by checking the brachial artery which is located under the bicep muscle of the upper arm.

Infant Chest Compressions

The correct landmark for chest compressions on an infant is the lower third of the sternum. In order to find this landmark, draw an imaginary line between his nipples, directly over the breastbone.

1. Using your index, middle, and ring fingers, place your index finger on the imaginary line between the nipples. The middle and ring fingers should be toward the infant's feet.
2. Center all three fingers directly over the sternum and then raise your index finger off the infant's chest. This position should then have your middle and ring fingers one finger-width below the imaginary line.
3. Use your free hand to maintain the infant's head position and open airway to facilitate ventilations.
4. Begin chest compressions at a depth of 1/2 to 1 inch.
5. The compression-to-ventilation ratio is 5:1, with a compression rate of at least 100 compressions per minute.

Infant Rescue Breathing

When performing ventilations on an infant guest, seal the infant's mouth and nose with your mouth or with an appropriate airway device. Adjust the ventilation volume to the size of the infant. Cheek puffs are the typical volume suggested during rescue breathing for the infant. The rescue breathing rate for infants is 1 ventilation every 3 seconds, or a ratio of 1:3 (20 times every minute).

INFANT FOREIGN BODY AIRWAY OBSTRUCTION

Conscious Infant with a Partial Airway Obstruction

Leave the infant alone! Let the infant attempt to dislodge the object naturally. A powerful gag reflex will usually do the trick in a few seconds.

Conscious Infant with a Complete Foreign Body Airway Obstruction

All infants naturally place foreign objects into their mouths. Common objects resulting in foreign body airway obstructions include: coins, peanuts, hot dogs, grapes, small toys and rocks, and hard candy. When you are assessing an infant for signs of choking, look for signs of anxiety (bulging eyes), cyanosis (blue skin), ineffective coughing, absence of crying, and decreased mental alertness. Pay attention to clues from the infant's surroundings. Ask yourself whether there are any objects lying around that the infant could have picked up and placed into his airway.

Once you determine that the infant has a complete airway obstruction, act rapidly:

1. Quickly place the infant in a face-down (prone) position on your forearm, using your thigh for support. Support the infant's head with your hand. With your other hand, deliver up to 5 back blows between the infant's shoulder blades. Raise your hand approximately 6 inches off the infant's back for each back blow.
2. If the object remains lodged in the infant's airway, place your free hand on his back and support his head.
3. Turn the infant into a face-up (supine) position and locate the chest compressions landmark. Remember to always keep the infant's head lower than his trunk. Deliver up to 5 chest thrusts.
5. After you complete the chest thrusts, place the infant on a hard surface and open his airway.
6. Remove any visible foreign objects. Do not attempt a blind finger sweep.
7. Attempt rescue breathing.
8. If your first ventilation is unsuccessful, slightly reposition the infant's head and give a second breath. If the airway remains completely obstructed, repeat steps 1-7. Continue this process until the object is relieved and ventilations are successful.
9. Check the infant's circulatory status (pulse) at the bracheal artery, and initiate chest compressions as necessary.

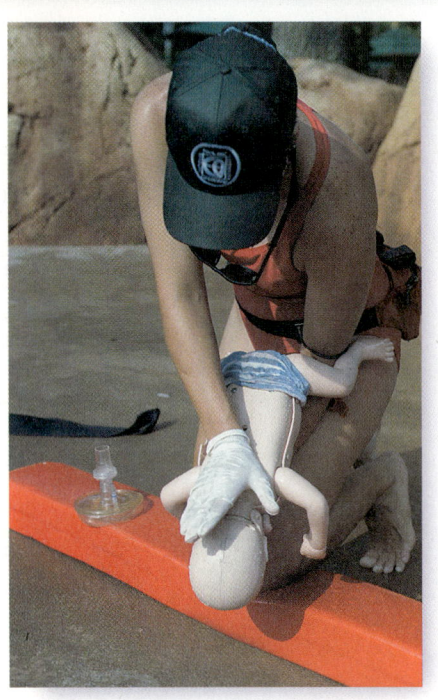

FIG 7.15 Back blows for an infant.

REVIEW QUESTIONS

1. (T) (F) CPR skills are easy to recall, even without practice.

2. Put the following steps of the adult initial assessment in the correct order, starting with the first step:
   a. If the guest does not respond, activate the EAS/EMS.
   b. Head-tilt/chin-lift, or jaw-thrust.
   c. Shake and shout, "Are you OK?"
   d. Look, listen, and feel.
   e. Check for a pulse.
   f. Give two slow breaths.
   g. Perform CPR.

3. If a guest has a pulse, but is not breathing, what should you do?

4. If a guest does not have a pulse, what should you do?

5. (T) (F) An infant's pulse should be checked at the carotid artery in the neck for 5 to 10 seconds.

6. (T) (F) When you are performing rescue breathing, if your first breath does not go in, reposition the guest's head and try again.

7. If repositioning the head does not open an obstructed airway in an unconscious adult or child, you should give _____ _____.

8. Match the age to the proper treatment:
   _____ Infant (birth to 1 year)   a. 1 breath every 5 seconds
   _____ Child (1 to 8 years)   b. 1 breath every 3 seconds
   _____ Adult (over 8 years)   c. 1 breath every 3 seconds

9. (T) (F) For a conscious adult guest who has a complete airway obstruction, you should perform the Heimlich Maneuver until the object is dislodged or the guest becomes unconscious.

10. (T) (F) For an unconscious infant with a complete airway obstruction, you should give 2 back blows and 5 abdominal thrusts.

Skill Sheet 8.a — CPR REVIEW

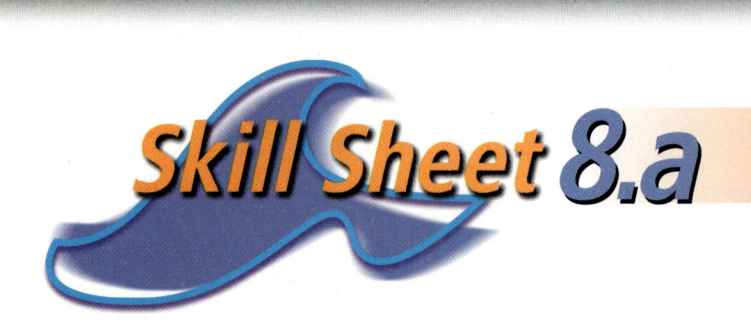

Item	Infant (0-1 year)	Child (1-8 years)	Adult (>8 years)
How to open airway?	Head-tilt/chin-lift	Head-tilt/chin-lift	Head-tilt/chin-lift
How to check breathing?	Look at chest and listen and feel for air (3 to 5 seconds)	Look at chest and listen and feel for air (3 to 5 seconds)	Look at chest and listen and feel for air (3 to 5 seconds)
How to breathe?	Slow, make chest rise and fall	Slow, make chest rise and fall	Slow, make chest rise and fall
Where to check pulse?	Brachial artery (5 to 10 seconds)	Cartoid artery (5 to 10 seconds)	Carotid artery (5 to 10 seconds)
Hand position for chest compressions?	1 finger's width below imaginary line between nipples	2 fingers width above the tip of the sternum	2 fingers width above the tip of the sternum
Compress with?	2 or 3 fingers	Heel of 1 hand	Heels of 2 hands, one hand on top of the other
Compression depth?	0.5 to 1 inch	1 to 1.5 inches	1.5 to 2 inches
Compression rate?	at least 100+ per minnute	100 per minnute	80 to 100 minutes
Compression:breath ratio?	5 : 1	5 : 1	15 : 2
How to count for compression rate?	1, 2, 3, 4, 5, breathe	1 and 2 and 3 and 4 and 5 and breathe	1 and 2 and 3 and 4 and 5 and 6 and... 15 and breathe, breathe
How often to reassess?	Every few minutes	Every few minutes	Every few minutes
After reassessment, resume CPR with?	Compressions	Compressions	Compressions
How often to give breaths during rescue breathing?	Every 3 seconds.; count one one-thousand, two one-thousand, (breathe)	Every 3 seconds; count one one-thousand, two one-thousand, (breathe)	Every 5 seconds; count one one-thousand, two one-thousand, three one-thousand, four one-thousand (breathe)

Skill Sheet 8.b — TWO-LIFEGUARD CPR

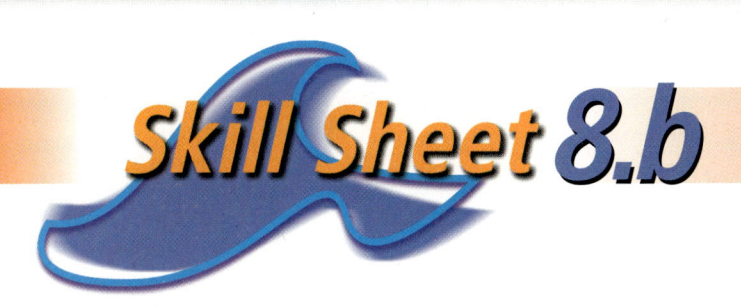

Entry of Second Trained Lifeguard to Perform Two-Lifeguard CPR	#1 #2 #1 #2 #1	Performing one-lifeguard CPR Says: • "I know CPR" • "EMS has been activated" • "Can I help?" • Completes CPR cycle (15 compressions and ends on 2 breaths) • Says, "Take over compressions" • Check pulse and breathing (5 seconds) • If pulse absent, #1 lifeguard says "No pulse, continue CPR" • Gives 5 compressions (at 80 to 100 per minute rate) • After every fifth compression, pauses for #1 lifeguard to give 1 slow breath • Gives 1 slow breath after every fifth compression given by #2 lifeguard • Feels carotid pulse during compressions
Two Lifeguards Starting CPR at the Same Time	#1 (Ventilator) #2 (Compressor)	• Assesses victim. If no breaths, gives 2 full breaths; if no pulse, tells #2 to start compressions • Gives 1 full breath after fifth compression given by #2 • Finds hand position and gets ready to give compressions • Gives 5 compressions after #1 says to start them • Pauses after every fifth compression for #1 to give 1 full breath
Switching During Two-Lifeguard CPR	#2 (Compressor) #1 (Ventilator)	• Signals when to change by saying "Change and, two and, three and, four and, five" or "Change after the next breath" • After #1 gives breath, #2 moves to victim's head and completes pulse and breathing check (5 seconds) and if absent, says "no pulse, begin CPR" • Gives 1 full breath after every cycle of 5 compressions • Gives 1 full breath at the end of fifth compression and moves to victim's chest • Finds hand position and gets ready to give compressions • Begins cycles of 5 compressions after every breath

KEY POINTS:

- Provide CPR for any guest who is not breathing and pulseless.
- Work as a team whenever possible.
- Use the Heimlich Maneuver to relieve an obstruction in a child or an adult
- Use back blows and chest thrusts to relieve an obstruction in an infant.

CRITICAL THINKING:

1. If an 11 month old infant is too large for you to support on your arm for backblows or chest thrusts, what should you do?
2. If the guest vomits while you are performing CPR, what should you do?
3. When should you stop CPR?

88 PART 2 • RESPONDING TO AN EMERGENCY

Skill Sheet 8.C

CPR FLOW CHART

Shout for help!
↓
Look Listen Feel — 3 to 5 sec.
↓
No breathing.
↓
Two Slow Breaths
↓
Air goes in.
↓
Check pulse 5 to 10 sec.
↓
There is a pulse.
↓
Continue Rescue Breathing.

Breathing → **Recovery Position: Monitor Secondary Survey.**

Air does not go in. → Retilt; try breaths again.

Air does not go in. ← Check for foreign matter.

Infant: 5 Back Blows.
↓
Infant: 5 Chest Thrusts.

Child / Adult: 5 Abdominal thrusts.

Infant: 1 breath every 3 seconds.

Child: 1 breath every 3 seconds.

Adult: 1 breath every 5 seconds.

Check pulse every few minutes.

KEY POINTS:
- Compress the chest smoothly and breath slowly.
- Keep the airway clear.
- Recheck the pulse every few minutes.

CRITICAL THINKING:
1. What do you do if you see fluid or vomit in the mouth?
2. Why is it so important to start rescue breathing as quickly as possible?
3. When should you do CPR?

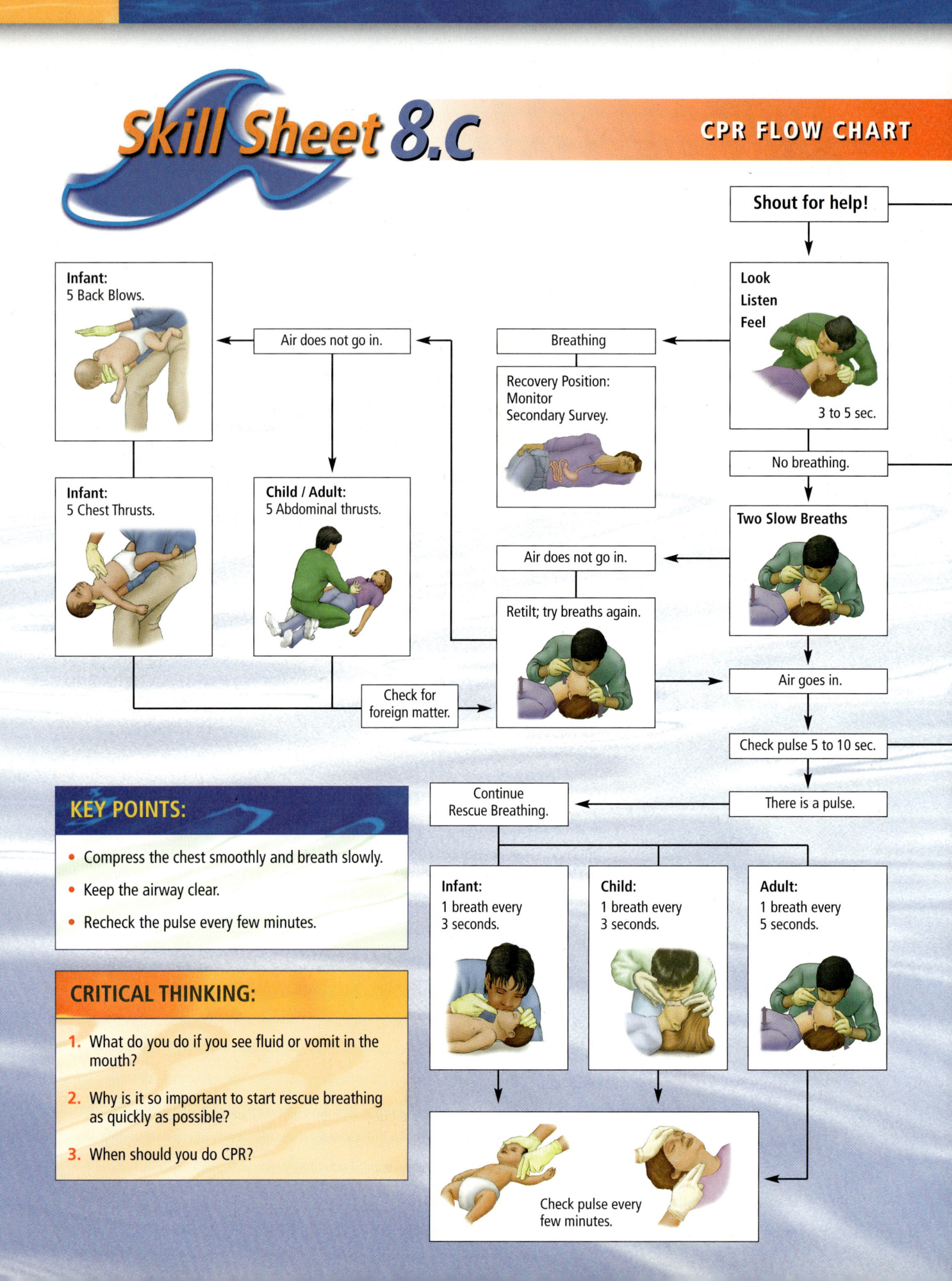

CHAPTER 7 • CPR AND AIRWAY OBSTRUCTION   89

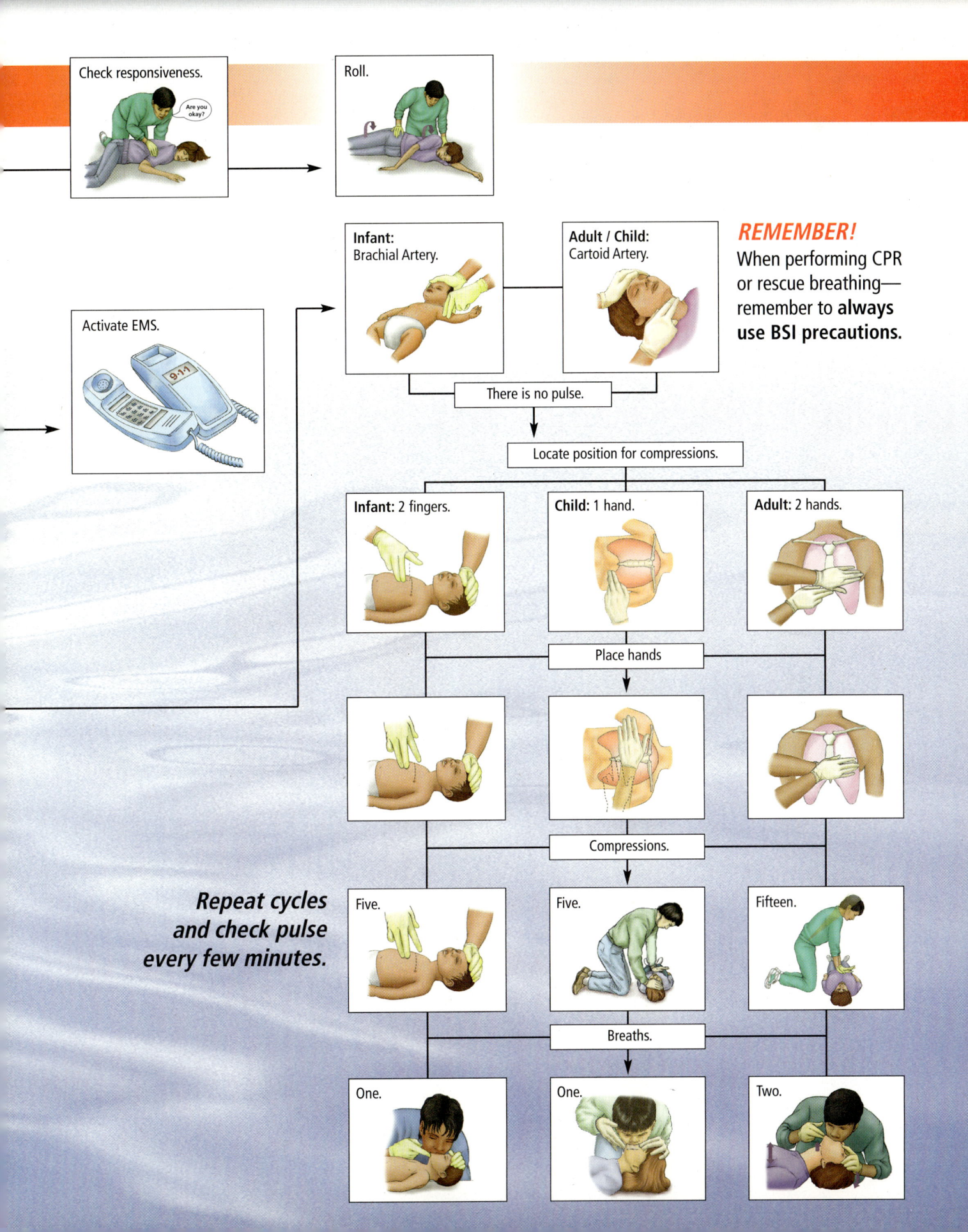

Check responsiveness.

Roll.

Activate EMS.

Infant: Brachial Artery.

Adult / Child: Cartoid Artery.

REMEMBER!
When performing CPR or rescue breathing—remember to always use **BSI** precautions.

There is no pulse.

Locate position for compressions.

Infant: 2 fingers.   **Child:** 1 hand.   **Adult:** 2 hands.

Place hands

Compressions.

Repeat cycles and check pulse every few minutes.

Five.   Five.   Fifteen.

Breaths.

One.   One.   Two.

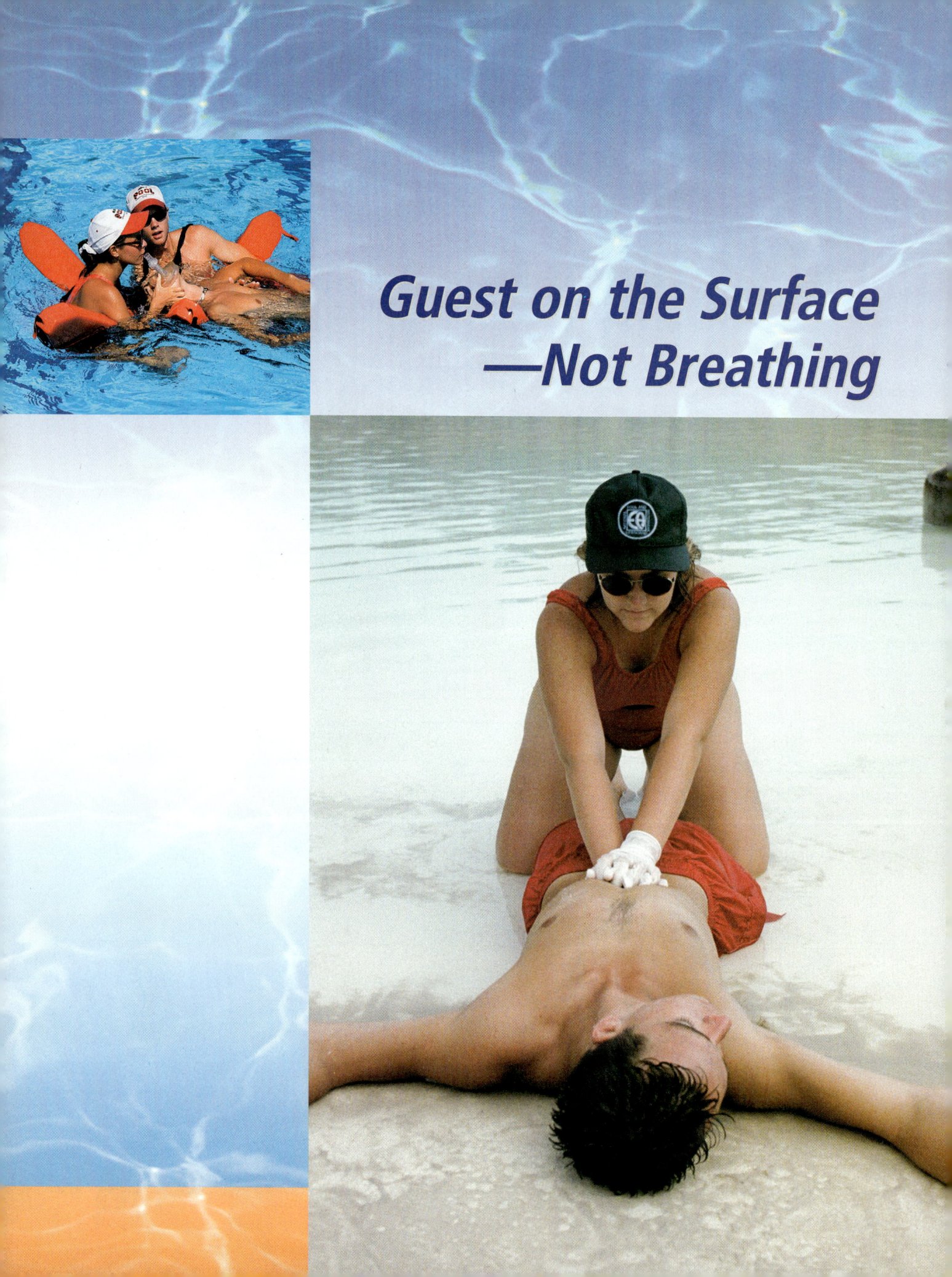

Guest on the Surface
—Not Breathing

chapter 8

OBJECTIVES

After reading this chapter and completing the related course work, you should be able to:

1. Explain the importance of Body Substance Isolation (BSI).

2. Adapt the rear huggie to the no-breathing guest.

3. Demonstrate how to provide care for a nonbreathing guest.

4. Demonstrate the Heimlich Maneuver sequence in the water.

5. Demonstrate the use of a resuscitation mask for rescue breathing in the water.

6. Safely and quickly remove a nonbreathing guest from the water.

7. Reassess a guest's condition after removal from the water and, if necessary, provide additional care.

Body Substance Isolation (BSI) precautions approach all body substances, including airborne, as potentially infectious.

The first few minutes of a water rescue are critical to the outcome of the emergency. As a professional lifeguard, you have the opportunity to improve the way immersion incidents are managed. In this chapter, you will learn simple, yet highly effective techniques for water rescue situations. The protocol presented in this chapter includes skills that have been adapted to allow for improved aquatic emergency management of an unconscious guest.

UNIVERSAL PRECAUTIONS

Universal Precautions refer to procedures for infection control that treat blood and certain bodily fluids as if they are capable of transmitting bloodborne diseases.

According to the concept of Universal Precautions, all human blood and blood-tinged fluids should be treated as if they are infectious for HIV, HBV and other bloodborne diseases. HIV is the human immunodeficiency virus which causes AIDS. HBV is the hepatitis B virus that attacks the liver.

Recently, the concept of "body substance isolation" (BSI) precautions has become the standard. This concept approaches all body substances, including airborne substances, as potentially infectious.

Following BSI precautions is the most important step in preventing the transfer of potentially infectious materials between victim and rescuer. You have no way of knowing in advance whether you will come in contact with body fluids, and if you do, whether they will be contaminated. Therefore, as a professional lifeguard, you must use some type of barrier to protect yourself when performing rescue breathing, whether in the water or on the deck. In addition, whenever you encounter blood or other bodily fluids, you should use a barrier, such as gloves.

Your facility will provide you with specific training about preventing bloodborne and airborne pathogens, and exposure control.

THE NONBREATHING GUEST

Lack of oxygen to the brain can rapidly lead to irreversible brain damage. That is why it is so important to begin rescue breathing as quickly as possible for an unconscious nonbreathing guest. In many cases, it will take you more than one minute to get the guest to the side of the pool and out of the water. That first minute can be critical.

The longer it takes to clear the airway, the less oxygen there is in the system to support the heart and brain functioning. The more oxygen that is depleted in the system, the closer the guest comes to cardiac arrest. Since the guest is likely to have water blocking his airway, the Heimlich Maneuver should be administered as quickly as possible on a nonbreathing guest in the water. If this is unsuccessful, and the guest is still not breathing, you will need to begin rescue breathing. Whenever possible, you should be moving toward the exit point in the pool, as you provide care.

Also of critical importance is your protection from possible disease transmission during rescue breathing. You should use a protective resuscitation mask at all times, when you administer breaths to a nonbreathing guest. The mask is designed to form an effective barrier and "seal," both in the water and on the deck. You must become very familiar with the specific type of resuscitation masks that are used at your facility. Practice is the only acceptable method for maintaining a high level of skill in using a resuscitation mask for rescue breathing.

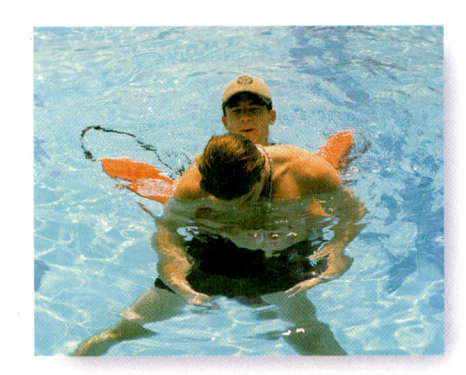

Rear Huggie—Nonbreathing Guest

The objectives of performing the rear huggie on a nonbreathing guest are to:

- Position the guest on a rescue tube to administer the Heimlich Maneuver.
- Position the guest across the rescue tube, in a face-up position, to administer rescue breathing, if necessary.

If a nonbreathing guest is in the water, he may be floating face down on the surface. As the first few minutes are so critical to the guest's survival, you must quickly position him in a vertical position, so that you can begin administering the Heimlich Maneuver. You may also have to position the guest across the rescue tube in order to administer rescue breathing.

When a guest is on the surface and not breathing, you will execute the *rear huggie*. This is the most effective way to maintain an open airway on the guest. However, there are some modifications you will need to make with the unconscious guest.

To execute the rear huggie on a nonbreathing guest:

1. Whistle and point to the guest, hit the E-Stop (if there is one), do a compact jump entry, and approach stroke toward the guest.

2. Swim to a position behind the guest, or to the side, depending on the buoyancy and the position of the guest.

3. Signal for assistance if a back-up lifeguard is available or you need a resuscitation mask.

4. Make contact. If the guest is in a vertical position, approach him and make contact the same way you did with a conscious guest on the surface—extend your arms under the guest's armpits, and wrap your hands around his shoulders.

If the guest is floating with his legs horizontal at or near the surface of the water, swim to a position behind and almost on top of him. This position will make it possible for you to put your arms under his armpits. After you extend your arms under the guest's armpits, wrap your hands around his shoulders. If the guest is floating very high in the water, you may need to push his hips down with one of your hands while you get into position.

5. Pull the guest backward to achieve a vertical position, keeping his face out of the water. Kick your legs to help you keep the guest's face above water. Remember to keep your face clear of the guest's head, which may snap back and strike you.

6. Position your hands just above the navel and perform the Heimlich Maneuver. Keep the guest vertical, with his face out of the water.

Practice is the only acceptable method for maintaining a high level of skill in using a resuscitation mask for rescue breathing.

FIG 8.1 Rear huggie–nonbreathing guest.

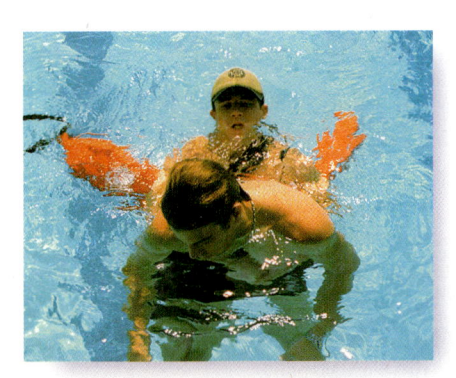

FIG 8.2 Pull the guest to a vertical position.

What's Being Said About the Use of the Heimlich Manuever in the Water

"The Heimlich Maneuver should be introduced immediately at the beginning of the ventilation sequence in the treatment of the drowning victim." John Hunsucker, Ph.D., P.E.

"The application of the Heimlich Maneuver as the initial and perhaps only step for opening the airway in all near-drowning victims has been proposed by Henry Heimlich, M.D. According to Dr. Heimlich, subdiaphragmatic pressure (Heimlich Maneuver) should be performed and repeated until no water flows from the mouth of the victim. In the event that spontaneous respiration does not occur, standard resuscitative methods should then be used immediately." Edward A. Patrick, M.D., Ph.D., FACEP.

"Your demonstration of the Heimlich Maneuver in deep water was most impressive, easily learned by the lifeguards, and appeared safe and logical." Henry Heimlich, M.D.

"Ellis & Associates has once again demonstrated their commitment to improving water safety and quality patient care. Utilizing protocol for unconscious victims that includes the application of the Heimlich Maneuver will effectively allow water safety experts from around the world to gather data on the most effective prehospital resuscitation procedure for drowning victims." Grant Goold, Center for Prehospital Research and Training, University of California, San Francisco Medical Center.

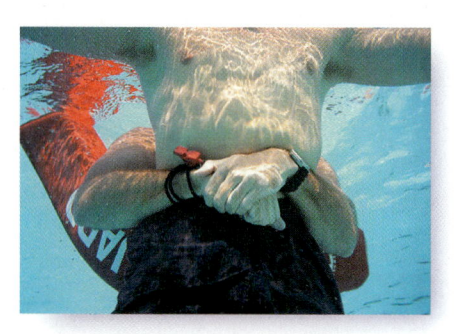

FIG 8.3 Performing the Heimlich Maneuver.

Heimlich Maneuver

The objective of the Heimlich Manuever in the water is to:

- Clear the guest's airway of foreign material to initiate spontaneous breathing or provide rescue breathing, if necessary.

Single-Lifeguard Rescue

1. If the guest is not breathing, administer a minimum of 5 sub-diaphragmatic thrusts (Heimlich Maneuver) as shown in Figure 8.3.

   - If fluid does not come out of the guest's mouth and he is still not breathing, begin rescue breathing in the water immediately.

   - If fluid comes out of the guest's mouth, continue to administer thrusts until fluid stops coming from the guest's mouth and he begins breathing, or you reach a point where other lifeguards are ready to remove the guest from the water.

2. If the guest is breathing, continue to make progress to the side, remove the guest from the water, and continue your assessment according to your Emergency Action System.

Two-Lifeguard Rescue

1. If the guest is not breathing and a second lifeguard is available, he should support the guest's head to keep his face out of the water. The lifeguard should not have his face, hands, or arms in front of the guest's face.

   As the second lifeguard supports the guest's head, you should administer thrusts.

2. If the guest is breathing, continue to make progress to the exit point, remove the guest from the water, and continue your assessment according to your Emergency Action System.

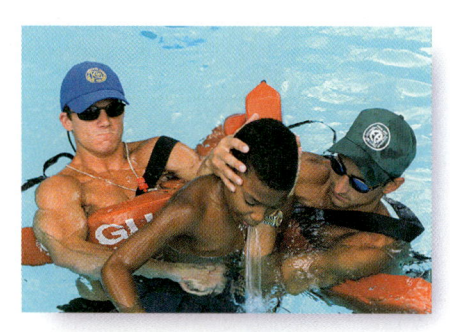

FIG 8.4 Two lifeguard rescue: One lifeguard supports the guest's head while the other lifeguard performs the Heimlich Maneuver.

MOUTH-TO-BARRIER RESCUE BREATHING

The objectives of mouth-to-barrier rescue breathing are to:

- Maintain an open airway for the guest.
- Position the resuscitation mask correctly on the guest's face.
- Maintain a good seal with the mask over the guest's face.
- Provide effective rescue breathing.

In some facilities, every lifeguard may enter the water with a resuscitation mask. You must be trained in how to control the rescue tube and the guest while you assemble the mask and place it properly on the guest's face. You must practice this skill as part of your inservice training.

In other facilities, the resuscitation mask will be brought to you by the second lifeguard. In these facilities, the Emergency Action System should designate which lifeguard should perform the rescue breathing.

1. To position the guest for rescue breathing, pull him backward, across the rescue tube. Kick your legs to help as you pull. Remember to keep your face clear of the guest's head as you pull him back. Be sure the rescue tube is under the guest's back. If the rescue tube has been placed properly, the guest's head will naturally fall back into an open airway position.

2. The lifeguard who will be administering rescue breathing must be in a position at the top of the guest's head. The guest's mouth should be open. You will have to protect it from going underwater or having water splash into it.

3. Shake any water out of the mask and valve and place the mask over the guest's nose and mouth with the valve directly over the guest's mouth.

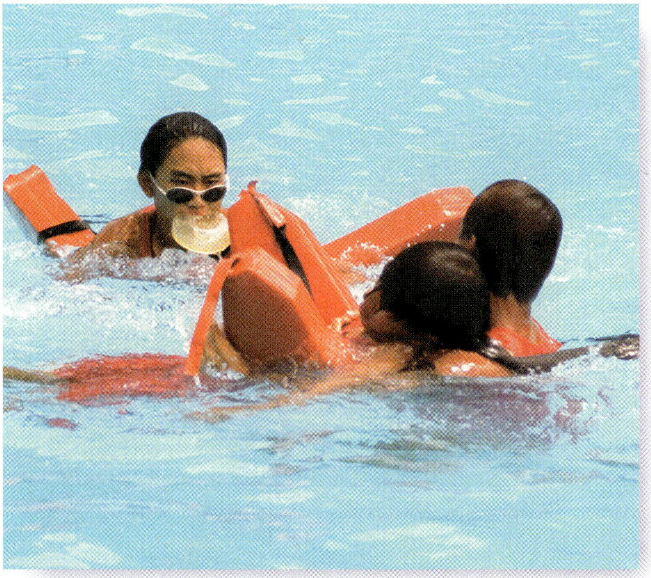

FIG 8.5 Kick and pull the guest back across the rescue tube.

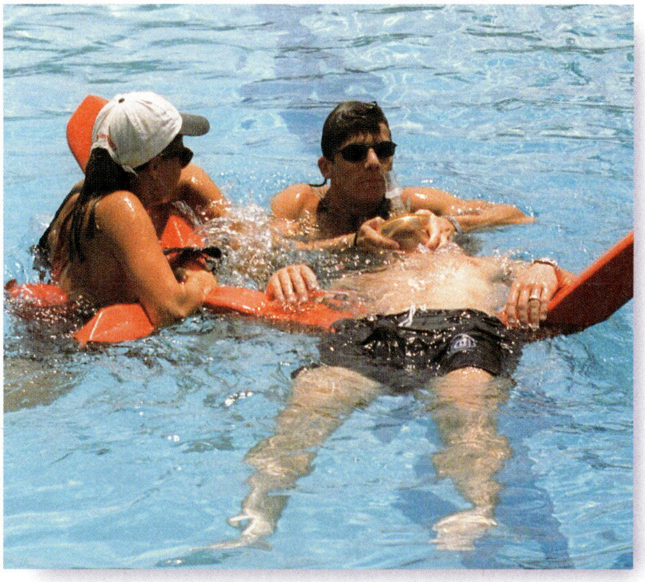

FIG 8.6 Open airway position on the rescue tube.

Blow just enough air into the guest to make the chest gently rise.

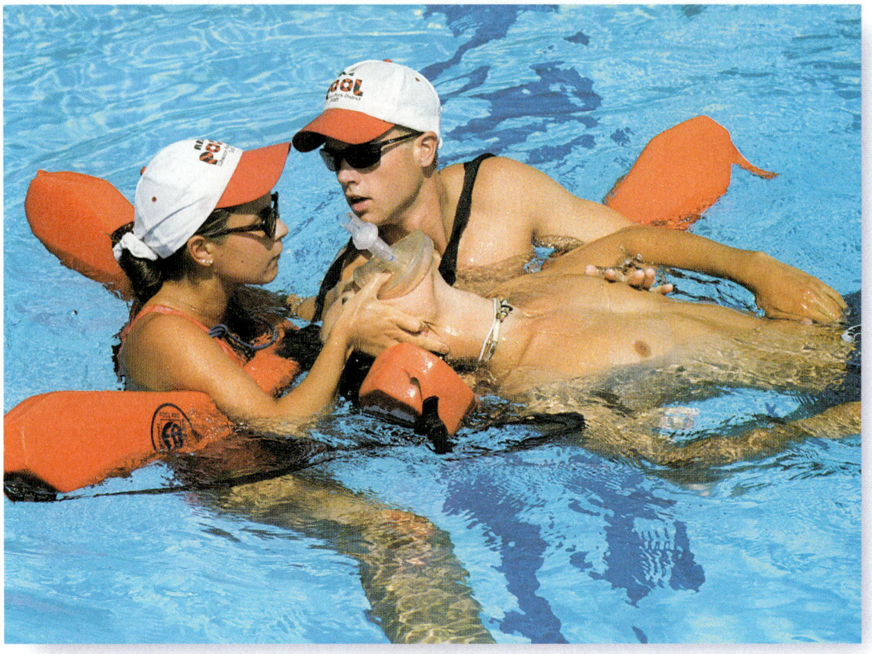

FIG 8.7 Place the resuscitation mask directly over the guest's mouth.

4. Place your palms over the mask, and press downward against the guest's cheekbones. Your thumbs should be pointed toward the guest's feet. Place your index fingers under the angles of the jaw on both sides of the guest's head and lift the jaw upward as you tilt the guest's head backward.
5. Place your mouth on the valve of the mask. To begin rescue breathing, take a deep breath and blow into the valve so that you make the chest gently rise. Slow ventilations prevent gastric distention.
6. As you perform rescue breathing, continue to move to the side of the pool where you will remove the guest from the water. The second lifeguard can assist by swimming alongside the guest and pulling or pushing the guest through the water.

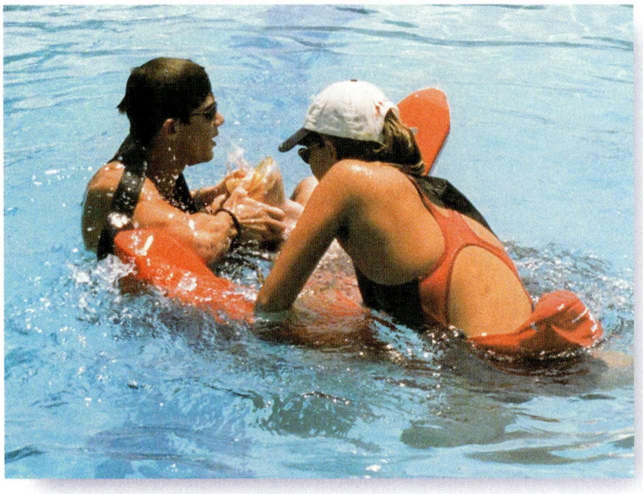

FIG 8.8 Take a breath and then seal your mouth on the one-way valve of the mask.

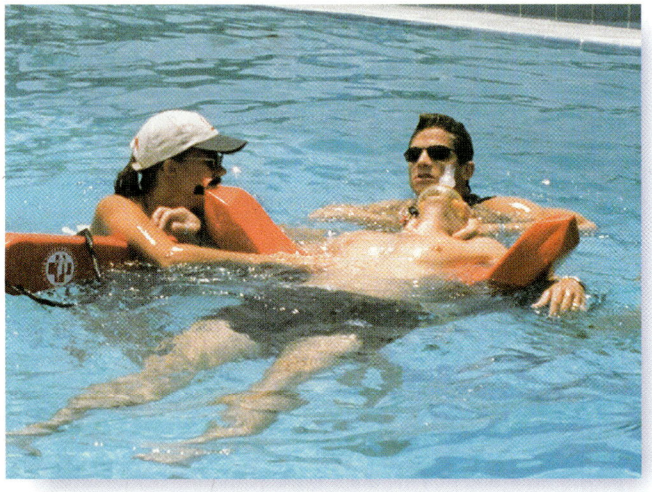

FIG 8.9 The second lifeguard should assist by swimming alongside the guest to guide him to the side of the pool.

CHAPTER 8 • GUEST ON SURFACE–NOT BREATHING

REMOVAL FROM THE WATER (EXTRICATION)

The objective of extrication is to:

- Rapidly and safely remove the guest from the water by using the backboard for support. This technique is used only when the guest is not breathing and you do not suspect a spinal injury.

Removing a nonbreathing guest from the water can be difficult and could cause injury either to the guest or to you. This is especially true if the guest is large. If you are in this situation, you can remove the guest quickly and safely from the water by using a backboard and a second lifeguard.

As with all rescue techniques, you must practice this skill at your facility with your lifeguard team and with your facility's equipment. You should familiarize yourself with the location of the backboard and the way the backboard performs in the water.

Each aquatic facility may have different water/deck levels or types of ledges or gutters. You will need to modify this technique according to your facility's design. Keep in mind that the number of lifeguards available will also affect the technique you use.

The rapid extrication technique is used only when the guest is not breathing and you do not suspect a spinal injury.

Two-Lifeguard Rapid Extrication Procedure

To use a backboard to remove a nonbreathing guest without a suspected spinal injury from the water, follow these steps:

1. As the primary lifeguard moves toward the side of the pool with the guest, a second lifeguard brings the backboard to the edge of the water and removes the head immobilizer. The second lifeguard puts on gloves and has an extra pair of gloves ready for the primary lifeguard when he exits the water. The second lifeguard places the board vertically in the water against the wall, getting the head pad of the board into the water whenever possible.

    The second lifeguard should also have all the resuscitation equipment on the deck ready for immediate use when the guest is removed from the water.

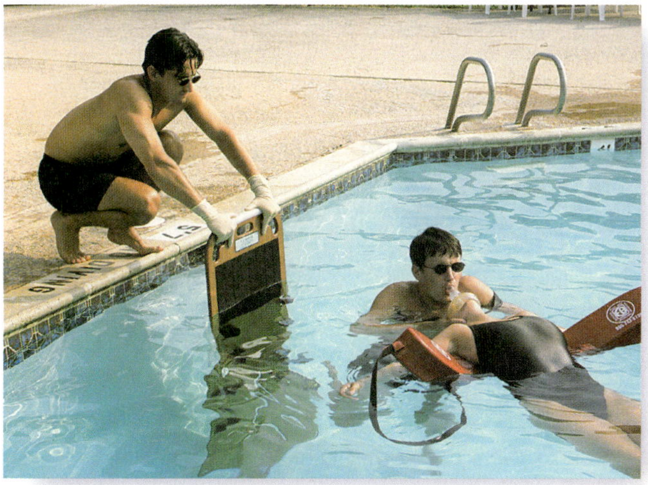

FIG 8.10 Second lifeguard assists with backboard.

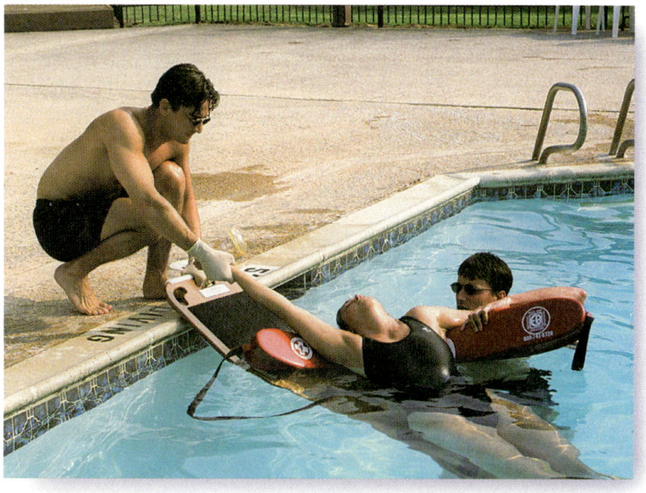

FIG 8.11 First and second lifeguards coordinate their efforts.

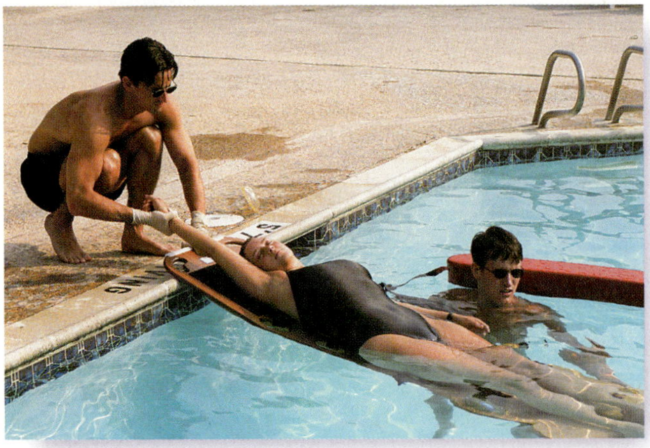

FIG 8.12 The second lifeguard grasps the guest's arm while the first lifeguard stabilizes the front of the backboard.

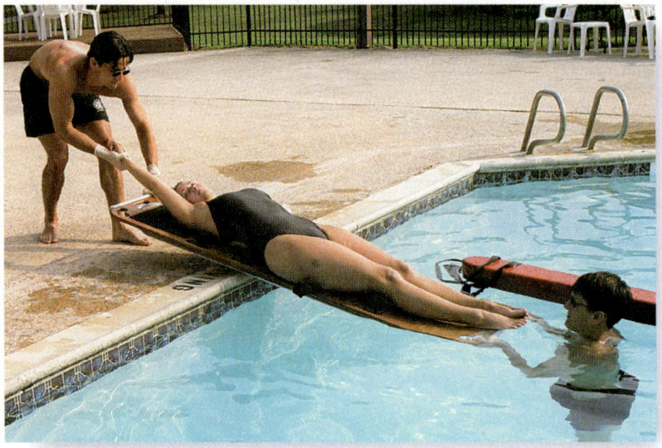

FIG 8.13 The first and second lifeguards smoothly transfer the guest from the water to the deck.

2. As the primary lifeguard approaches the backboard, one last breath is given and the mask is placed on the deck. The primary lifeguard then moves into position at the side of the guest, and raises the guest's arm, so the second lifeguard can grasp it.

3. Slide the rescue tube out from under the guest before contact is made with the backboard.

4. The second lifeguard should now be holding the backboard with one hand and the guest's arm with the other. The primary lifeguard should be alongside the backboard holding onto the deck or gutter with one hand and the backboard with the other.

5. With the guest positioned properly on the backboard, the second lifeguard signals that he or she is ready to remove the guest. As the second lifeguard pulls the backboard and guest onto the deck, the primary lifeguard pushes the backboard from the water. **Do not try to lift the backboard. Slide it up onto the deck.**

If three lifeguards are available, the primary lifeguard makes the initial Heimlich Maneuver and rescue breathing for the nonbreathing guest. The second lifeguard positions the guest's face above water while the thrusts are given, and helps move the guest to the removal point. The third lifeguard brings the backboard and other resuscitation equipment. The two lifeguards in the water position themselves on opposite sides of the backboard and help push as the third lifeguard pulls the victim and the backboard onto the deck.

Special Situation: Large Victim

The removal of a guest from the water using a backboard should be safe, quick, and efficient. If the guest is very large or the distance from the water line to the deck is great, you may need to modify your technique. You can do this by fastening a strap around the guest's chest to secure him to the backboard. While the second lifeguard holds the guest's arm, the primary lifeguard fastens the strap high on the guest's chest and under his armpits.

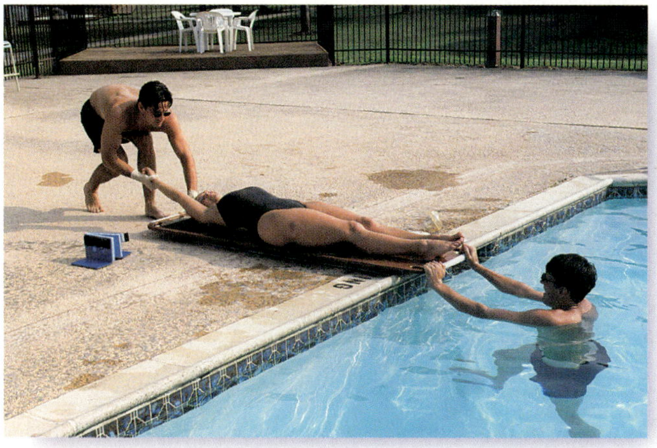

CHAPTER 8 • GUEST ON SURFACE—NOT BREATHING

FIG 8.14 Once the guest is safely on deck, continue care.

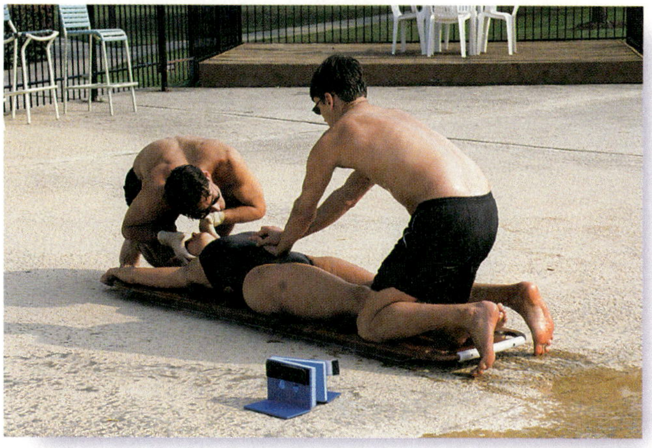

FIG 8.15 Take personal protection precautions before giving proper care.

Once the chest strap is secured, the second lifeguard can release the guest's arm.

On a signal, the second lifeguard can pull the backboard with both hands while stepping backwards and sliding the backboard onto the deck. The primary lifeguard can push the backboard or climb out of the water and help the second lifeguard pull the backboard up onto the deck.

Communication between the lifeguards is very important during removal of the guest from the water.

CARING FOR THE GUEST ONCE ON THE DECK

Once you have moved the backboard to a level area at least six feet away from the water's edge, check to see if the guest has begun breathing spontaneously. If the guest is not breathing, turn her head to the side and administer a minimum of 5 thrusts (Heimlich Maneuver).

- **If no fluid comes out of the guest's mouth**, check for breathing. If the guest is still not breathing, attempt to ventilate and follow rescue breathing/CPR?AED protocols immediately.

- **If fluid comes out of the guest's mouth**, continue to administer thrusts (Heimlich Maneuver) until the fluid stops flowing from the guest's mouth.

- **Once fluid has stopped flowing from the guest's mouth**, check for breathing. If the guest is not breathing, attempt to ventilate and follow rescue breathing/CPR/AED protocols immediately.

If the guest begins breathing, place her in the recovery position, continue supplemental oxygen support, keep her warm, and monitor her until EMS Personnel arrive.

REVIEW QUESTIONS

1. List three things you may have to do to adapt a rear huggie for use with an unconscious guest:

   a. _____

   b. _____

   c. _____

2. Why is it important to start rescue breathing in the water?

3. (T) (F) BSI precautions regard all body fluids as if they are contaminated.

4. (T) (F) Placing an unconscious guest on the rescue tube, with the rescue tube under the guest's back, is usually an ideal way to open the airway.

5. Name two reasons for using mouth-to-barrier rescue breathing in the water:

   a. _____

   b. _____

6. (T) (F) When removing an unconscious guest from the water, it is important to do it quickly with minimal risk of injury to the guest or to you.

7. (T) (F) Another word for removal is extrication.

8. (T) (F) A method of removing a nonbreathing guest that is both quick and safe, is to use a backboard.

CHAPTER 8 • GUEST ON SURFACE–NOT BREATHING   101

Skill Sheet 9

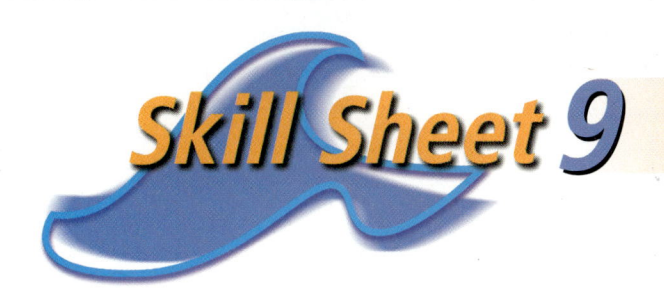

NONSPINAL EXTRICATION

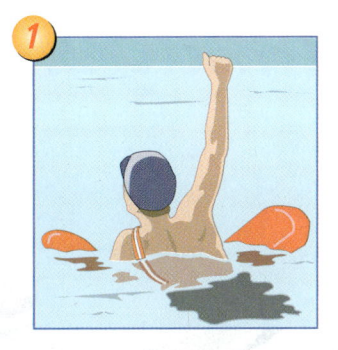

1. Primary lifeguard signals for help.

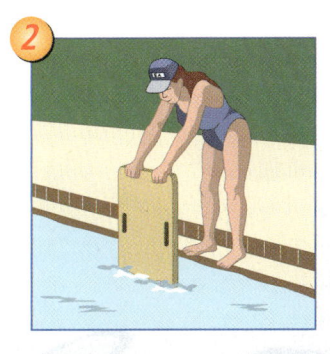

2. Second lifeguard places backboard.

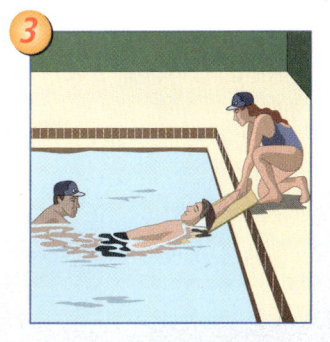

3. Primary lifeguard removes rescue tube and places guest on backboard. Second lifeguard grasps the guest's arm.

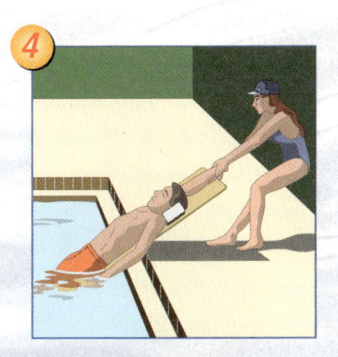

4. Second lifeguard maintains contact with guest's arm and pulls backboard onto deck, while primary lifeguard pushes backboard onto the deck.

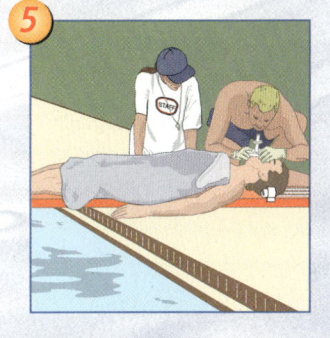

5. Reasses the guest and provide care as needed.

KEY POINTS:

- Respond quickly!
- Communicate your needs.
- Maintain contact with guest.
- Work as a team to remove the guest.
- Use the backboard and side of pool as a support

CRITICAL THINKING:

1. When would you use the non-spinal extrication technique?

2. What if, for some reason, your backboard was not readily available, and it would take a minute or so for it to arrive? What are your options?

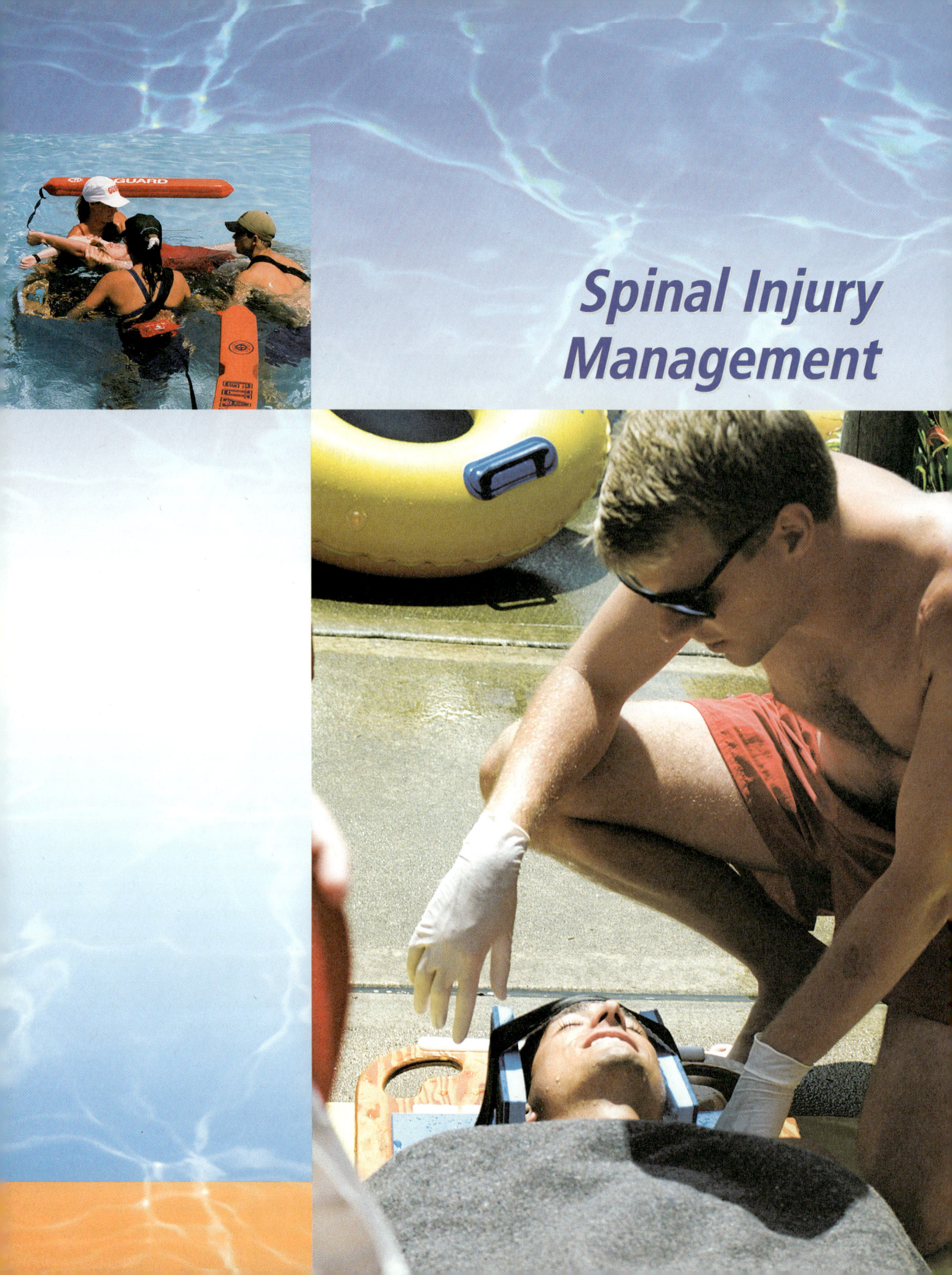

Spinal Injury Management

chapter 9

NINE

OBJECTIVES

After reading this chapter and completing the related course work, you should be able to:

1. Identify situations that could result in a spinal injury in aquatic facilities.

2. Identify signs and symptoms of a spinal injury.

3. Demonstrate how to stabilize a guest's head and neck if you suspect a spinal injury.

4. Demonstrate how to use a backboard to remove a guest with a suspected spinal injury from the water.

A spinal injury is one of the most devastating incidents that can happen at an aquatic facility. In the aquatic environment, there are many ways that a person can injure the spinal cord, including:

- Direct blows to the spine.
- Head-first entries into shallow water.
- Falls from a height.

As a professional lifeguard, you must be skilled in the recognition and handling of a suspected spinal injury. The only way to positively identify a spinal injury and determine the extent of the damage is through x-rays. Since you cannot know the extent of the injury, you must treat all suspected spinal injuries as if there is spinal cord damage.

As a lifeguard, you can affect the final outcome of the injury. You should regularly practice the skills described in this chapter during your in-service training sessions, because you will use these skills every time you suspect a spinal injury. You can make the difference between life and death, or life-long paralysis or normal limb use for guests with a spinal cord injury.

UNDERSTANDING THE SPINE

The **spine** is composed of a column of 33 vertebrae that extend from the base of the head to the tip of the coccyx (tailbone). **Vertebrae** are circular or irregularly shaped heavy masses of bone.

Intervertabral discs are circular cushions of cartilage that separate the vertebrae. The **spinal cord** is a group of nerve tissue that carries messages from the brain to the rest of the body. The spinal cord runs through, and is protected by, the vertebrae.

NPWLTP Position Statement

The National Pool and Waterpark Lifeguard Training Program (NPWLTP) recognizes the importance of providing care for injured guests suspected of having a spine-related injury while in, on, or about the water. These guests require care that should be provided by medical professionals (emergency medical technicians, paramedics, nurses, and/or physicians) who have received extensive training in the proper management of such injuries.

The National Pool and Waterpark Lifeguard Training Program believes that devices, such as cervical collars, should only be applied by qualified medical professionals who have received extensive training in this specialty. Accordingly, we believe that the role of the lifeguard should be focused on basic stabilization of the guest and preventing further injury until these qualified medical professionals arrive on the scene.

The rescue skills you learn in this chapter will minimize the risk of unnecessary movement in the water, until medical professionals assume care of the guest.

In some instances, it may be necessary to extricate the guest from the water prior to the arrival of medical professionals. The extrication skills you learn in this chapter minimize the risk of unnecessary movement to guests during that procedure.

Care for guests suspected of having a spinal injury requires well-planned protocols. These protocols should be developed in joint cooperation with your local EMS provider, aquatic facility administrator, and lifeguard staff. As NPWLTP lifeguards, you should be thoroughly familiar with these protocols. You should attend frequent in-service training sessions, which include EMS personnel, to review these protocols and maintain technical competence in executing them.

The spine is divided into five regions:
- **Cervical**—the neck area. This is the area of the spinal column most susceptible to injury because it has the least amount of protection.
- **Thoracic**—the middle back area.
- **Lumbar**—the lower back area.
- **Sacrum**—the pelvic area.
- **Coccyx**—the tailbone, including the final three or four vertebrae.

Unlike many other body parts, the spinal cord cannot be repaired once it is damaged, and even slight movement of one vertebrae or disc could pinch or shear the spinal cord. This could mean the difference between normal function and permanent paralysis for the guest.

For every guest suffering a serious head injury, you must proceed as if he has a spinal cord injury. You must not allow the guest to move his neck. The techniques you use in the water and on the deck are designed to minimize movement, thereby limiting the extent of further injury.

SIGNS AND SYMPTOMS OF SPINAL INJURY

Lifeguards must be able to recognize signs (physical features) and symptoms (complaints of the guest) that indicate the possibility of a spinal injury.

The signs suggesting possible spinal injury include:
- Deformity
- Bruises, lacerations, or cuts
- Altered level of consciousness
- Vomiting
- Blood or blood-tinged fluid in the ears or nose

The symptoms suggesting possible spinal injury include:
- Pain with or without movement
- Numbness, tingling, or paralysis
- Weakness

When these signs or symptoms are present in a person who has been injured, you should activate the Emergency Action System and treat the injured guest for a possible spinal injury.

You must also become skilled at asking **qualifying questions** of the guest so that you can get enough information to determine if you should suspect a spinal injury. Two important areas of questioning are:
- **The mechanism (cause) of the injury.** Ask the guest or witnesses about the incident to determine what happened.
- **How the guest feels.** Ask the guest about areas of pain, numbness, and mobility.

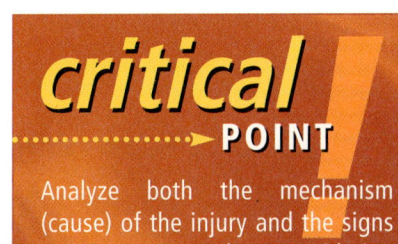

> **critical POINT**
> Analyze both the mechanism (cause) of the injury and the signs and symptoms when considering the possibility of spine injury.

critical POINT!

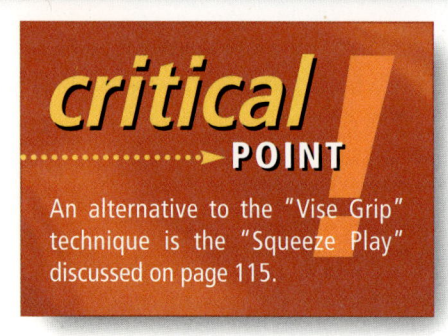

An alternative to the "Vise Grip" technique is the "Squeeze Play" discussed on page 115.

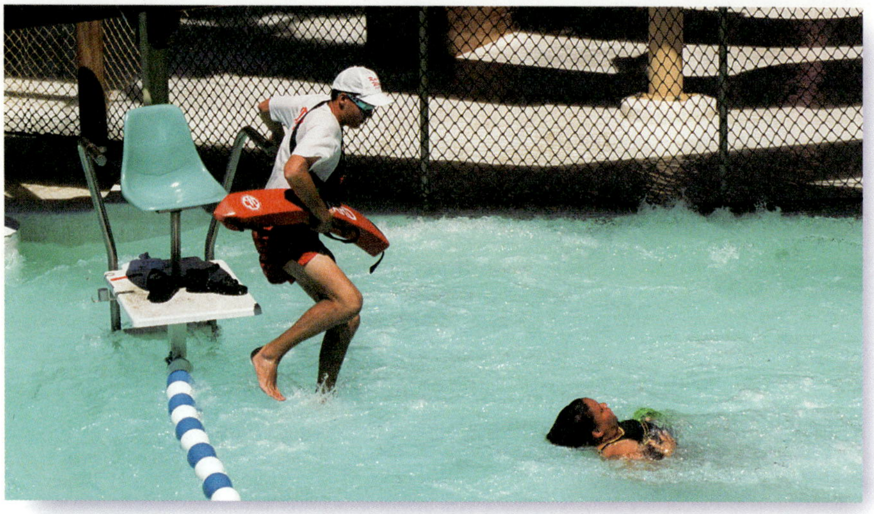

FIG 9.1 Consider the mechanism of the injury as you approach the guest.

CARING FOR GUESTS WITH SPINAL INJURIES

Ellis & Associates safety statistics indicate that the overwhelming number of spinal rescues in the aquatic environment involve conscious and sometimes active guests. You should practice the spinal management skills you learn in this course on simulated conscious and unconscious guests, so you will be prepared to address a catastrophic incident.

While the technical skill is the same for both conscious and unconscious guests, additional support is necessary when a guest with suspected spinal injury is conscious. In this situation, additional communication, calmness, and reassurance are needed. If the guest is unconscious, you must provide additional care to manage the airway.

Your spinal injury management begins with the way you enter the water. If you enter calm water near the injured guest, use an entry that will not significantly disturb the surface of the water. Sit on the edge of the pool and ease in; then move toward the guest. If the injured guest is further away or in moving water, you can enter the water as you would normally.

Vise Grip

The technique you will use in the water to minimize movement is called the vise grip. It can be performed in shallow or deep water, on a conscious or unconscious guest, if the guest is submerged or on the surface, and if the guest is face-up or face-down.

The objectives of the vise grip method of care for spinal injuries are to:

- Provide stabilization and support to the head and neck of a guest with a suspected spinal injury by pressing the arms of the guest alongside his or her head.
- Position the guest face-up for breathing.

To perform the vise grip in shallow water, follow these steps:

1. Whistle: signal to stop dispatch/waves, if necessary, and signal for help. Enter the water.
2. Carefully approach the guest.

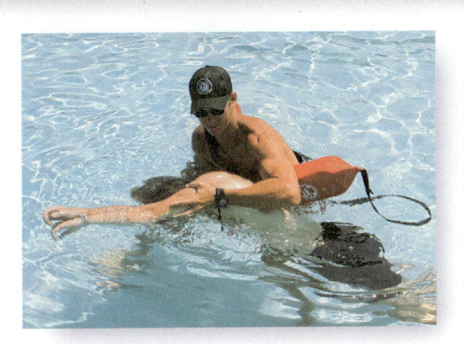

FIG 9.2 Pull up on outside arm. Press down on near arm.

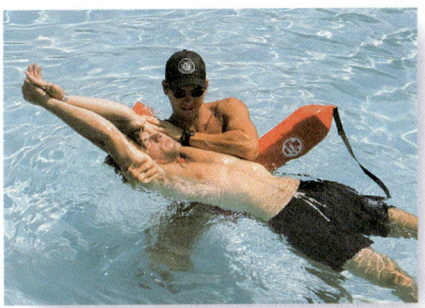

FIG 9.3 Move forward while you roll and lower yourself into the water.

3. Use the overarm vise grip to grasp the guest's arm just above the elbow.
4. Slowly move the guest's arms up alongside his head. Press his arms firmly against his ears.
5. Apply pressure firmly on both arms to secure his head.
6. If the guest is face down, use the underarm vise grip to roll him to a face-up position. You can do this by:

    Positioning the guest's arms next to his head. Grasp the guest's right arm with your right hand. Maintain firm pressure against the guest's head during the turn, and roll the guest toward you. If there is room in front of the guest, you can move forward while you roll the guest. This will cause the guest's legs to rise slightly, and will make the roll easier.

    As you roll the guest, lower yourself in the water. This will help you to avoid lifting the guest during the roll.

7. Once the guest is face-up, check him for consciousness and breathing.
    - If the guest is conscious, talk calmly to him as you move toward the backboard or wait for your team to bring it to you.
    - If the guest is unconscious and not breathing, begin rescue breathing. This is discussed at the end of this chapter. Be sure to keep the guest's face above water at all times.

To perform the vise grip in deep water, follow these steps:

1. Whistle, point to the guest, hit the E-Stop (if there is one), and signal for help.
2. Enter the water and carefully approach the guest.
3. Keep your rescue tube under your arms. This will position you higher in the water.
4. Apply the vise grip.
5. If the guest is face down, roll him in the same manner as you would in shallow water. The rescue tube will support you and the guest and allow you to maintain firm pressure on his arms.
6. With the guest face-up, check him for consciousness and breathing, and move to the backboard.

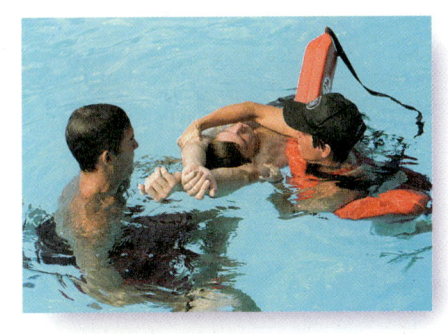

FIG 9.4 Deep water vise-grip.

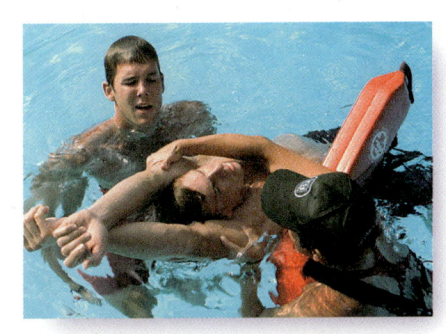

FIG 9.5 Move to the backboard.

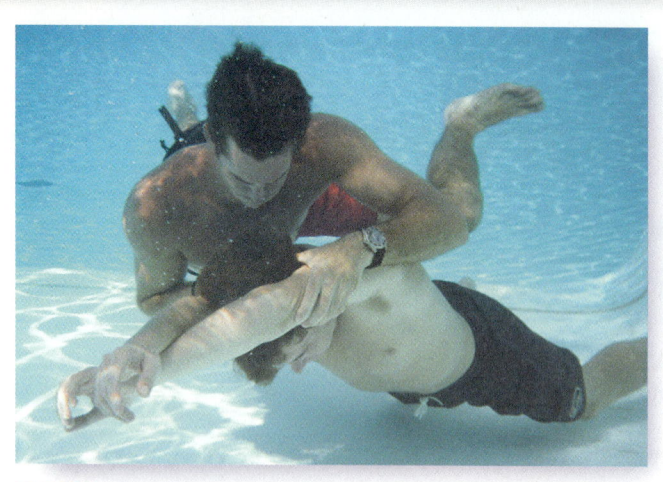

FIG 9.6 When the guest is submerged, position yourself alongside and just above him.

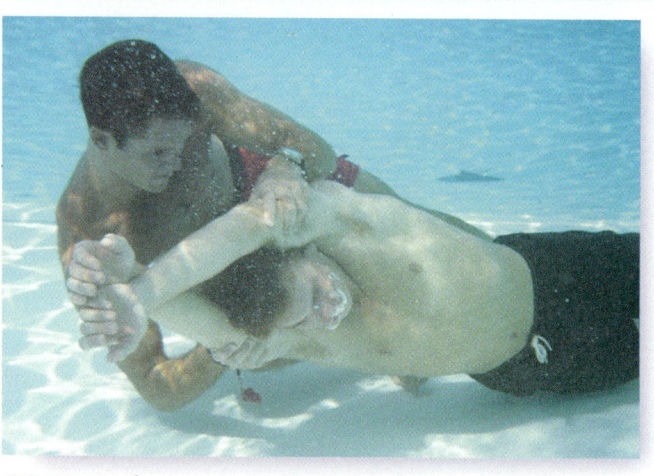

FIG 9.7 Apply vise-grip to submerged guest.

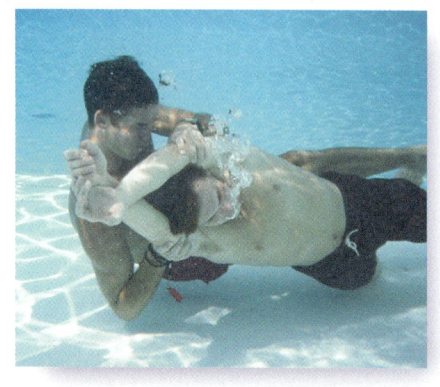

FIG 9.8 Keep the guest's head pinned between your arms.

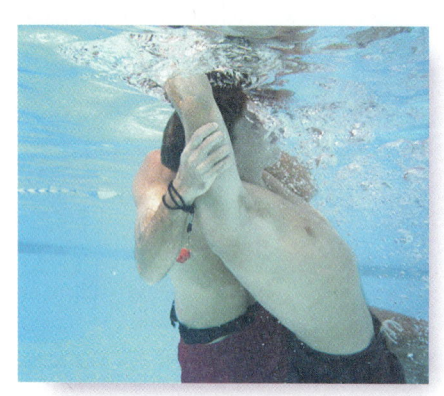

FIG 9.9 Start toward the water's surface on a diagonal path.

To perform the vise grip if the guest is submerged, follow these steps:

1. Carefully move to a position alongside, and just above, the guest. If you are in deep water, do a feet first surface dive to a position alongside him.
2. Apply the vise grip in the same manner as previously described.
3. Move forward, maintaining firm pressure on the guest's arms. Keep his head pinned between his arms.
4. Lift the guest by his arms. In deep water, start toward the surface on a diagonal approach to help minimize excessive bending of the spine.
5. Roll the guest. If you are in very shallow water, you may bring the guest to the surface and then roll him to a face-up position. If you are in deep water, you may roll the guest before you break the surface. Then, as you break the surface, the guest will already be in a face-up position.

Backboarding

The objectives of backboarding are to:

- Secure the guest to a long backboard, in preparation for removal from the water by:
    - Placing the long backboard under the guest.
    - Strapping the guest to the backboard.
    - Securing the head and neck of the guest with a head immobilizer.
- Maintain control of the guest and the backboard.

Backboarding is performed by two or more lifeguards, who will act quickly and efficiently to remove the guest from the water. You will learn procedures for backboarding a guest when two or more lifeguards are available at your facility.

It is important that you practice being both the initial lifeguard and a member of the lifeguard support team. You need to know your responsibilities for every position on the team.

Spinal injury management equipment includes backboards, head immobilizers, and straps. This equipment comes in all shapes and sizes. You will learn the basics of spinal injury management during this course. Once you begin working at your aquatic facility, you must become thoroughly familiar with the specific equipment and procedures used at that facility.

The protocols you use will be based on the equipment, staff size, and input from the facility management and local EMS providers.

The key components for any backboarding protocol are:

- **Communication**—between the lifeguard team and a conscious guest.
- **Minimizing unnecessary movement**—of the guest throughout the entire backboarding procedure.
- **Careful removal**—to avoid further injury to the guest or the lifeguard.
- **Protection from hypothermia**—spinal injury makes a guest more likely to suffer hypothermia, even in warm climates.

Overarm Vise Grip

Depending on how you initially stabilized the guest, it may be necessary to remove your arm from under him to place him on a backboard. However, you must continue to stabilize the guest's head. You can change from an underarm vise grip to an overarm vise grip by simply switching the position of the hand that you are supporting the guest with.

To transfer to the overarm vise grip:

1. Apply firm pressure with your outside hand. Pull the guest toward your chest. This presses the guest's arm that is closest to you against your chest.
2. Release your hand that is holding the arm against your chest. Reach over the guest with this hand and grab his outside arm, next to your other hand.
3. Apply firm pressure against the guest's outside arm, pulling him toward your chest.
4. Release your hand that is under the guest and move it to the guest's arm that is against your chest. Continue to apply pressure on both of the guest's arms against his head.
5. You now have the guest's head pressed between his arms, with neither of your arms under the guest.

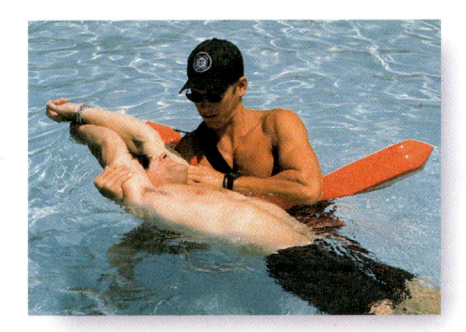

FIG 9.10 When performing the overarm vise grip, press the guest toward your chest.

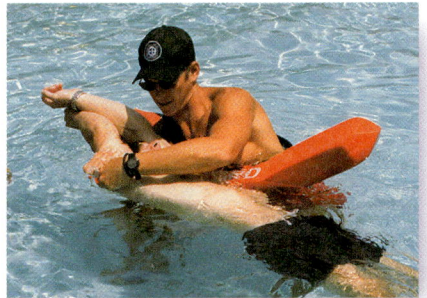

FIG 9.11 Release the guest's arm, reach over him, and grasp his outside arm.

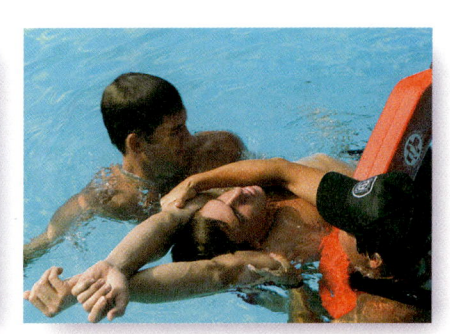

FIG 9.12 Example of the overarm vise grip in deep water.

Two-Lifeguard Backboarding

Two-lifeguard backboarding techniques are performed at the side of the pool. The following steps describe the procedure from the initial recognition of a guest with a suspected spinal injury, through extrication from the water.

1. **Recognition and reaction**
   - The first lifeguard whistles, signals the situation, enters the water carefully, and approaches the guest. He assumes the correct position, applies the vise grip, moves the guest to the pool edge, checks for consciousness and spontaneous breathing, and calls out findings.
   - The second lifeguard clears the pool, makes sure 911 is called, and brings the backboard to the edge of the pool for extrication. He removes the head immobilizer, prepares the backboard and straps, and inserts the backboard into the water. He should place the head immobilizer near the side of the pool, where he can easily reach them.

2. **Bring injured guest to the side**
   - The lifeguard on the deck puts the backboard into the water, keeping the foot end of the backboard on the bottom of the pool. The head of the board should be in the water. He slides the foot end out so that the lifeguard in the water can step on it. He then presses the head of the backboard against the wall with his forearms.
   - The lifeguard in the water switches to the overarm vise grip as he nears the backboard. He steps on the end of the backboard or in one of the handholds to keep the backboard down.

3. **Place the guest on the backboard**
   - The lifeguard in the water follows the direction of the guard on the deck to place the guest correctly on the backboard.
   - The lifeguard on the deck directs the lifeguard in the water to position the guest on the backboard, making sure that the guest's head is positioned in the center of the head space on the backboard.

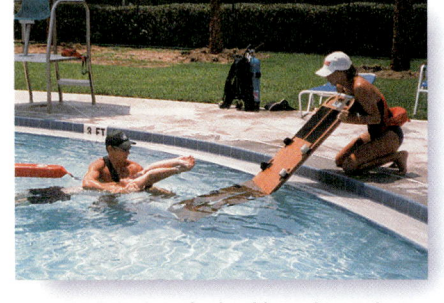

FIG 9.13 Insert the backboard into the water.

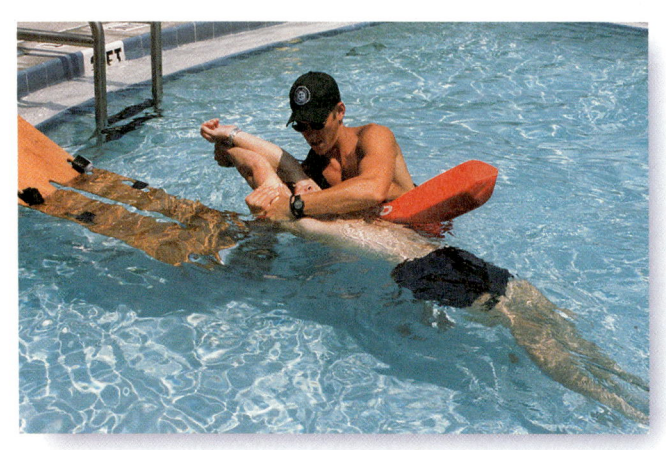

FIG 9.14 Step on the foot end of the backboard to keep it down in the water.

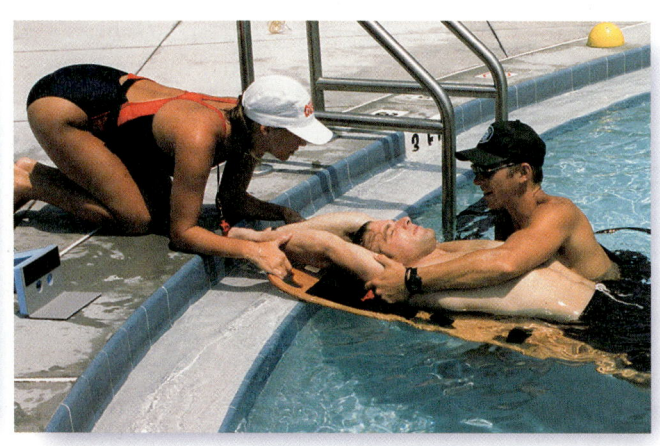

FIG 9.15 Position the guest on the backboard.

CHAPTER 9 • SPINAL INJURY MANAGEMENT   111

4. **Transfer control of the head**

    - The lifeguard on the deck grasps the guest's armpits, and presses his forearms against the sides of the guest's head. He maintains pressure and tells the lifeguard in the water that he has control of the head.

    - The lifeguard in the water releases the guest's arms. He removes his foot from the backboard and guides it up to the guest. He then checks the guest's airway, breathing, and circulation.

   If the guest is not breathing or does not have a pulse, he should be immediately removed from the water, with precautions taken to minimize movement. Rescue breathing and/or CPR can most successfully be performed on the deck.

5. **Secure the guest's chest**

    - The lifeguard in the water tightly secures the chest strap, high on the guest's chest under his armpits.

    - The lifeguard on the deck maintains firm pressure with his forearms against the guest's head.

6. **Secure the rest of the body**

    - The lifeguard on the deck monitors the guest's condition and stabilizes the guest's head and the backboard.

    - The lifeguard in the water straps the rest of the guest's body to the backboard. He may also place a rescue tube under the backboard for flotation and stability during the rest of the strapping procedure, remembering that the rescue tube will have to be removed before the extrication begins. The remaining straps should be placed across the guest's hips, which may include hands, thighs, and lower legs. Securing the lower legs is good for extra support if it is a large guest, or if you need to remove the backboard.

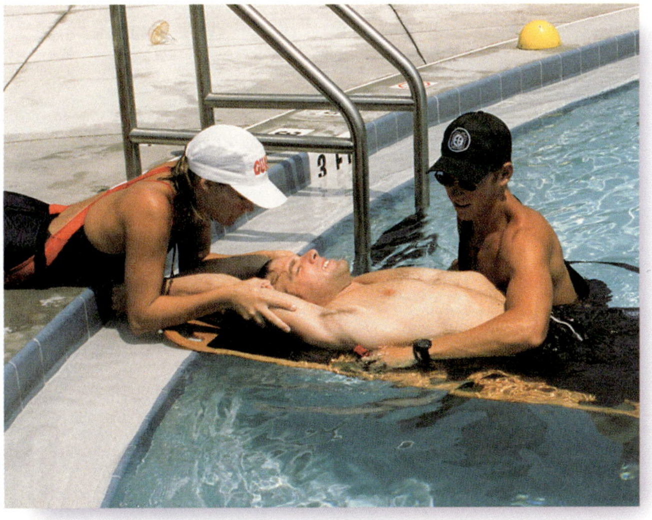

FIG 9.16 Lifeguard on deck supports guest's head while lifeguard in water locates the chest strap.

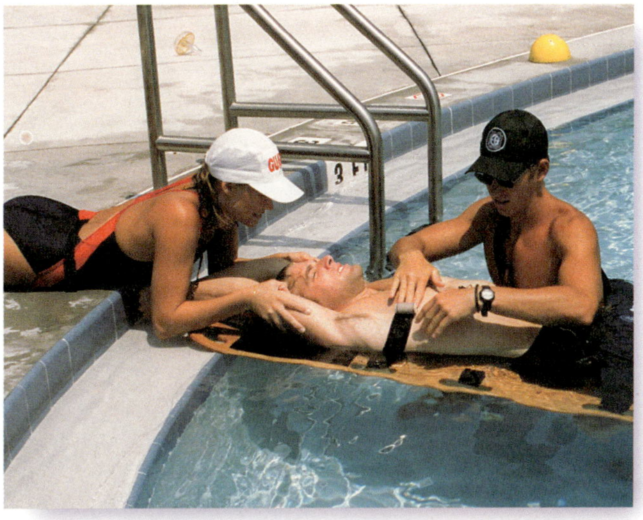

FIG 9.17 Lifeguard on deck maintains firm pressure while the lifeguard in water secures the straps, beginning with the chest.

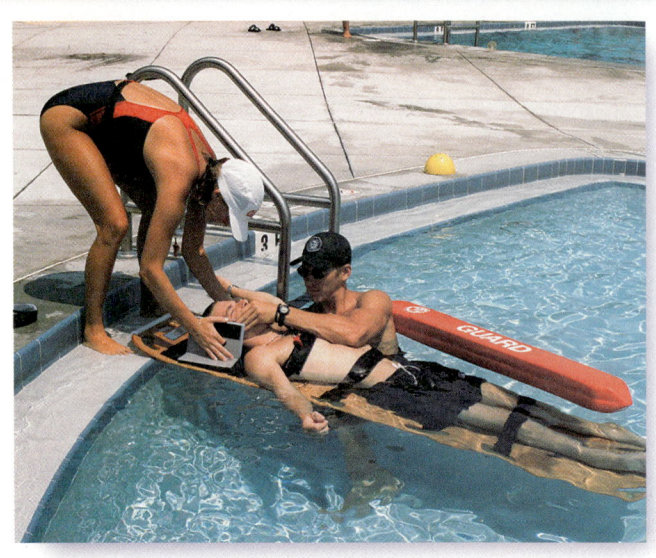

FIG 9.18 The initial lifeguard in the water holds the guest's head while the head immobilizer is applied.

7. **Secure the head**
   - The lifeguard in the water places one hand under the backboard and controls the guest's head with his other hand. He places his thumb and index finger on the guest's cheekbones, covering but not blocking, his mouth. He tells the lifeguard on the deck that he has control of the guest's head. He continues to stabilize the backboard.
   - The lifeguard on the deck releases the head and moves any hair off the guest's face and lowers the guest's arms. He then applies the head restraints. Depending on the type of head immobilizer that is used, the head restraints may be applied one-at-a-time or simultaneously. Next, the lifeguard attaches the head strap, applying even pressure on both sides. He tells the lifeguard in the water that the head is secured.

8. **Remove the guest from the water**
   - The lifeguard in the water moves to the foot end of the backboard. He lowers the foot end of the backboard down in the water.
   - The lifeguard on the deck lifts the head of the backboard onto the deck, making sure that the runners of the backboard are on the deck. As the foot end of the backboard is submerged, the water will help lift the guest's head out of the water.
   - The lifeguard on the deck pulls as the lifeguard in the water pushes the backboard up onto the deck. The backboard is then slid onto the deck.

9. **Care for the guest**
   - Both lifeguards use BSI precautions and monitor the guest's ABC's.
   - Watch for vomiting. If the guest does vomit, roll the entire backboard to the side. Do not attempt to turn the guest's head. Clear the guest's airway. Place the backboard down on the deck, and continue to monitor the guest's ABC's.
   - Cover the guest to prevent hypothermia.

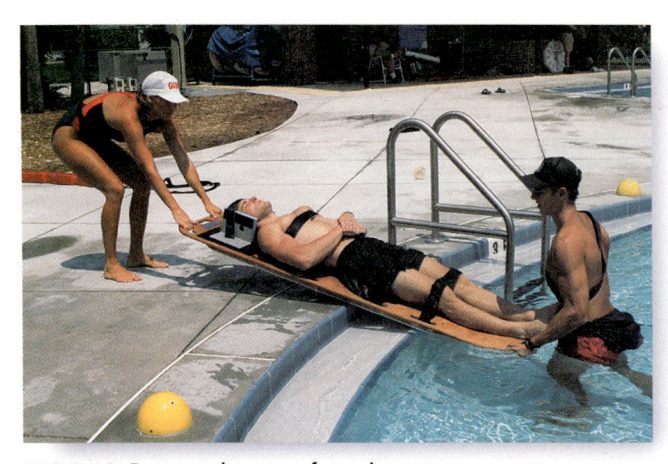

FIG 9.19 Remove the guest from the water.

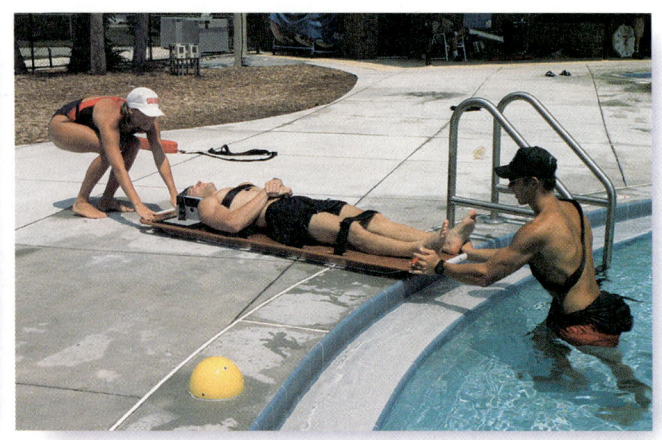

FIG 9.20 Slide the backboard onto the deck.

Team Backboarding

In some situations, multiple lifeguards will be available to assist the initial lifeguard making the rescue. The original lifeguard should be talking to the injured guest, assessing consciousness and breathing, and communicating to the lifeguard team. By this time, the lifeguard team should have cleared the activity area, called for emergency personnel, brought the backboard and resuscitation equipment to the extrication point, and be ready to assist the original lifeguard. As with any team activity, communication among the lifeguards is very important during this procedure. The lifeguard at the head of the guest has the best position to monitor all activity. This lifeguard is usually the one who will be in control of the rescue. However, each facility Emergency Action System will designate which lifeguard has the control (i.e., the head lifeguard or a higher trained lifeguard).

The following steps describe the team backboarding procedures for a guest with a suspected spinal injury from the water. If the procedure is being done in deep water, rescue tubes can be inserted under the backboard once it is in position. Remember that you will have to remove the rescue tubes before beginning the extrication.

> **critical POINT**
>
> As with any team activity, communication among the lifeguards is very important during this procedure.

1. **Move into position**
   - The initial lifeguard uses the overarm vise grip position.
   - Other lifeguards position themselves to help the initial lifeguard.
   - One lifeguard is on the same side of the guest as the initial lifeguard. This lifeguard slowly and gently raises the guest's body to a horizontal position.
   - Two lifeguards on the opposite side of the guest move the backboard into place.

2. **Place the backboard**

   Submerge the backboard so that it is underneath, but not touching, the guest. Lifeguards on both sides of the guest can position the backboard so that it is centered under the guest.

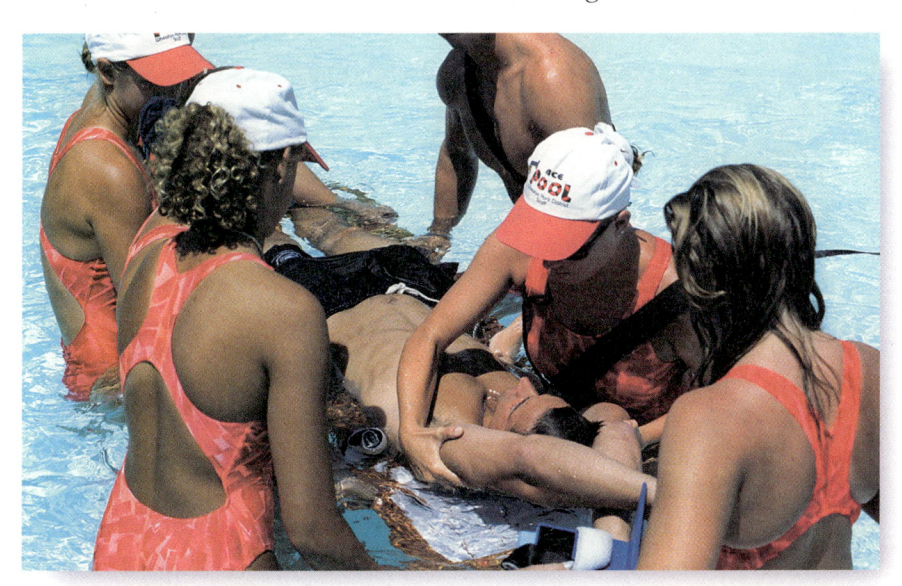

FIG 9.21 When positioning the backboard, lifeguards on both sides can check to see that it is centered and that the guest's head is positioned correctly.

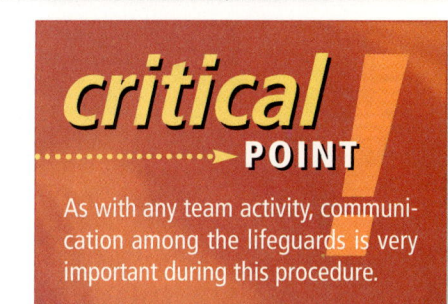

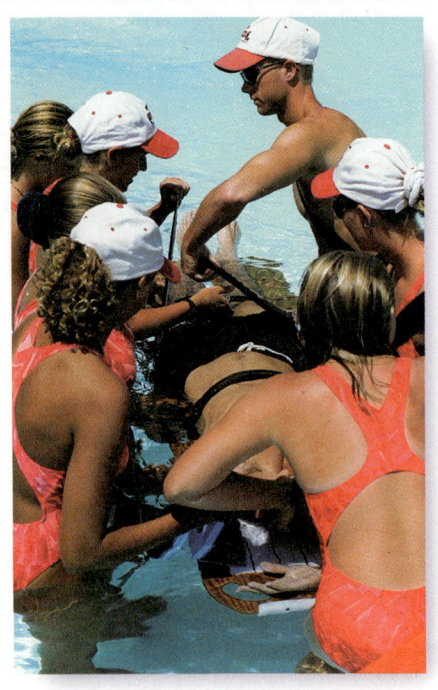

FIG 9.22 Secure the rest of the body.

3. **Transfer control of the head**
   - The lifeguard nearest the head of the backboard moves near the guest's head. He grasps the guest's armpits and presses his forearms against the side of the guest's head. The pressure should be firm and even.
   - The initial lifeguard releases the vise grip once the other lifeguard has control of the guest's head. He now becomes a member of the support team and takes a position alongside the guest. He continues to talk to the guest and monitor the ABC's.

   After the position change, the backboard is gently raised underneath the guest.

4. **Secure the chest**

   Secure the chest strap, tightly, high on the guest's chest, under his armpits.

5. **Secure the rest of the body**

   The lifeguard at the guest's head continues to monitor the guest's ABC's. The other lifeguards strap the rest of the guest's body as previously discussed.

6. **Secure the head**

   Place the head restraints.

7. **Remove the guest from the water**

   Carefully lift the backboard from the water and slide it onto the deck.

8. **Care for the guest**

   Watch for vomiting. If the guest vomits, roll the entire backboard to the side and clear his airway. Do not just turn the guest's head. Lay the backboard down on the deck, and continue to monitor the ABC's. Cover the guest to prevent hypothermia.

Handling Spinal Injuries in Speed Slides

Because of the small space available at the bottom of a speed slide in the run-out, the usual procedure of managing a suspected spinal injury is modified.

After stopping dispatch and activating the EAS, the initial lifeguard will need to evaluate the position in which the guest is lying in the slide. If the guest's arms can be brought over his head without excessive movement of the head and neck, the lifeguard can use the overarm vise grip, as previously described.

If there is risk of movement, the lifeguard can stabilize the guest's head by simply holding the guest's head in line with his body.

The procedure you use will depend on the height of the sides of the run-out, the amount of room in the run-out, other physical features of the area, and the position of the guest.

As the lifeguard support team arrives to assist, position them along the outside of the walls, with an equal number on each side. The team then quickly positions their hands over the guest, to assure they will be in the correct position. Their positions will be based on the body size of the guest. The lifeguards should alternate their arms with one another.

The arm/hand position of the lifeguards should be spaced to provide maximum support along the length of the guest's body, from the shoulders to the feet. Once any position adjustments have been made, the lifeguards slide their hands under the guest in the slide. The lifeguards' arms and elbows should be **inside the wall of the slide**.

While the lifeguards are getting their arms and hands in the proper positions, another lifeguard should be placing the backboard in the slide, at the guest's feet, making sure that all the straps will be clear when the backboard is moved under the guest.

The lifeguard stabilizing the head will give the commands during this procedure and maintain the pressure against the guest's head at all times.

On the command to lift, the lifeguard team lifts the guest. It is only necessary to lift the guest far enough to allow the backboard to be inserted under him. As the guest is lifted, the other lifeguards slide the backboard under the guest.

The lifeguard at the head watches for alignment of the backboard. He must be sure that the guest's head will be positioned in the center of the head pad. Communication is very important.

On the command to lower, the lifeguards lower the guest to the backboard. Clear all straps, if any are in the way, and place them on top of the guest. The lifeguards now get into position to lift the backboard out of the slide.

Again, on the command to lift, the lifeguards lift to a complete standing position—lift with your legs, not your back.

Rotate the backboard carefully, step over the sides of the slide and move to safety.

Slowly lower the backboard and the guest down. In some facilities, the guest and backboard may be placed across the top of the slide walls. In other facilities, you may place the guest and the backboard down on the deck. Secure the guest to the backboard, monitor his ABC's, and follow your facility's Emergency Action System.

Spinal Injury Management with a Guest Standing or Sitting

There may be times when a guest will walk out of the pool or slide and exhibit the signs and symptoms of a neck injury. In these situations, it is necessary to take the same precautions as previously described. To stabilize a standing or sitting guest, use the technique known as the *squeeze play*.

- Stand at the guest's side.
- Place one forearm along the guest's spine. Place your hand against the back of the guest's head.
- Place your other forearm in front of the guest, in line with his sternum. Place your thumb and index finger against the guest's cheekbones.
- Apply pressure with your forearms against the guest's chest and back. Hold the guest's head steady.

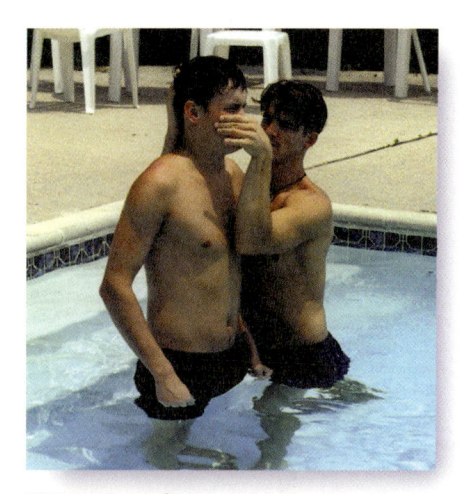

FIG 9.23 Performing the Squeeze Play with a standing guest.

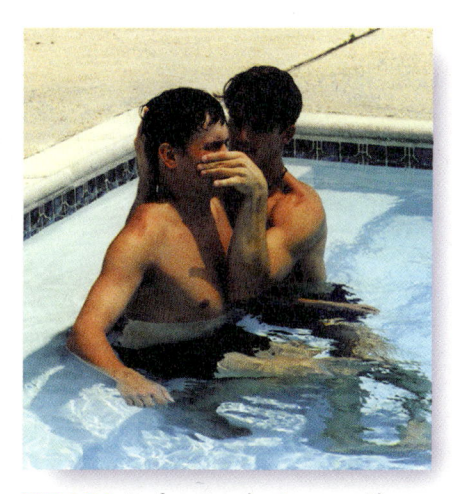

FIG 9.24 Performing the Squeeze Play with a sitting guest.

If there will be a delay in EMS arrival, or if the guest becomes faint or tired, you will need to sit or lie him down.

If the guest is seated in a position where you can place a backboard behind him, do so and then slowly lower him to it.. With the assistance of the lifeguard team, transfer control of the guest's head to another lifeguard. Other lifeguards should slide the guest onto the backboard. If the guest is standing and faints or becomes tired, several lifeguards will be needed to safely lower him to the ground.

RESCUE BREATHING AND CPR

There may be situations where a guest who has sustained a spinal injury requires rescue breathing or CPR. Once the lifeguard has applied the vise grip, he can quickly check for consciousness and breathing. Look for the chest to rise and fall, and listen for breathing. With the vise grip being applied, it will be impossible for the initial lifeguard to check the pulse or perform rescue breathing. It will be necessary for a second lifeguard to do this.

If a guest stops breathing or loses his pulse, he should immediately be removed from the water. Place the guest on the backboard, but do not take the time to strap him in. The guest's ABC's are your top priority in this type of situation. You should follow spinal management precautions, but begin rescue breathing or CPR immediately.

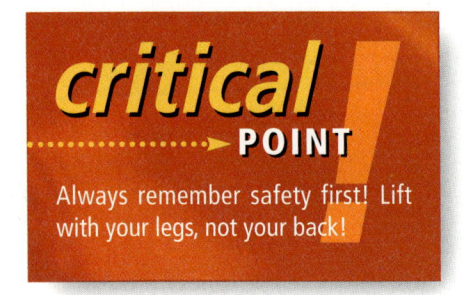

ADDITIONAL SPINAL INJURY MANAGEMENT ISSUES

If there are not enough lifeguards available to form a rescue team, and you do not wish to use the two-lifeguard technique, you may use the aid of other facility staff or even guests at your facility, making certain you tell them exactly what to do at each step.

It is important that you perform spinal management rescues only when circumstances indicate that these protocols are warranted. Otherwise, you may spend extensive time on backboarding, instead of on managing near-drowning problems. For example, if you discover an unconscious nine-year-old guest lying on the bottom of the pool, in the center, at a depth of ten feet, and there is no diving board, this is not a likely situation for a spinal injury. You should survey the entire scene of the incident before you determine what rescue technique you will use.

> **critical POINT**
> Always remember safety first! Lift with your legs, not your back!

REVIEW QUESTIONS

1. Which of the following is a sign of possible spinal injury?
   a. Pain in the neck or back.
   b. Inability to move.
   c. Bruising or deformity.
   d. All of the above.

2. (T) (F) The technique used to minimize movement of a guest's head and neck in the water is called the spine splint.

3. Which of the following is true of the vise grip procedure?
   It requires:
   a. The guest's arms to be positioned at his sides.
   b. Two or more lifeguards to perform the technique.
   c. The lifeguard to place the guest's arms next to his ears.
   d. The lifeguard to keep the guest face-down in the water.

4. The vise grip can be performed:
   a. In shallow or deep water.
   b. On a conscious or unconscious guest.
   c. On a victim who is at the surface or who is submerged.
   d. All of the above.

5. (T) (F) When applying a backboard, it is acceptable to release the support of the guest's head to remove the guest from the water.

Skill Sheet 10

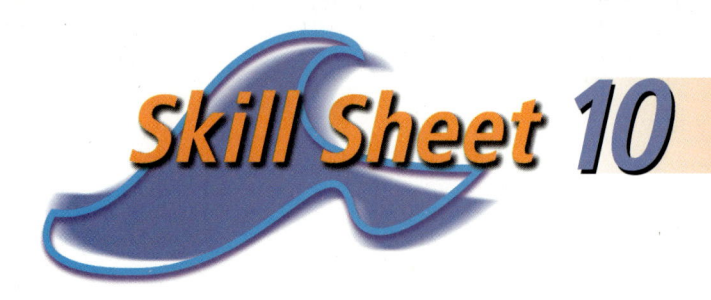

VISE GRIP

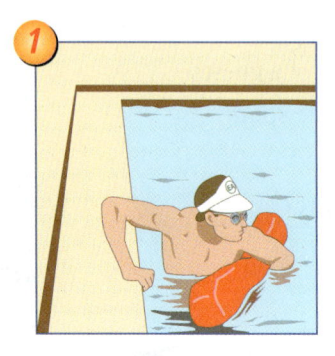

1. Activate EAS and enter the water.

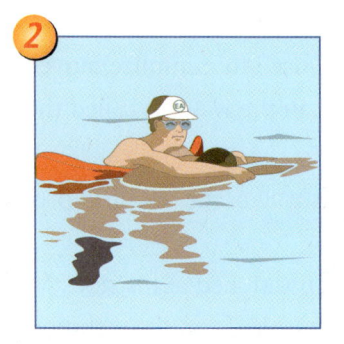

2. If the guest is face down in deep water, reach over tube and guest.

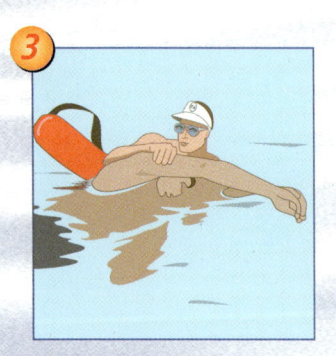

3. Hands on upper arms; press arms to head.

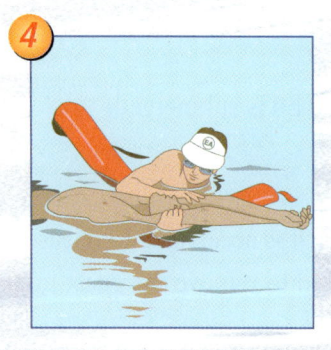

4. Roll the guest face up.

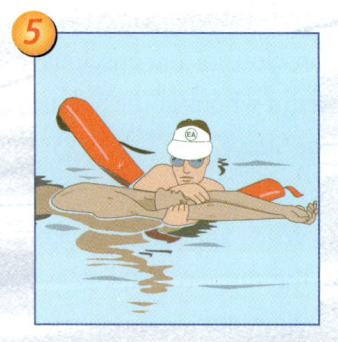

5. Assess breathing; progress to backboard.

KEY POINTS:

- Maintain firm pressure.
- Roll the body gently as a unit.

CRITICAL THINKING:

1. In what situations would this skill be used?
2. What could you do if the injured guest is already face up?
3. How could you provide care if a guest was:
   a. sitting on the side of the pool, or
   b. standing in the water?

CHAPTER 9 • SPINAL INJURY MANAGEMENT   119

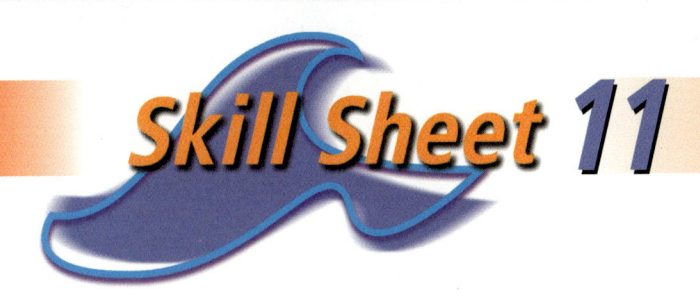

Skill Sheet 11

TWO-LIFEGUARD TEAM BACKBOARDING

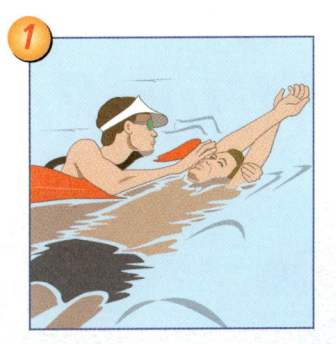

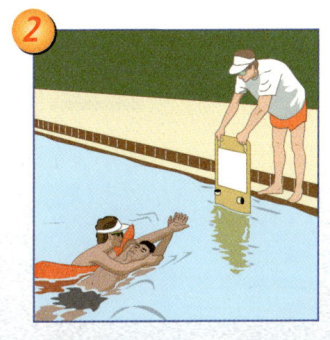

1. Vise grip.

2. Assess breathing; move guest to side; switch to overarm vise grip (first lifeguard). Slide backboard in water (second lifeguard).

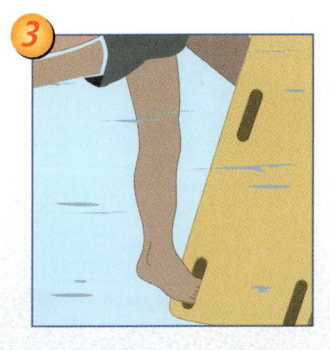

3. Grab backboard end with foot (first lifeguard).

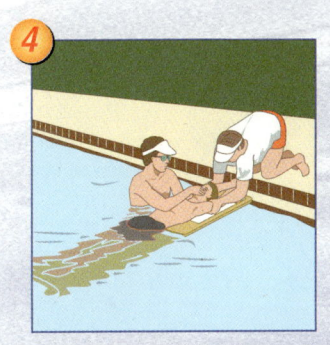

4. Place injured guest on backboard; transfer control of head (second lifeguard).

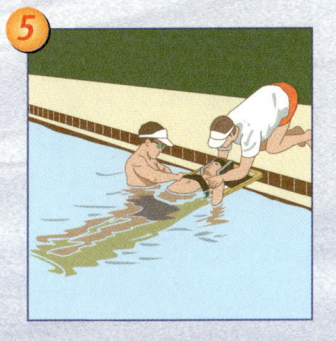

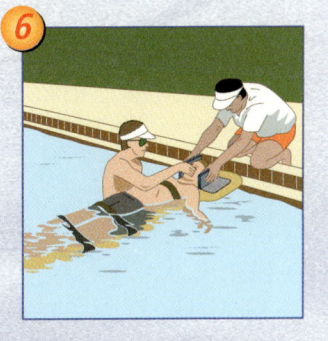

5. Apply straps.

6. Apply head immobilizer.

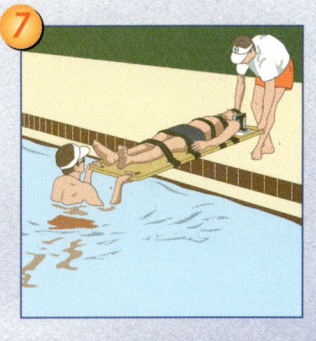

7. Remove guest from water: Lower foot end (first lifeguard). Lift head end; slide onto deck; assess/follow EAS plan.

KEY POINTS:

- Communicate with conscious guest and with other lifeguards.
- Constantly minimize unnecessary movement.
- Maintain proper board alignment.
- Carefully remove guest.
- Protect guest from hypothermia.

CRITICAL THINKING:

1. If you had to perform this skill in deep water, what could you do to make it work?

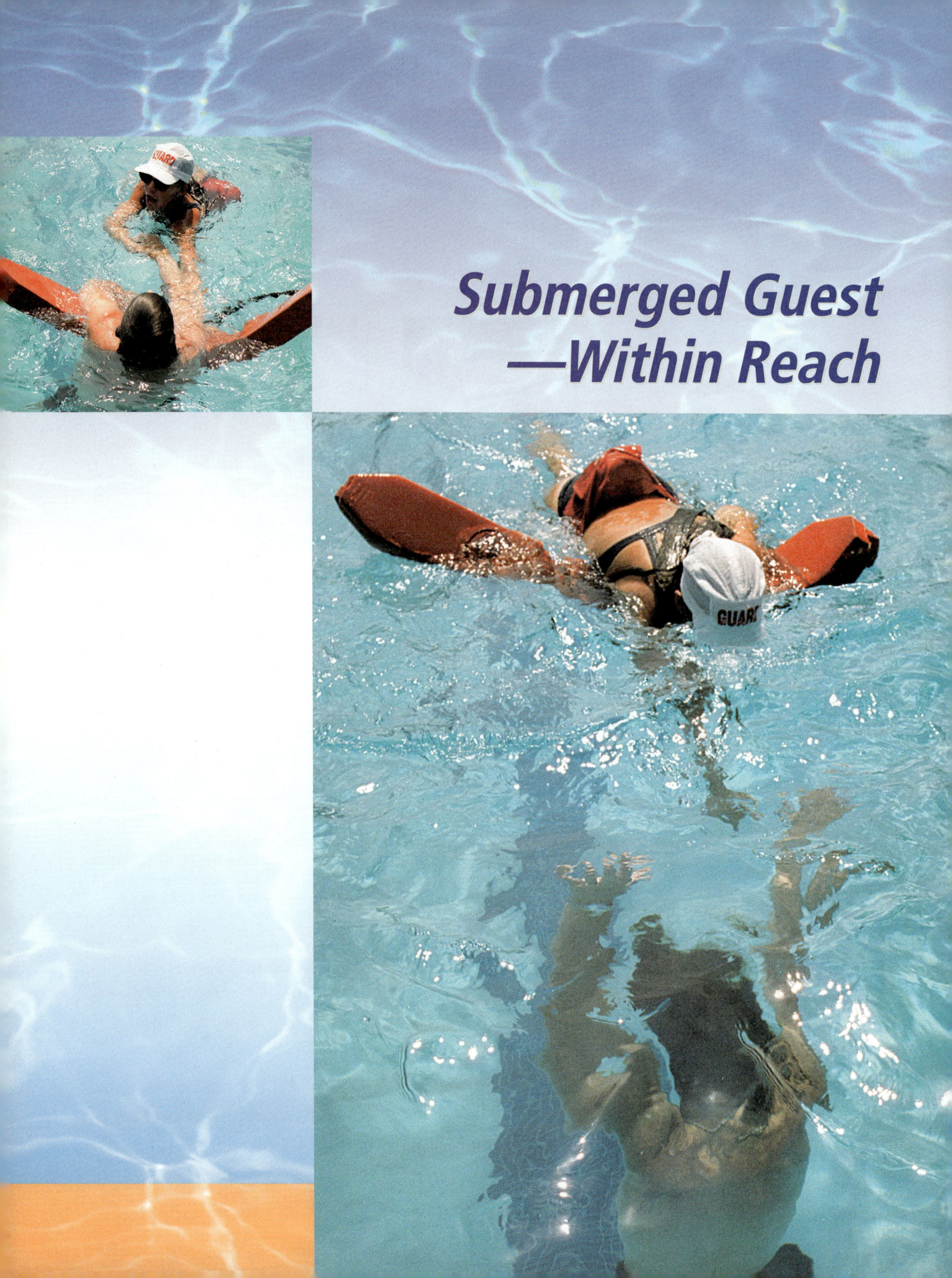

Submerged Guest —Within Reach

chapter 10
TEN

OBJECTIVES

After reading this chapter and completing the related course work, you should be able to:

1. Demonstrate the "duck pluck" procedure used to recover a conscious or unconscious guest below the surface of the water.

2. Demonstrate the duck pluck on an unconscious guest and give follow-up care, which includes:
    a. Heimlich Maneuver
    b. Rescue Breathing
    c. Extrication
    d. Supplemental Oxygen Administration
    e. CPR

There are times when a guest will be just a few feet underwater, and may be unable to get back to the surface. An example of this is when a guest exits a free-fall, or "shotgun" slide. The guest enters the water at a high velocity and goes to the bottom in water that may be 7 to 8 feet deep. The guest may be conscious or unconscious. For whatever reason, the guest makes no effort to return to the surface. This reinforces the need to scan your entire area, including below the surface.

GUEST WITHIN REACH

Even though a guest may be standing on the bottom in 7 or 8 feet of water, you may be able to reach him without going completely underwater yourself. The most effective way of doing this is to use the duck pluck. The duck pluck allows you to remain on the surface of the water, with your rescue tube between you and the guest. The guest could be active, and as a professional lifeguard you must protect yourself as you assist him.

DUCK PLUCK FOR A CONSCIOUS GUEST

The objectives of the duck pluck for a conscious guest are to:

- Recover a guest and provide support while in the water by reaching across the rescue tube, grabbing the guest's arm or hand, and pulling him to the surface.
- Maintain control of the rescue tube and the guest.

You should execute the duck pluck when the distressed guest is below the surface and within reach. The duck pluck can be executed in either deep or shallow water.

To execute the duck pluck on a conscious guest:

1. Whistle, point to the guest, hit the E-Stop (if there is one), do a compact jump entry, and approach stroke toward the guest.
2. Stop swimming when you are slightly in front of and above the guest.
3. Hold your rescue tube with one hand in the middle of the tube. With the other hand, reach across the rescue tube and down to the guest. You may need to submerge your head to look down into the water.
4. Grab the guest's arm or hand. It makes no difference which hand or arm you grab. It may be helpful to you to push your rescue tube underwater as you grab the guest. Steady yourself on the rescue tube.
5. Pull the distressed guest to the surface. With the hand that is controlling the rescue tube, push the tube under the guest's armpits and into his chest. Push the rescue tube with one hand while you

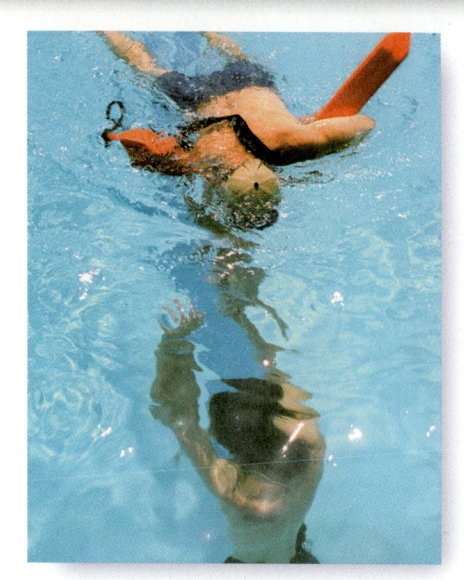

FIG 10.1 Position yourself above the guest.

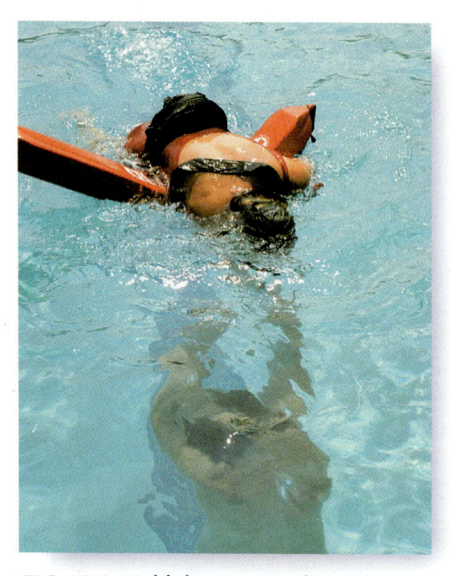

FIG 10.2 Hold the rescue tube with one hand, and reach across and down to the guest with your other hand.

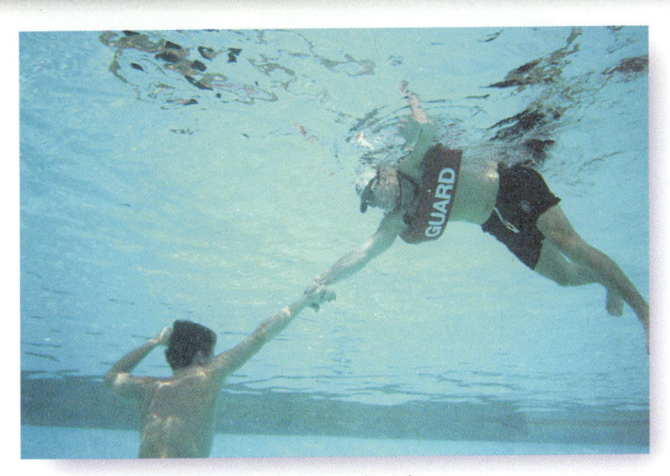

FIG 10.3 Grasp the guest's arm or hand.

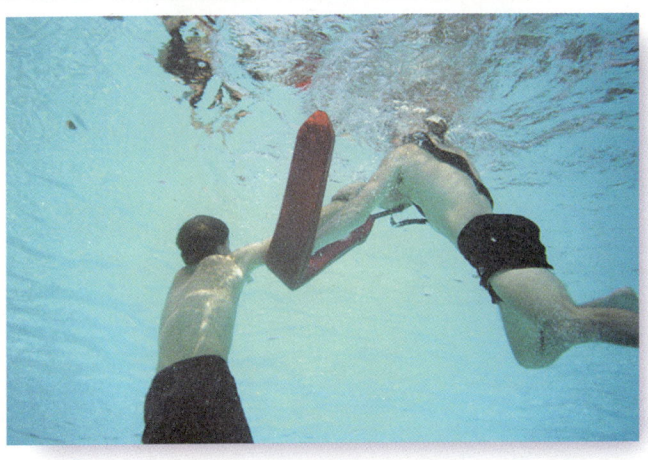

FIG 10.4 Pull the guest to the surface, push the rescue tube under the armpits and into his chest.

   are pulling the guest up with your other hand. This will keep you from colliding with the guest, or pulling yourself over the top of your rescue tube.

6. Keep your arm holding the rescue tube straight, and your elbow locked. Talk to the guest while you continue to move toward the side of the pool or an exit point.

7. Assist the guest from the water, making sure that he is alright before you leave. Your Emergency Action System should explain exactly what procedure you should follow at this time. Fill out the rescue report.

DUCK PLUCK FOR AN UNCONSCIOUS GUEST

The objectives of the duck pluck for an unconscious guest are to:
- Recover the guest, provide support, administer the Heimlich Maneuver, and rescue breathing, if necessary.
- Maintain control of the rescue tube and the guest.

When the distressed guest is below the surface, within reach, and unconscious, execute the duck pluck, administer the Heimlich Maneuver, and, if necessary, administer rescue breathing. This can be done in either deep or shallow water.

To execute the duck pluck on an unconscious guest:

1. Perform the same sequence of skills that you performed for a conscious guest. When you reach the surface with the guest, if he is not struggling or breathing spontaneously, position him so that you can administer the Heimlich Maneuver.

2. Hold onto the guest's arm or hand with one hand, and roll him to a face-up position.

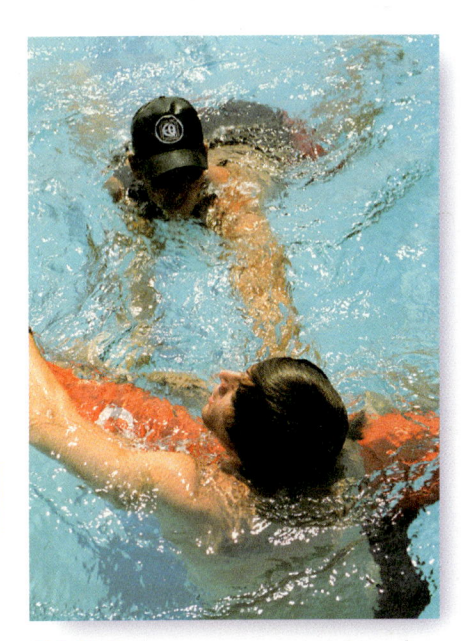

FIG 10.5 Keep your arms straight and talk to the guest.

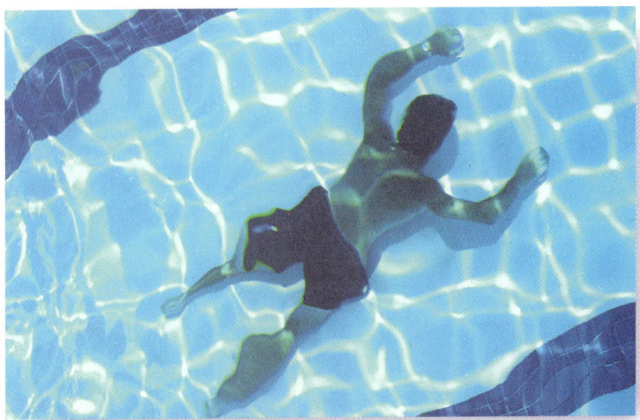

FIG 10.6 Unconscious guest on bottom of pool.

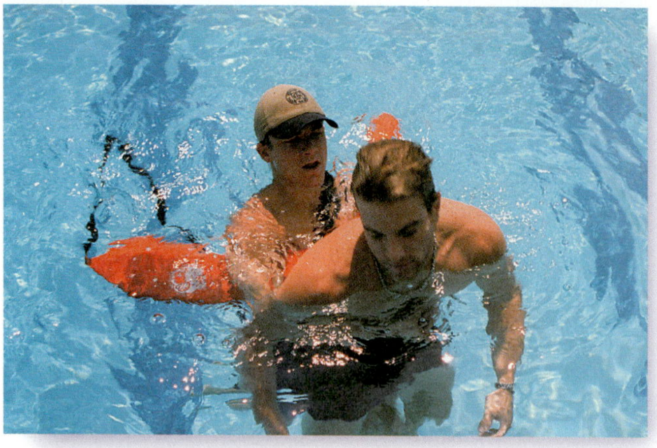

FIG 10.7 Bring the unconscious guest to a vertical position and perform the Heimlich Maneuver.

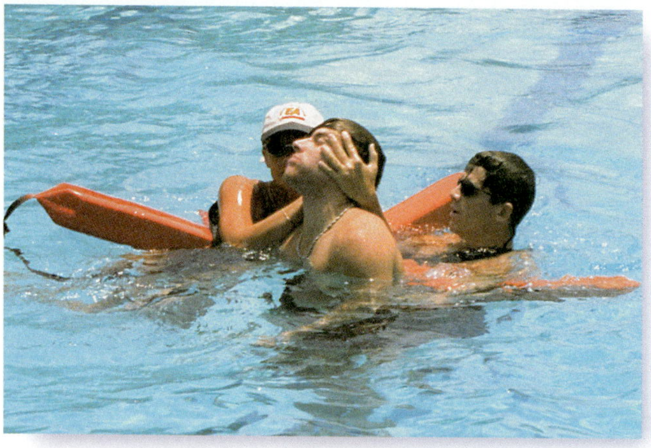

FIG 10.8 Two-lifeguard Heimlich Maneuver.

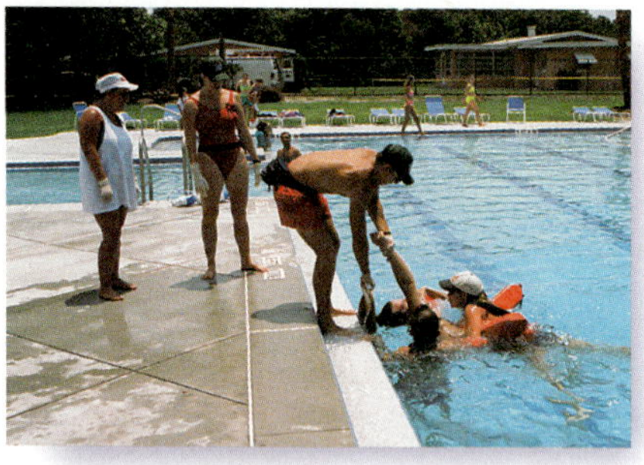

3. Reach over the rescue tube with both of your hands and under the guest's armpits. Bring the guest to a vertical position. Be sure to keep his face out of the water.
4. Position your hands properly and perform the Heimlich Maneuver.

Follow the same protocols you learned for the single-lifeguard or two-lifeguard rescues. If the guest remains unconscious and water or fluid no longer flows from his mouth, position the guest for rescue breathing. Perform rescue breathing while moving to the nearest exit point. Remove the guest from the water and continue to provide care.

FIG 10.9 Extrication.

REVIEW QUESTIONS

1. (T) (F) Guests may be submerged just a couple of feet, but they are unable to get to the surface.

2. To help keep you from pulling yourself into the guest or pulling yourself over the top of the rescue tube, you can

   _____.

3. The procedure used to rescue a submerged guest within reach is known as the _____ _____.

4. (T) (F) An unconscious guest could be face down on the surface of the water or on the bottom of the pool.

5. (T) (F) An unconscious, submerged guest should be given the Heimlich Maneuver.

CHAPTER 10 • SUBMERGED GUEST - WITHIN REACH   125

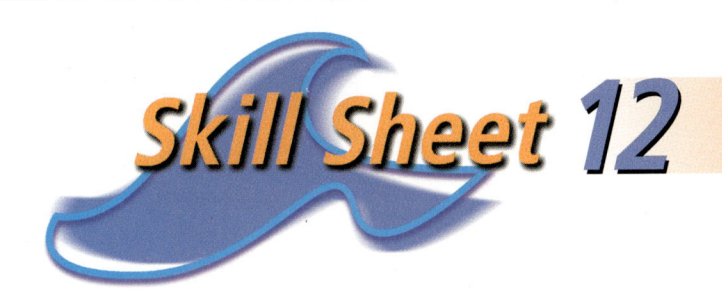

Skill Sheet 12

DUCK PLUCK

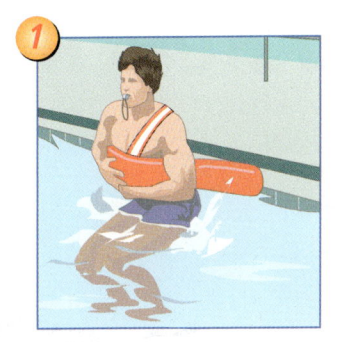

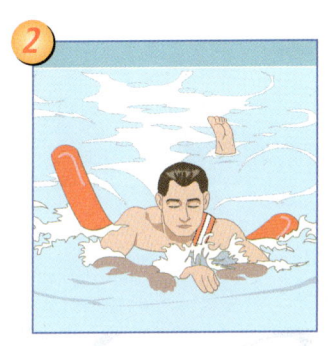

1. Compact jump.

2. Approach stroke.

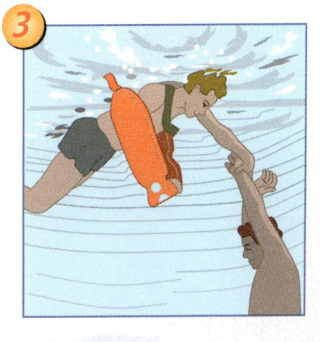

3. Reach over rescue tube; grasp guest's arm.

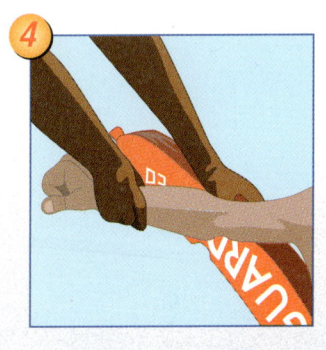

4. "Push-pull" the guest up, rescue tube in armpit.

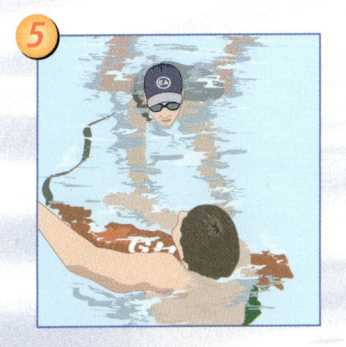

5. If conscious, talk to guest; kick toward side.

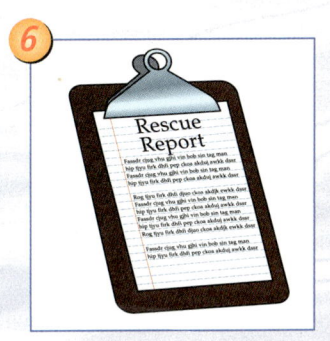

6. Secure guest; remove guest from pool; complete rescue report.

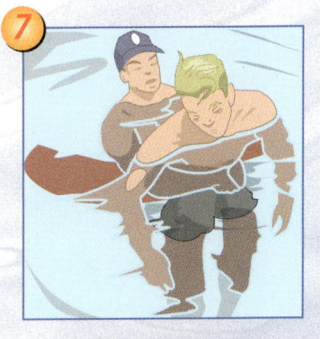

7. If unconscious, bring guest to a vertical position; execute Heimlich Maneuver.

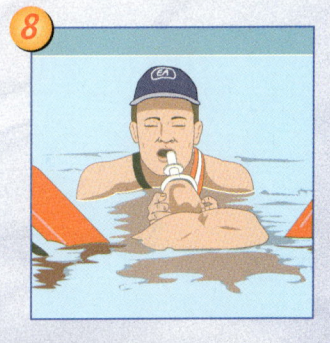

8. If still not breathing, begin rescue breathing with pocket mask; bring guest to side; extricate guest; assess; follow EAS protocol.

KEY POINTS:

- Keep driving forward.
- Grab and go.
- Keep hips up.
- Submerge rescue tube while pulling guest.

CRITICAL THINKING:

1. What if the guest grabs your arm when you reach down to duck pluck?
2. What do you do when you can't reach the guest?

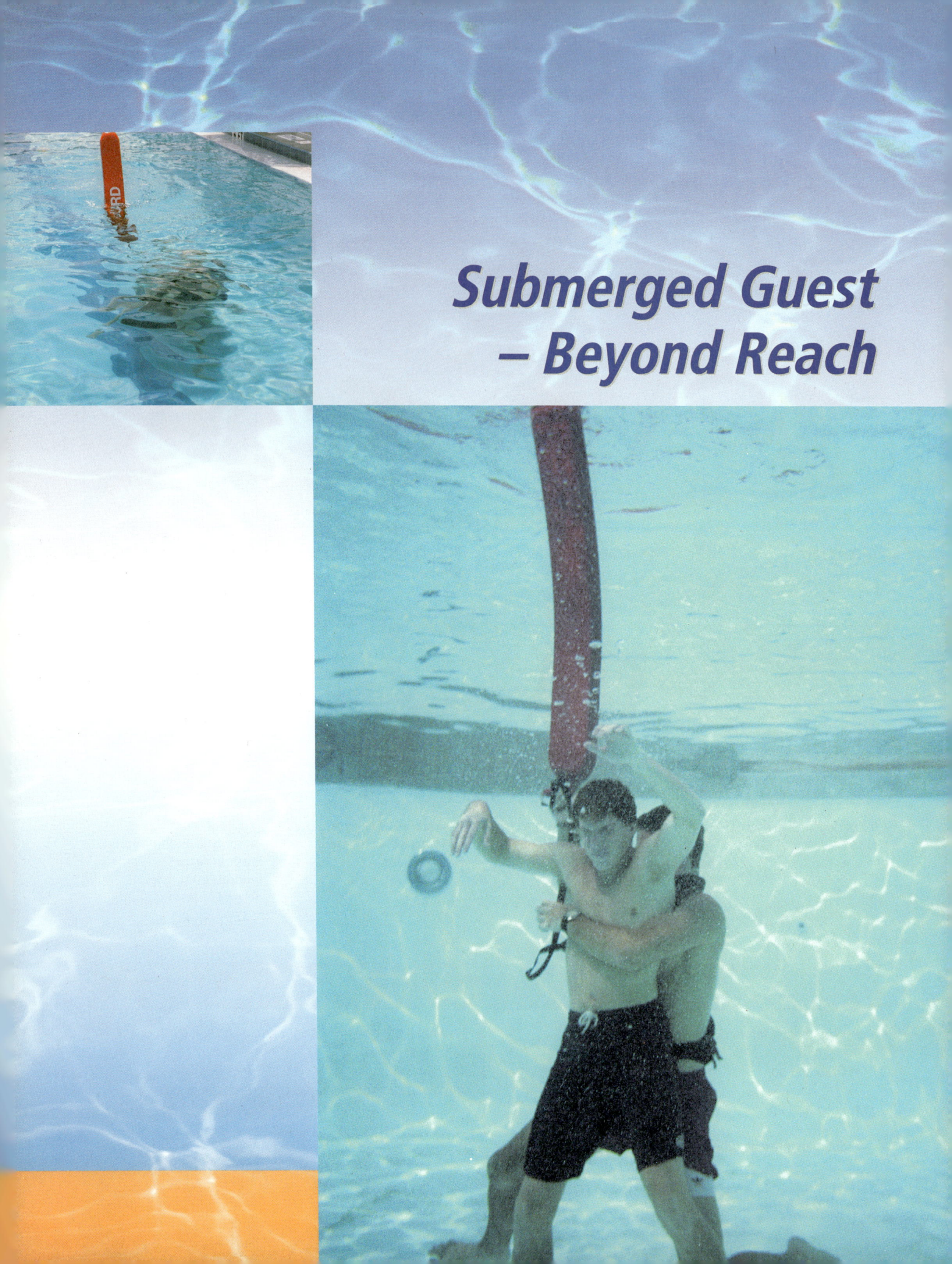

Submerged Guest – Beyond Reach

chapter 11
ELEVEN

OBJECTIVES

After reading this chapter and completing the related course work, you should be able to:

1. Demonstrate a deep water rescue on a conscious guest.

2. Demonstrate a deep water rescue on an unconscious guest, with follow-up care which includes:
    a. Heimlich Maneuver
    b. Rescue Breathing
    c. Extrication
    d. Supplemental Oxygen Administration
    e. CPR

A guest who is submerged and beyond your reach from the surface must be managed with special techniques. The guest may be either active or passive, conscious or unconscious. Regardless of the guest's condition, he or she needs to be returned to the surface as quickly as possible.

DEEP WATER RESCUE—SUBMERGED CONSCIOUS GUEST

The objectives of a deep water rescue of a conscious guest are to:

- Bring the guest to the surface.
- Place the rescue tube in front of the guest.
- Maintain control of the rescue tube and the guest while moving to an exit point.

When the distressed guest is below the surface, beyond your reach, and conscious, execute a deep water rescue, as follows:

1. Whistle, point to the guest, hit the E-Stop (if there is one), do a compact jump entry, and approach stroke toward the guest.

2. When you are directly above the guest, stop, and release the rescue tube from under your armpits. Be sure the strap is still across your chest and over your shoulder. Hold onto the rope of the rescue tube with one hand.

3. Do a feet first surface dive so that you come to a position directly behind the guest.

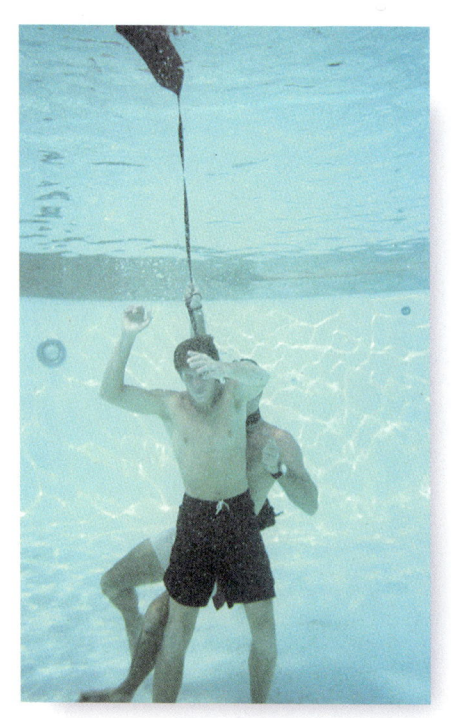

FIG 11.1 Hold onto the rope and come to position directly behind the guest.

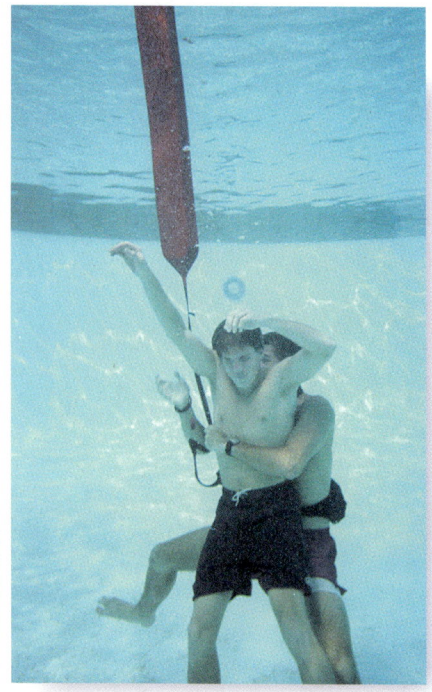

FIG 11.2 Reach across the guest's chest and feed the rope into your other hand.

CHAPTER 11 • SUBMERGED GUEST–BEYOND REACH   129

4. With your free hand, reach across the guest's chest. If possible, move your hand up under his armpit.

5. As you bring the guest to the surface, "feed" the rope of the rescue tube into the hand that is around the guest's chest. Do not let go of the rope with both hands at any time.

6. As you come to the surface, you will be holding the guest and the rope of the rescue tube with one hand. Your other hand is now free to position the rescue tube in front of the guest. The rescue tube will support both you and the guest on the water's surface. To place the rescue tube in front of the guest, grasp it with your free hand, close to the middle of the rescue tube, and position the rescue tube in front of the guest, while continuing to hold onto him.

7. An alternative approach you may want to use, is to position the rescue tube behind the guest, and move your hands and arms into the rear huggie position. This will provide better control on a stuggling guest. Remember to protect your face in case the guest involuntarily snaps his head back. Move to the side of the pool or an exit point, while maintaining a firm hold on the guest, and reassuring him by immediately beginning to talk to him. Assist the guest from the water, making sure that he is all right before you allow him to leave. Your Emergency Action System should explain exactly what procedure you should follow at this time. Fill out the rescue report.

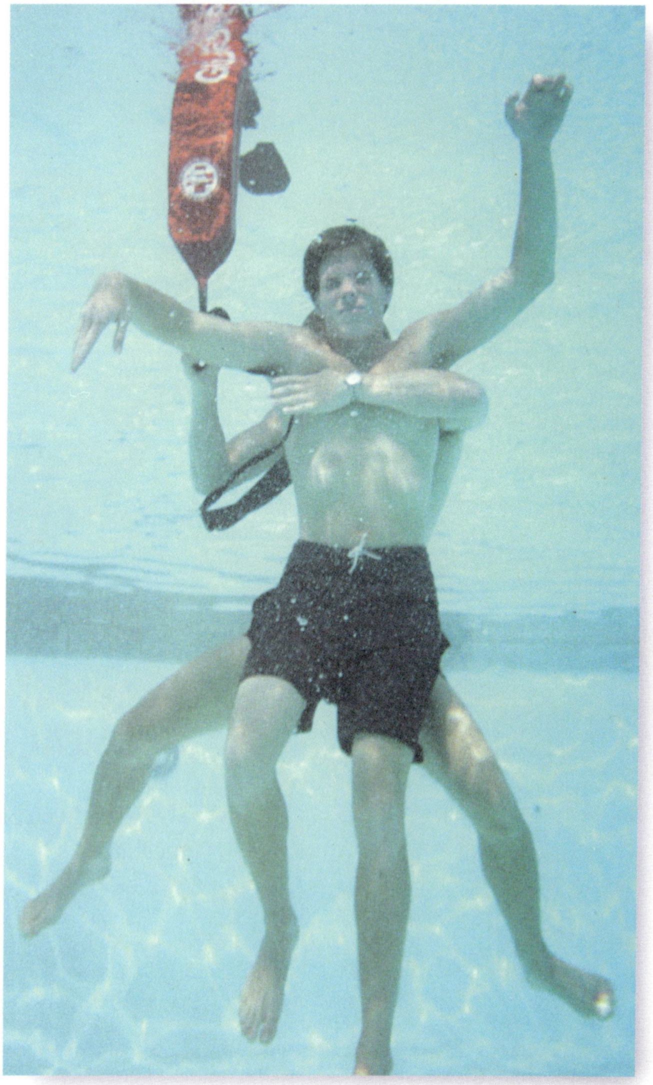

FIG 11.3 Feed the rope into your hand and hold guest and rope of rescue tube.

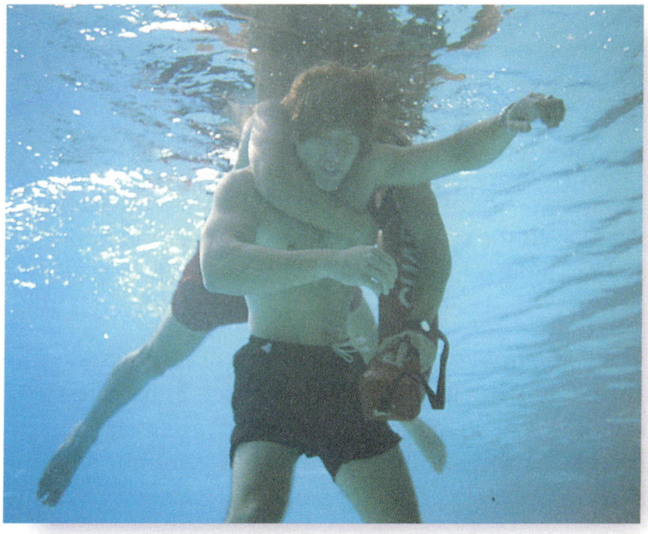

FIG 11.4 Shove rescue tube in front of the guest.

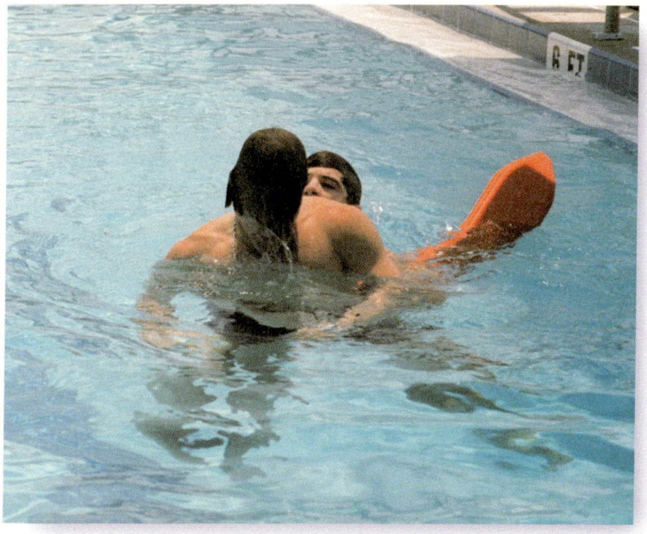

FIG 11.5 Alternative: Move to Rear Huggie position.

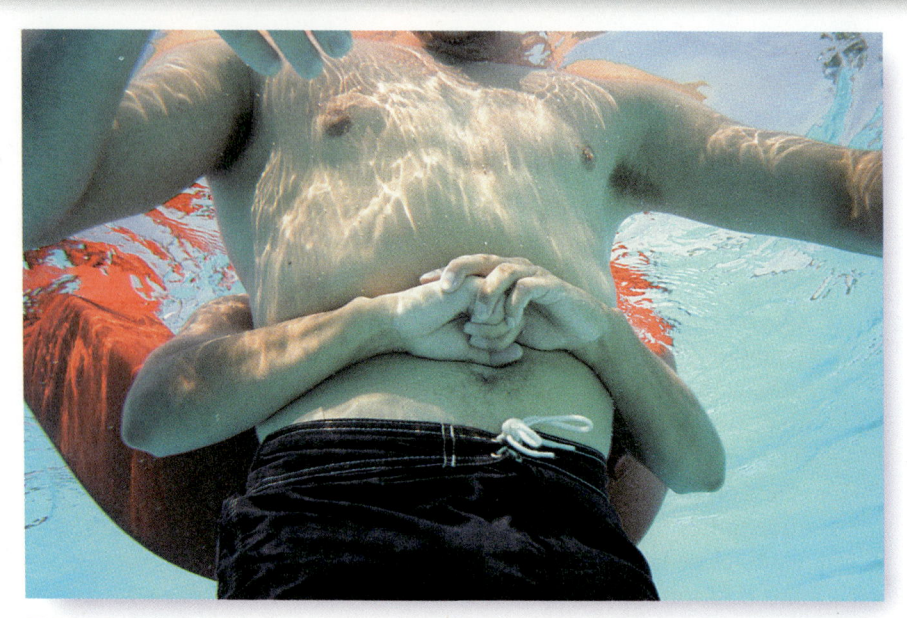

FIG 11.6 Pull the guest to a vertical position, and administer the Heimlich Maneuver.

DEEP WATER RESCUE—SUBMERGED UNCONSCIOUS GUEST

The objectives of a deep water rescue of a submerged unconscious guest are to:

- Bring the guest to the surface.
- Perform the Heimlich Maneuver to clear the guest's airway.
- Properly position the guest on the rescue tube.
- Maintain an open airway.
- Properly perform rescue breathing if it is needed.
- Maintain control of the rescue tube and the guest while moving to an exit point.

When the distressed guest is below the surface, beyond your reach, and unconscious, you will execute the deep water rescue, administer the Heimlich Maneuver, and, if necessary, administer rescue breathing.

To execute the deep water rescue on a submerged unconscious guest:

1. Perform the same sequence of skills as you would for a conscious guest. When you reach the surface, if he is motionless and not spontaneously breathing, administer the Heimlich Maneuver at least five times.

2. If fluid does not come from or ceases to come from the guest's mouth, and the guest is still not breathing, position him for rescue breathing. Perform rescue breathing as you move toward an exit point. If fluid does come out of the guest's mouth, continue administering the Heimlich Maneuver until it stops.

3. Extricate the guest with the assistance of the lifeguard team, and continue to provide the guest with the appropriate care once on the deck.

REVIEW QUESTIONS

1. (T) (F) In a deep water rescue, your rescue tube will help you bring even a very large guest to the surface.

2. When surface diving to the bottom, you should descend _____ first.

3. After surface diving to the bottom, you should position yourself _____ the guest.

4. If a guest is submerged in deep water and is conscious, you will place the rescue tube _____ the guest's body when you break the surface of the water. If the guest is unconscious, you will place the rescue tube _____ the guest's body.

5. If the guest is unconscious and not breathing when you reach the surface, you should perform _____.

6. Once fluid no longer exits the guest's mouth, and if the guest is still not breathing, you should perform _____.

PART 2 • RESPONDING TO AN EMERGENCY

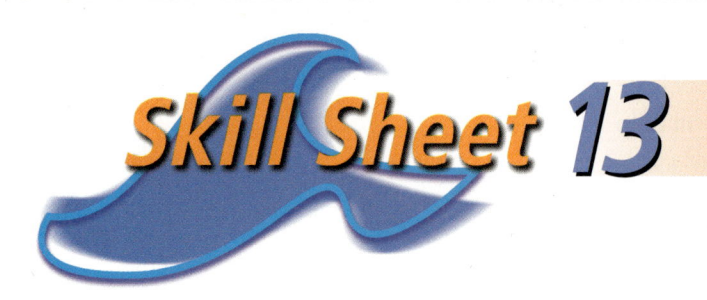

Skill Sheet 13

DEEP WATER RESCUE

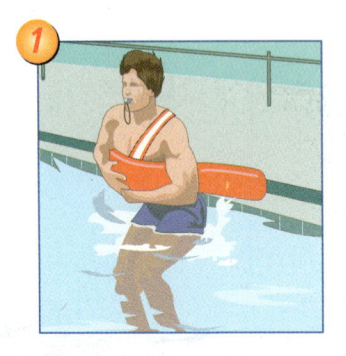

1. Compact jump entry; approach stroke.

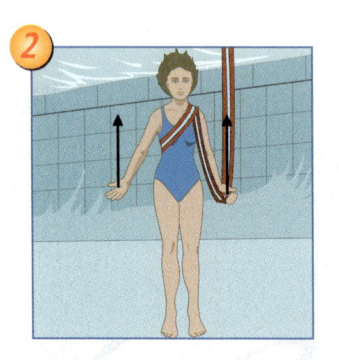

2. Feet first surface dive to position behind guest.

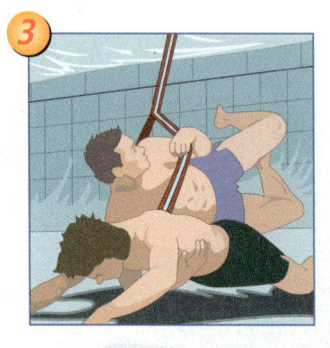

3. Roll to side; reach across body, hand under armpit.

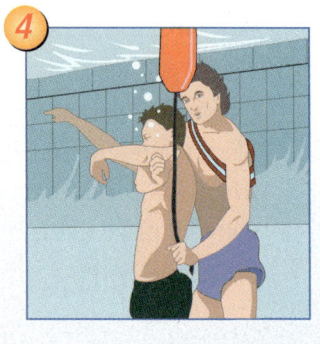

4. Feed rescue tube strap to other hand while surfacing.

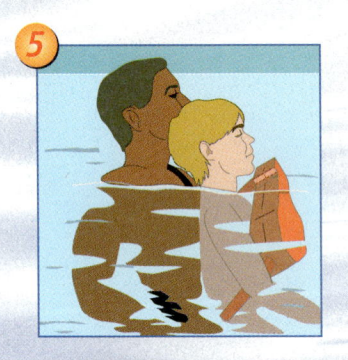

5. If conscious, place rescue tube in front of guest; talk to him; progress to exit.

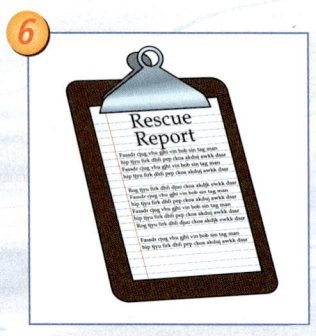

6. Exit the water; evaluate the guest; complete report.

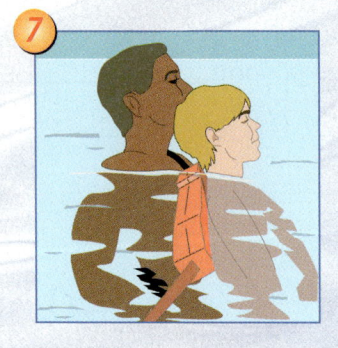

7. If unconscious, place rescue tube behind guest, across shoulders. Administer Heimlich manuever.

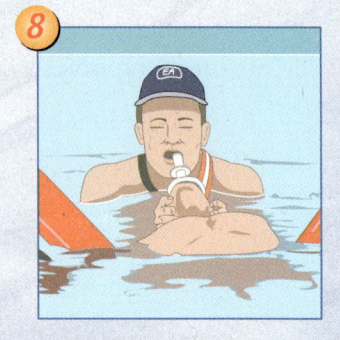

8. If guest is still not breathing, begin rescue breathing; progress to side; extricate guest; assess; perform CPR or rescue breathing as needed. Complete report.

KEY POINTS:

- Perform a feet first surface dive in a vertical position.
- Use the rescue tube to pull yourself and the guest to the surface.
- Have the rescue tube in place before breaking the surface.

CRITICAL THINKING:

1. What would you do if a guest became unconscious after you had placed the rescue tube in front of him?
2. What would you do if a conscious guest struggled with you?

part THREE
3

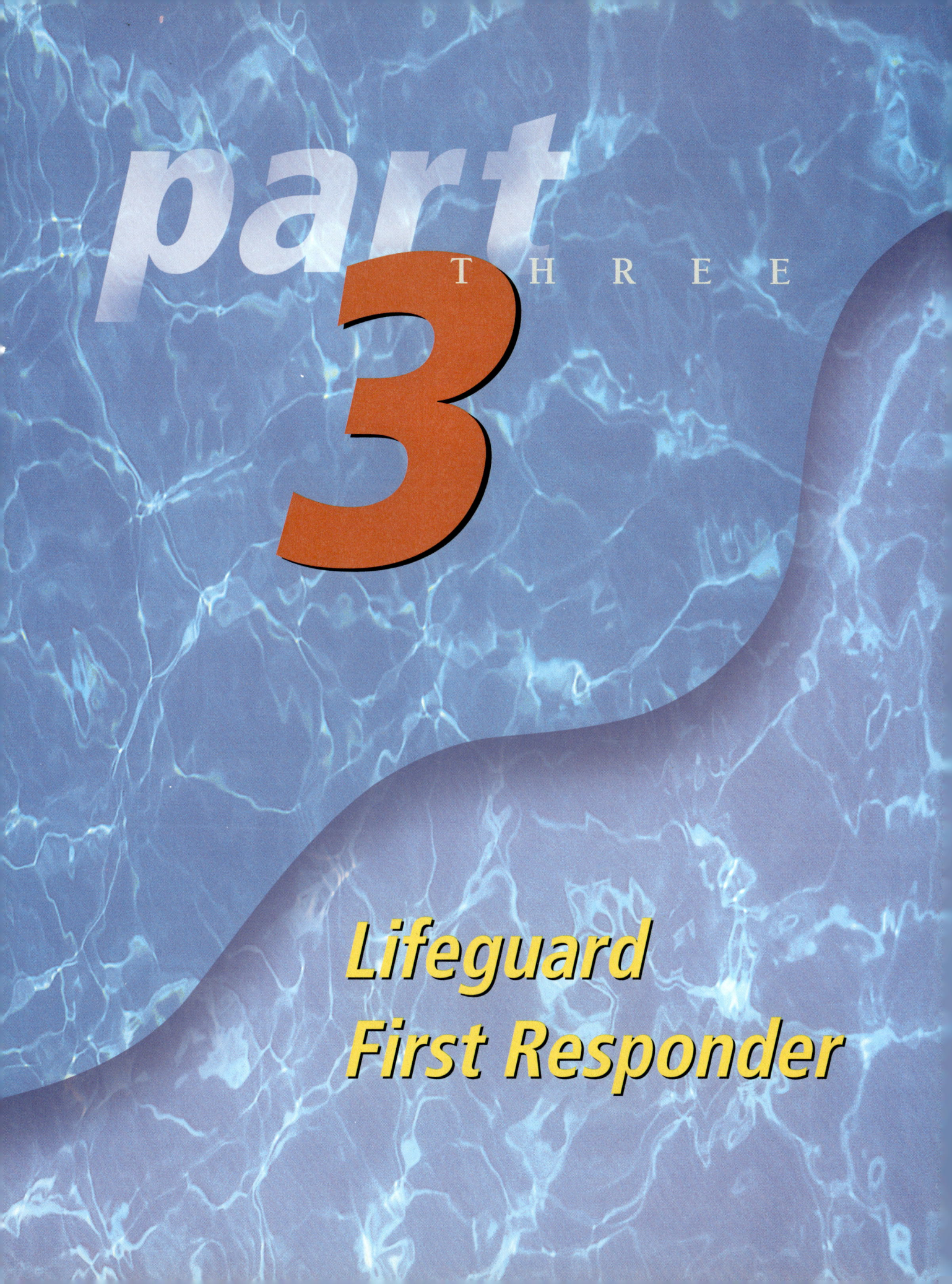

Lifeguard First Responder

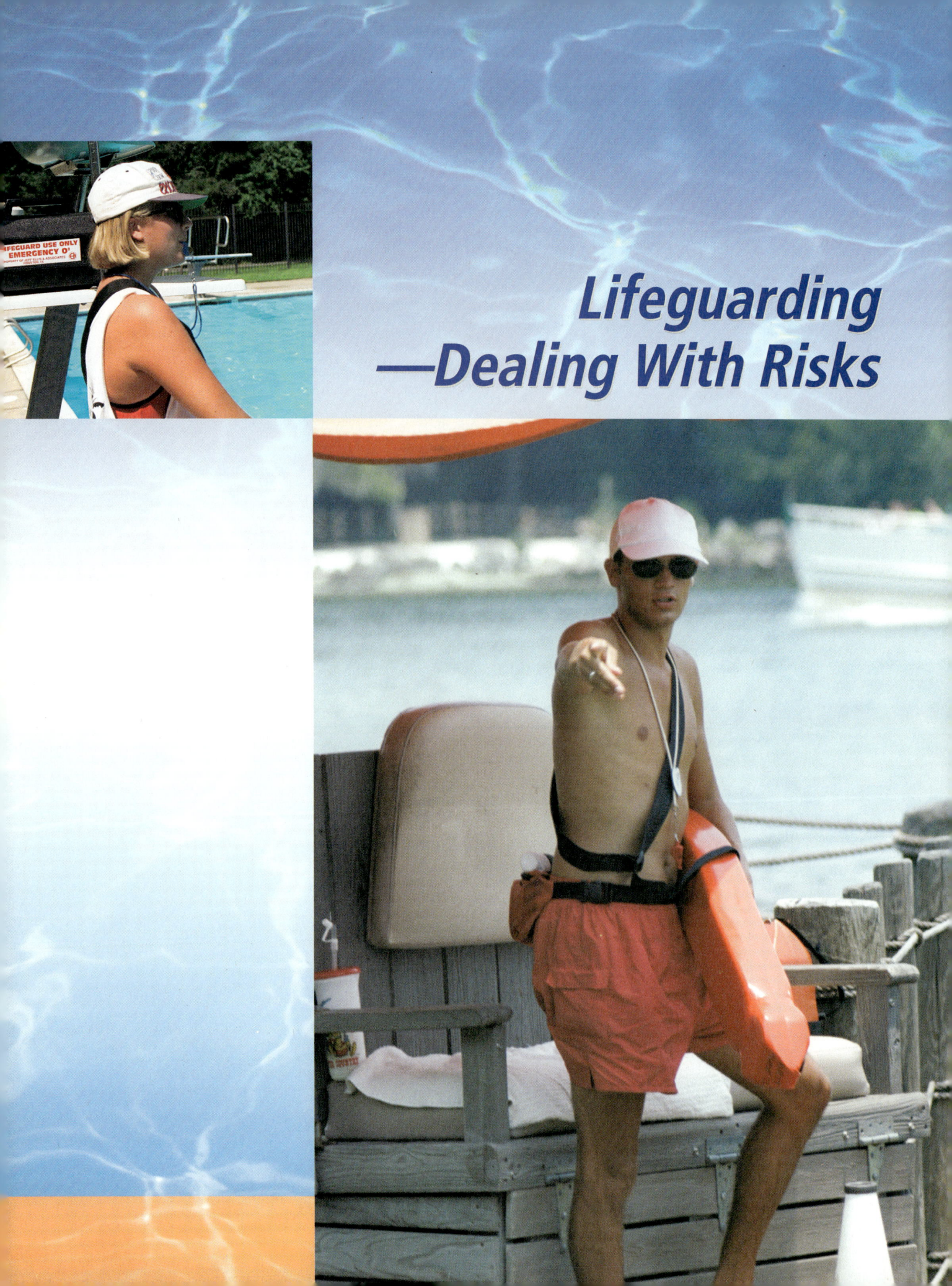

Lifeguarding —Dealing With Risks

chapter 12

OBJECTIVES

After reading this chapter and completing the related course work, you should be able to:

1. List eight health and safety risks you will encounter as a lifeguard, and ways you can work to reduce those risks.

2. Identify ten strategies for dealing with the emotional impact involved in the management of a drowning or a near-drowning incident.

3. Describe the concept of legal liability and standard of care.

Being a lifeguard can affect your life in many ways. Every day, you are putting yourself at risk, both physically and emotionally. This chapter discusses the more significant of these risks, as well as strategies to use to protect yourself.

HEALTH RISKS

Health risks you will experience as a lifeguard, and ways you can protect yourself from these risks include:

- Dehydration and heat-related illness—drink plenty of water; sit or stand in the shade whenever possible; cool down often; eat small, light meals.
- Eye damage—wear polarized ultraviolet sunglasses.
- Skin irritation—remove wet suits after work and use talcum powder.
- Skin aging—lubricate your skin with moisturizer regularly.
- Exposure to bloodborne pathogens such as human immunodeficiency virus and hepatitis B virus—use BSI precautions, treating all body fluids as if they are infectious.
- Bodily injury or drowning—stay trained; practice your facility's Emergency Action System (EAS) and attend in-service training sessions; practice your rescue techniques; and stay in good physical condition.
- Chemical burns and inhalation—handle any pool chemicals carefully, and learn their use. Be prepared for an emergency.
- Electrical shock—use extreme care when using electrical equipment near the pool. Seek safe shelter during storms.

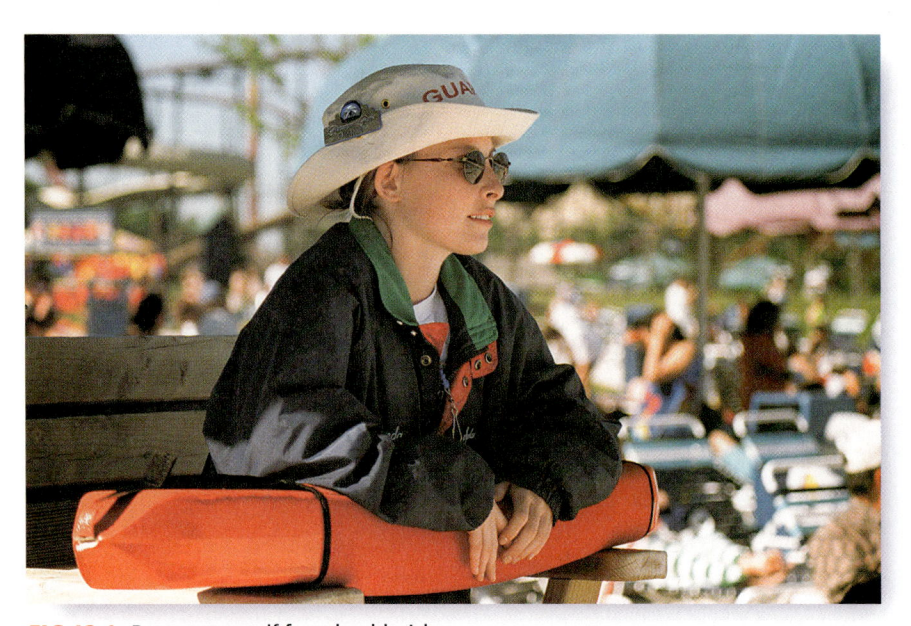

FIG 12.1 Protect yourself from health risks.

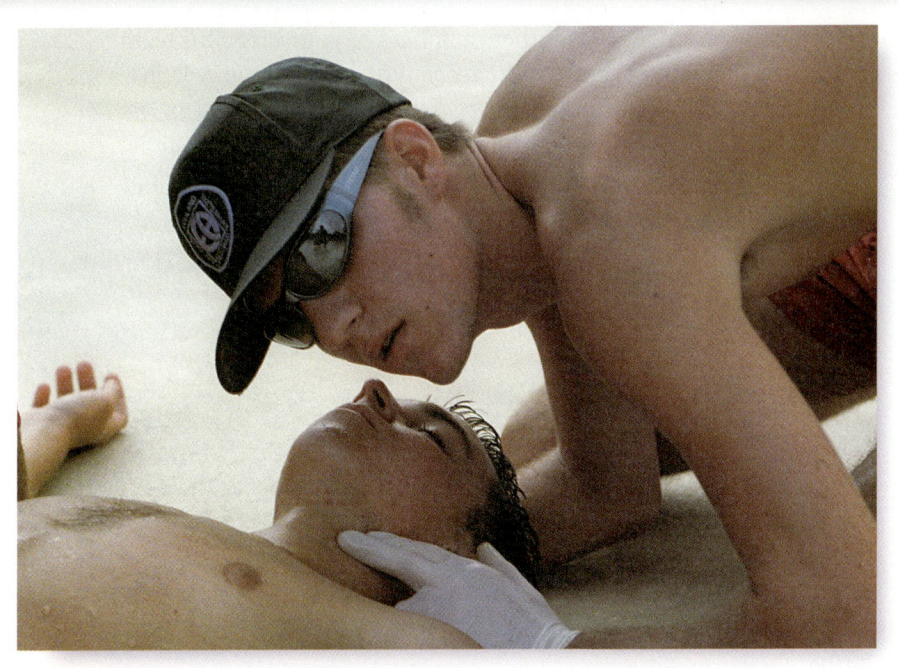

FIG 12.2 Drowning and near-drowning incidents can be emotionally traumatic.

EMOTIONAL RISKS

In addition to physical risks, you are also putting yourself at risk of experiencing events that could have a tremendous psychological impact on you. As the person or lifeguard team member who brings a drowned guest to the water's surface and to the deck, you are involved in a traumatic experience. It is traumatic at the time, and can have some long-term effects. Knowing you did everything correctly and well does not lessen the impact of the incident.

The emotional effects of such a traumatic experience can never be completely eliminated, but here are some things you can do or keep in mind that will help reduce them:

- Fill out your incident report accurately and completely.
- As soon as possible, work out in the water.
- Think about what happened, and emphasize in your mind the things you did correctly and well.
- Even though you did everything as well as possible, the questioning session with authorities could be intimidating. Just remember that this questioning is a necessary part of "the system."
- Put the incident behind you; guilt is the least beneficial of all human emotions.
- Be prepared for media coverage that might distort some of the facts. Try not to let it bother you. Putting yourself on the defensive can be frustrating and emotionally draining.
- Hang in there! Keep up your schoolwork and your job. Familiar routines help, and they are important to you.

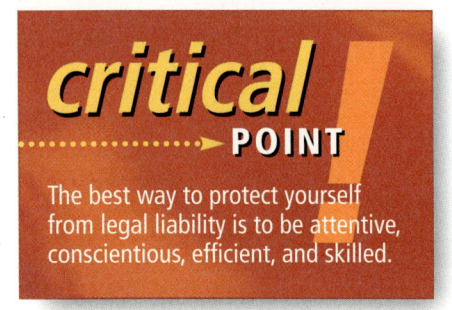

> **critical POINT**
>
> The best way to protect yourself from legal liability is to be attentive, conscientious, efficient, and skilled.

- Be supportive of the other members of your lifeguard team; they are going through the same type of experience. Don't hesitate to ask for their support, either.
- Take advantage of trained individuals in your area who can help you and your lifeguard team deal with stress after you have been involved in a catastrophic incident.
- Realize that you won't forget what happened, but you don't have to keep remembering it constantly either.

LEGAL RISKS

If you are a lifeguard, there is always the possibility that you will be involved in a drowning incident. If there is a lawsuit over the incident, it is not likely to be quickly resolved. Your own involvement in the litigation could be time consuming (most litigation in America lasts two to five years), and have a serious negative impact on your future—if you are starting in a new career or on a new educational path, or in financial terms.

Is safety maintained because people are afraid of a lawsuit? While many people believe that society has gone "lawsuit crazy," just keep in mind that the system was designed to protect the welfare of every citizen.

People have a right to expect that they will be adequately protected by competent and attentive lifeguards while they are swimming at public facilities. It is disturbing that some people in the industry suggest that the only reason safety is a priority is to protect themselves from a lawsuit. If you recognize this attitude as existing in society today, then you can understand why it is important to believe in and fully support civil jurisprudence. The future of the aquatic industry (and many other things) would be in jeopardy if such a system were not in place. It is true that providing a "reasonable standard of care" is costly. However, the cost of not providing a reasonable standard of care is beyond measure, when weighed against the lives and welfare of people in general.

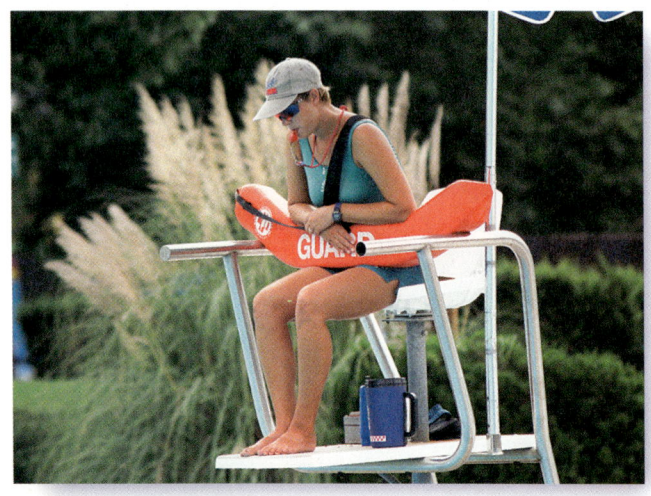

FIG 12.3 Attentiveness is the best safeguard against drowning incidents.

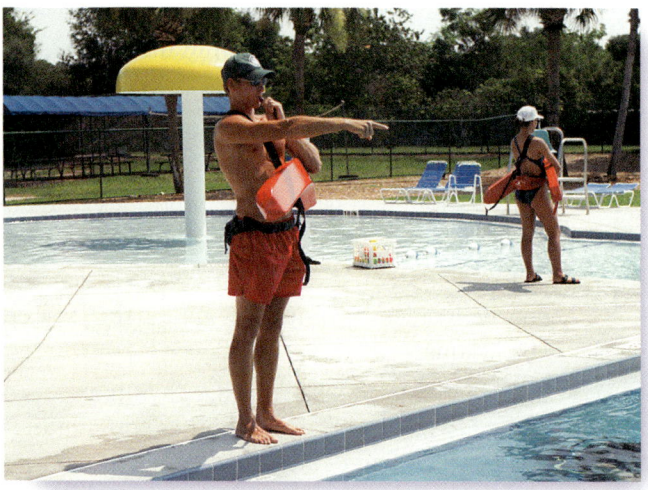

FIG 12.4 Take immediate action if you see guests engaging in potentially hazardous behavior.

As a lifeguard, you assume responsibility for guest safety and for maintaining a reasonable standard of care. If you are required to give aid, you must do so promptly and efficiently without endangering the guest, other swimmers, or yourself.

Your performance during your rescue efforts will be measured according to the standards of care currently expected of the aquatic industry. These standards reflect the knowledge and skills expected of others working as professional lifeguards in the same position.

Your actions when you give follow-up aid, such as CPR, will be measured against the actions of health care professionals. This is because lifeguards are categorized by the Department of Labor, the American Red Cross, and the American Heart Association as "health care professionals." Thus, you will be held accountable for performing technical skills commonly performed by first responders.

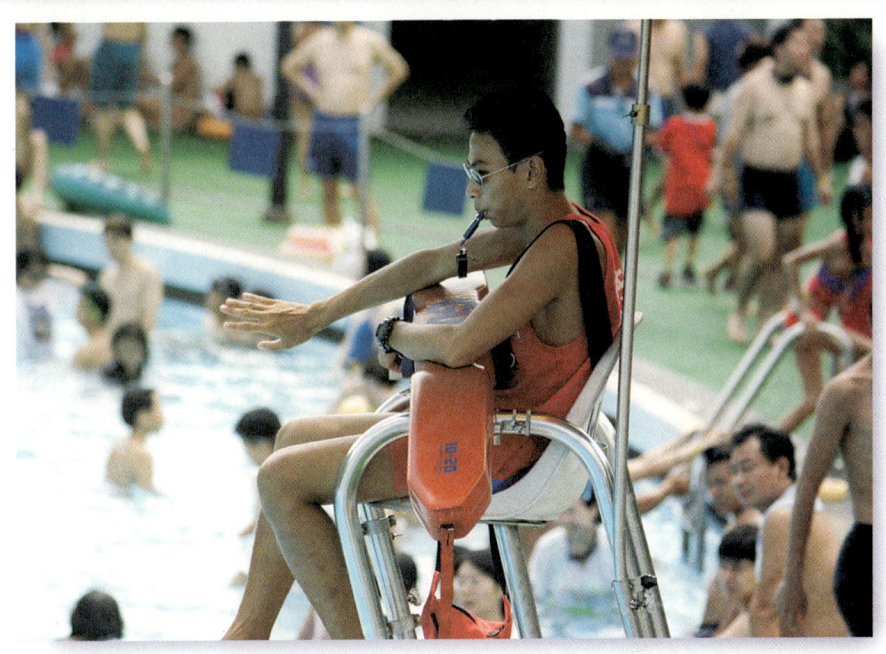

FIG 12.5 Maintaining the 10/20 Protection Rule at all times is the best way to account for your level of attentiveness.

The word *professional* is meaningful. Society has two different views of lifeguards. The first view is of a physically fit young person who enjoys getting a suntan and who is active among peers—a "fun in the sun" person taking a seasonal or part-time job to help finance his or her way through school. The second view is usually taken after a catastrophic incident involving a lifeguard occurs. Society has historically taken on the role of judge and jury, asking questions such as "How could such an accident happen?" "Were the lifeguards performing their lifesaving duties correctly?" In effect, they are asking if the lifeguard acted professionally during the emergency. Regardless of which view is taken, society expects lifeguards to be professionals in the way they perform their duties, and in the manner in which they handle emergencies.

Some lifeguards who have been involved in liability litigation were unable to establish their attentiveness prior to the accident, and were unable to confirm basic facts. Additionally, some of the lifeguards who were questioned in such instances were not able to remember the date and location of their lifeguarding course, or the name of their lifeguarding instructor. This makes a person wonder how well they remembered what to do when responding to an emergency. Actively maintaining the 10/20 (or 10/3 minute) Protection Rule at all times when you are lifeguarding is one of the best ways for you to establish the level of your attentiveness if you are ever questioned about it.

Many lifeguards have also been unable to establish their skill level at the time of an aquatic incident. You should spend at least four hours per month participating in in-service training sessions. By attending regular

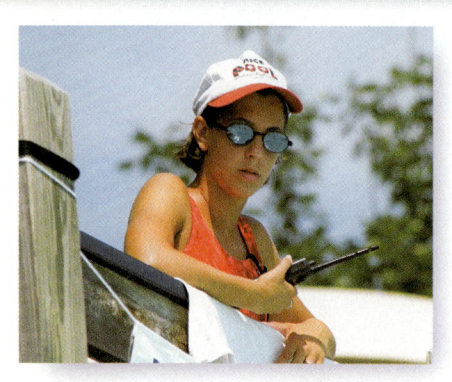

FIG 12.6 As a professional lifeguard supervisor, you are responsible for your guest's safety.

in-service training sessions, you will show that you are maintaining your skills—competency is directly related to the reinforcement of skills through practice.

As a lifeguard concerned with liability risk, you must:
- Assume responsibility for guest safety.
- Assume accountability for upholding reasonable standards of care as a health care professional.
- Learn and maintain your skills through regular documented in-service training.
- Take into consideration the consequences of litigation and its impact on your future.
- Act maturely even while associating with and confronting people your own age.
- Accept potential risk to your personal safety.

REVIEW QUESTIONS

1. For each of the physical conditions listed, name one action you can take to minimize the effects.
    a. Dehydration
    b. Skin damage
    c. Eye damage

2. (T) (F) Standard of Care refers to the skills and care that would normally be known and given by others working as professional lifeguards in the same position.

3. (T) (F) If you are involved in a lawsuit, it could take many years to resolve, and be financially draining.

4. (T) (F) You should attend 1 hour of in-service training per month.

5. (T) (F) The best way to protect yourself from legal liability is to be attentive, conscientious, efficient, and skilled.

6. List at least four things you can do to reduce the emotional effects of being involved in a near-drowning incident.
    a. _____
    b. _____
    c. _____
    d. _____

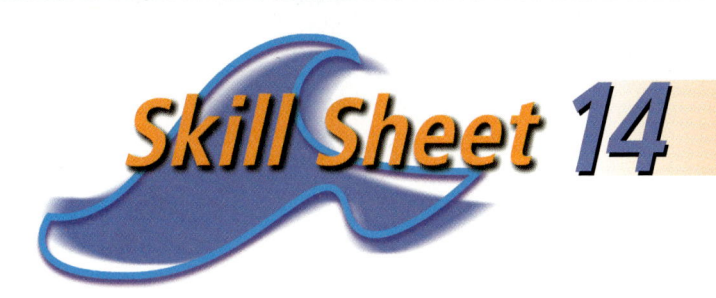

CHAPTER 12 • LIFEGUARDING - DEALING WITH RISKS   141

Skill Sheet 14

RISK AND LIABILITY

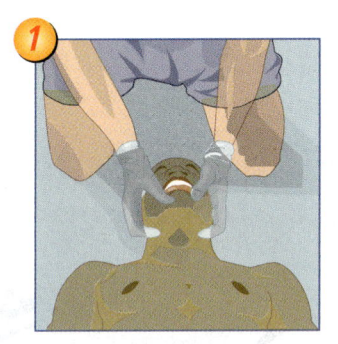

1. Take personal health and safety precautions.

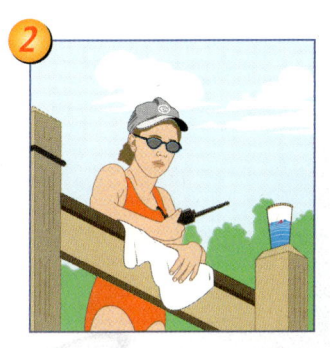

2. Reduce legal liability by remaining attentive to your guests and staff.

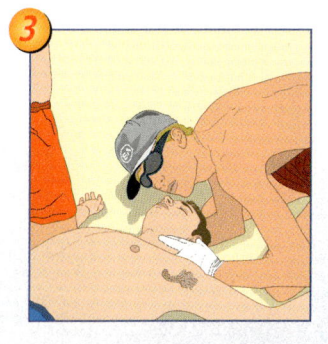

3. The emotional impact of an incident can be difficult to deal with in the aftermath of the incident.

KEY POINTS:

- Be attentive at all times.
- Take corrective action promptly, when needed.
- Maintain your skill level.
- Always act in a professional manner.

CRITICAL THINKING:

1. How could a lawsuit affect you, even if you were not the primary lifeguard performing a rescue?

2. How might your failure to drink an adequate amount of fluid or wear appropriate sunglasses, become factors in a lawsuit against you?

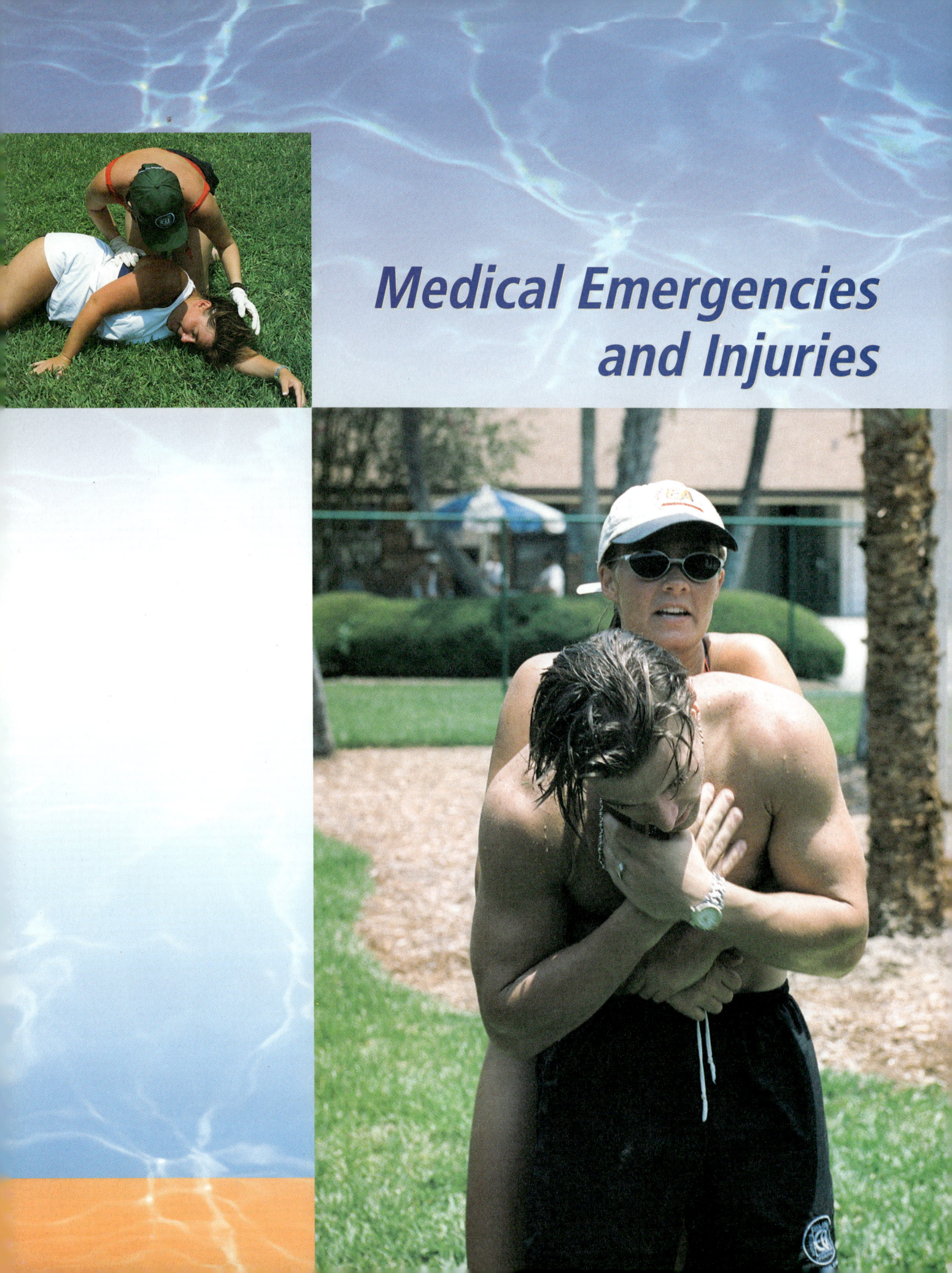

Medical Emergencies and Injuries

chapter 13

OBJECTIVES

After reading this chapter and completing the related course work, you should be able to:

1. Explain your role as a lifeguard first responder.
2. Demonstrate how to assess an ill or injured guest.
3. Recognize the signs, symptoms, and causes of emergencies you are likely to encounter in an aquatic environment.
4. Describe how to provide care for these emergencies until EMS personnel arrive.

THIRTEEN

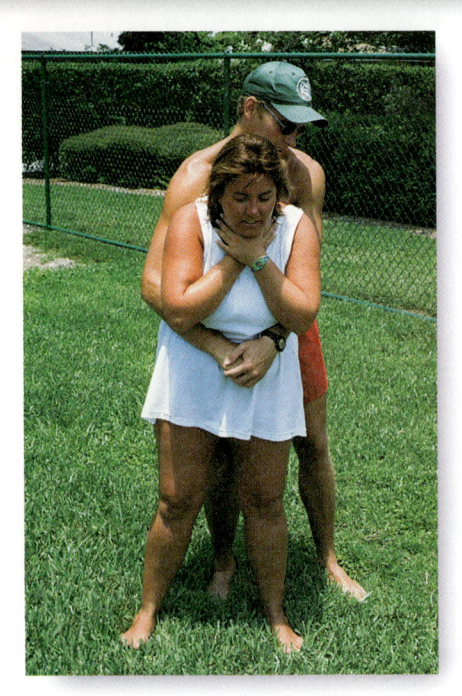

FIG 13.1 Universal choking sign.

Professional lifeguards play a key role in local Emergency Action Systems (EAS), and in the Emergency Medical Services (EMS) System. The care that a lifeguard provides in the first few minutes of an emergency is frequently credited with saving lives. However, occasionally a lifeguard may begin to believe that his basic medical knowledge allows him to function alone, without the support of the more highly trained members of the EMS. This attitude is incorrect and unacceptable, and can lead to inadequate care and significant personal liability. As a professional lifeguard, you must possess the ability to quickly determine when you should activate EAS/EMS, and what care you must provide until more advanced personnel arrive.

This chapter provides basic first aid information that enables you to provide care for common problems you encounter during the first few minutes of an emergency. The primary objective in the following pages is to reinforce the basic life-saving skills necessary for you to perform your job in a safe, consistent, and competent manner. The information that appears in this chapter may be supplemented by more advanced training offered by your aquatic facility.

Despite the basic nature of this material, you must realize that if basic skills are not performed quickly and efficiently, the result can be additional injury and possible death. Every lifeguard must perform skills with the belief that his emergency actions will make a positive difference for the patient.

RESPONSIBILITIES OF THE FIRST RESPONDER

As a lifeguard you will have many important responsibilities. Those related to providing life-saving first aid are among the most significant. Your responsibilities include being able to:

- Recognize and respond to aquatic emergencies.
- Recognize when to activate the EAS/EMS.
- Safely and appropriately rescue the guest.
- Provide appropriate emergency care until EMS personnel arrive and assume care.
- Work as a team player in every emergency situation.
- Provide the arriving EMS professionals with critical information regarding the emergency event.

Each aquatic facility will have specific policies and procedures for activating the EAS, accessing the local EMS, and handling facility emergencies. You must become thoroughly familiar with these procedures before you provide any lifeguarding services. Unfamiliarity with these procedures can place you and your employer at risk for costly litigation.

In almost every emergency situation, you should simultaneously activate the EAS/EMS and begin providing basic care. Remember, highly trained EMS professionals are a quick phone call away. Let EMS professionals arrive and assume medical care as soon as possible.

Additional responsibilities you may have could include:
- Training new staff members in EAS/EMS policies and procedures.
- Developing injury prevention programs for guests and employees.
- Maintaining or improving a safe working environment.
- Documenting each rescue/emergency event.
- Practicing first aid skills frequently.
- Purchasing and maintaining basic rescue and first aid equipment.
- Participating in rescue incident investigations.

LIFE-THREATENING EMERGENCIES

As a lifeguard, you can expect just about any type of medical emergency to occur within an aquatic facility. Life-threatening emergencies are those that compromise a guest's airway, breathing, or circulation (heartbeat or bloodflow).

Assessing An Ill or Injured Guest

The objectives of an assessment are to:
- Identify and perform the components of the initial assessment (primary survey), including Airway, Breathing, and Circulation.
- Recognize the importance of maintaining airway, breathing, and circulation in an unresponsive guest.
- Perform a complete focused physical exam (secondary survey).
- Identify the proper sequences for activating the EAS/EMS, given various medical emergencies.

Initial Assessment

Regardless of the severity of the emergency, you must give every ill or injured guest a complete initial assessment. The assessment is divided into two basic parts: the initial assessment and the focused physical exam. The initial assessment is designed to assess and treat conditions that are immediately life-threatening. The focused physical exam is designed to reveal conditions or problems that, while potentially serious, can wait minutes or hours for treatment.

Your assessment skills are the foundation for all first aid/CPR techniques you will provide. Without proper assessment skills, you may treat the most obvious or visually disturbing problem(s), while neglecting more serious or immediately life-threatening conditions. During your lifeguarding career, always remember that in every emergency situation, you must immediately give all guests a complete and competent initial assessment.

The components of the initial assessment include:

1. Form a general impression. Look around, listen to conversations, and look for signs of objects that are out of place. Begin to formulate your ideas of what may have caused the accident or injury.
2. Check for scene safety. Ask yourself: Is the area safe to enter, and could I become ill or injured by entering? If you believe the scene is unsafe, do not enter or allow others to enter it. Wait until the appropriate authorities determine that the area is safe.

In the initial assessment, you must remember that guests can be breathless and still have a pulse. But, guests without a pulse will be breathless.

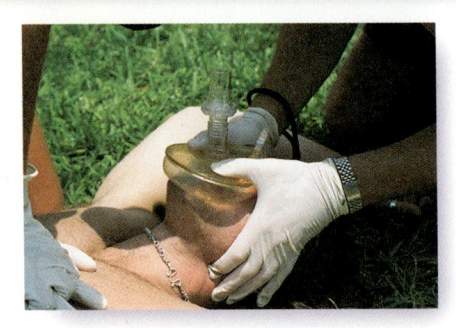

FIG 13.2 Lifeguard protection.

Check the ABCs

A = Airway
B = Breathing
C = Circulation

3. Take all necessary BSI precautions prior to any contact with the guest. This means donning latex gloves, and eye protection, if necessary, as soon as possible.
4. Determine the guest's level of consciousness (Shake and shout, "Are you O.K.?"). Place the guest's response into one of these four categories:

   A = Alert and responding appropriately

   V = Verbal, responds only to loud verbal stimulus

   P = Pain, responds only to painful stimulus

   U = Unresponsive, no response

If the guest has an altered level of consciousness, (anything falling in the VPU categories), immediately activate the EAS/EMS.

Check and correct any problems you find with the guest's **A**irway, **B**reathing, and **C**irculation (pulse and severe bleeding). Open the guest's airway using either the head-tilt/chin-lift or the jaw-thrust maneuver. If you do not suspect a spinal injury, use the head-tilt/chin-lift maneuver. If you do suspect a head or spinal injury, use the jaw-thrust maneuver. Once the guest's airway is open, assess his breathing.

Assess the guest's breathing by placing your head and face close to his mouth and nose. Look (at his chest), listen, and feel for breathing. This should take you 3 to 5 seconds to complete. If the guest is not spontaneously breathing, begin rescue breathing. As a lifeguard, you will normally begin rescue breathing with a resuscitation mask. You must become thoroughly familiar with the device used by your facility, and practice frequently to maintain a high skill level. Practice using airway devices on guests of different sizes.

Once you have opened the guest's airway, and he is either breathing spontaneously or you are providing rescue breathing, check the status of his circulation (pulse). If there is more than one rescuer on the scene, you may be able to check the guest's pulse simultaneously with previous assessment steps. Assessing circulation should take you 5 to 10 seconds. If the guest no longer has a pulse, begin CPR.

Occasionally, you may encounter a guest who is bleeding. If you find significant bleeding during the initial assessment, immediately apply direct pressure over the wound. If you can, elevate the area above the level of the patient's heart. If you are alone, remember to check the guest's ABCs before controlling any bleeding.

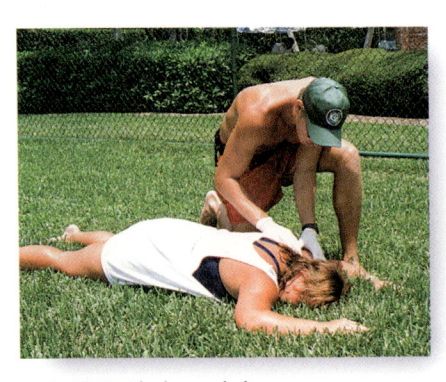

FIG 13.3 Shake and shout.

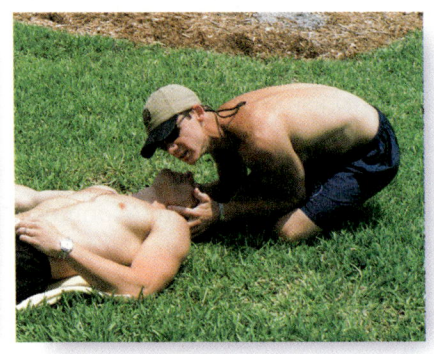

FIG 13.4 Head-tilt/chin-lift.

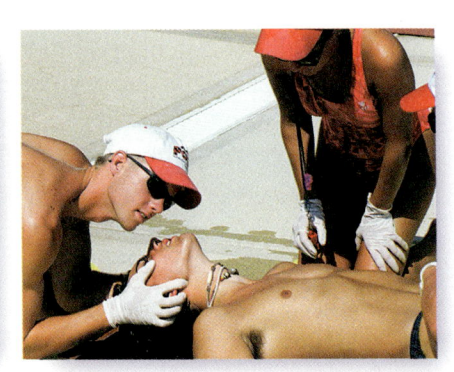

FIG 13.5 Jaw-thrust.

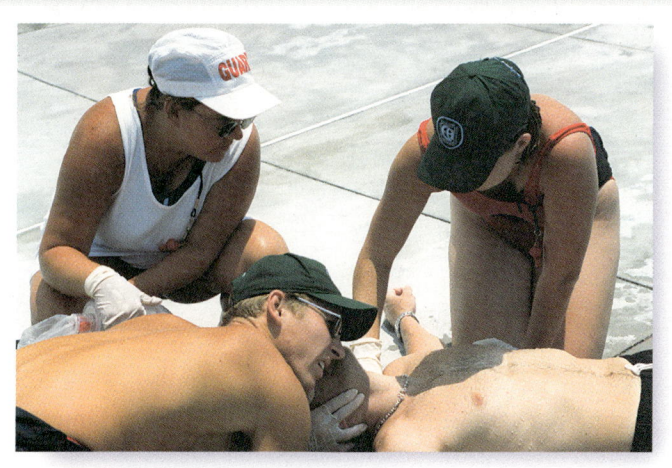

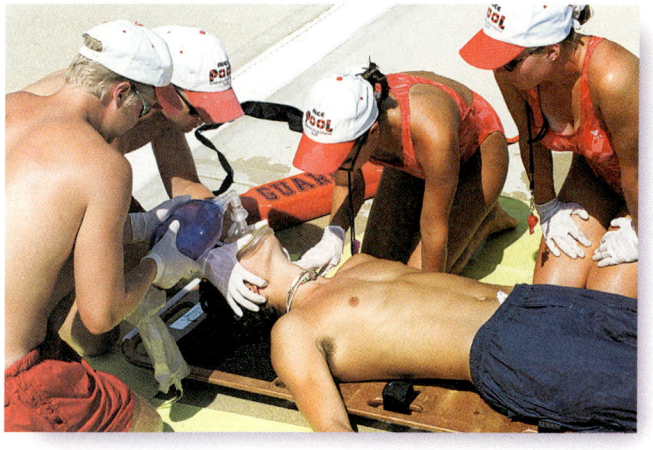

FIG 13.6 Breathing assessment.

FIG 13.7 Pulse check.

Focused Physical Exam (Head to Toe Assessment)

After you complete your initial assessment and have any treated life-threatening conditions, begin a focused physical exam. This is also a good time to make sure the EAS/EMS have been notified. Remember, at no time should you perform a focused physical exam while problems still exist with the ABC's. The focused physical exam requires you to quickly look and feel for additional injuries.

The following steps are used in performing the focused physical exam:

1. Starting at the head and ending at the toes, look and feel for areas of pain, tenderness, and obvious injury, such as deformity, bruising, etc.

2. During this assessment, constantly communicate with the guest, and attempt to find out what happened. Ask the guest or bystanders what caused the injury. This information helps describe the **mechanism of injury**. You can ask the guest to describe any pain or injuries she feels. You can also ask questions related to her chief complaint (biggest problem), medical history (i.e., heart condition, diabetes), and other necessary information. Make sure you provide the information you gather to the EMS providers.

At no time should you perform a focused physical exam while problems still exist with the ABC's

SPECIFIC EMERGENCIES AND TREATMENT PROCEDURES

In this section you will learn about the causes, signs and symptoms, and general treatment guidelines for some of the more frequent illnesses or injuries found in the aquatic environment. In addition to these guidelines, always make sure to follow the procedures specifically established for your aquatic facility.

Signs and Symptoms of Serious Head/Spinal Injuries

- Pain
- Tenderness
- Deformity

- Cuts and bruises
- Paralysis
- Black eyes
- Altered levels of consciousness (knocked unconscious, garbled speech)
- Vomiting
- Blood from ears or nose

Head Injuries

A major factor in deciding if a guest is suffering from a serious head injury, is to find out if he has had any loss of consciousness. If a guest has lost consciousness, even briefly, then assume the head injury is serious until proven otherwise. Remember, in the aquatic environment, there are very limited tools to tell us the seriousness of a closed head injury.

Also, look for additional signs and symptoms of serious head injury even if the guest has not reported a loss of consciousness. Always activate the EAS/EMS for any patient who has lost consciousness, regardless of the length of time involved. In some situations, a guest with a head injury may initially appear fine, and then suddenly collapse.

Spinal Injuries

For any guest with a serious head injury, always assume that he may have a spinal cord injury too. In these instances, do not allow the guest to move his neck. Even accidental spinal movement can make the difference between full recovery and total paralysis. The water rescue and on-deck treatment must also take this into consideration.

As the First Responder on the scene, your primary goal for a guest with a head and/or spinal injury is to maintain his ABCs while simultaneously preventing him from moving. The only instance where you should move a guest whom you suspect has a head or spinal injury is if he vomits. If a guest vomits while lying on his back, he may inhale the vomit into his lungs.

Remember that a guest without a clear airway will most likely die. Always have your suction unit available when you are treating a guest—think of the alternative if you need to suction the airway without your manual suction unit!

If you need to move a guest with a spinal injury, use the logroll technique. The logroll technique allows you to maintain head and neck alignment, using the vise grip. Work as a team to roll the guest to his side.

Heat-Related Emergencies (Hyperthermia)

As a professional lifeguard, it is likely that you will come in contact with guests who are suffering from heat-related problems. Heat-related emergencies can occur from a person spending too much time in a hot environment without taking in enough fluid to maintain the body's equilibrium. The guest's recovery from heat-related conditions will be directly related to your ability to recognize the different signs and symptoms of a heat-related emergency, and give the appropriate care.

Signs and Symptoms of Hyperthermia

- Muscle cramps, most commonly in the legs, calves, and abdomen
- Dizziness
- Nausea/vomiting
- Fatigue
- Hot and sweaty skin
- Severe headache
- Diarrhea
- Extreme thirst
- Extremely hot skin, which can be either wet or dry
- Rapid pulse
- Mental confusion (including unconsciousness)
- Seizures

Emergency Treatment for Mild Hyperthermia (Heat Cramps)

1. Have the guest stop any strenuous activity and rest in a cool location.
2. As long as the guest is not nauseous, have him drink cool water, about one half glass every 15 minutes.
3. Have the guest gently stretch any muscles that are affected.
4. If the guest's condition does not quickly improve, activate the EAS/EMS.

Emergency Treatment for Moderate Hyperthermia (Heat Exhaustion)

1. Remove the guest from the heat source and begin to cool him. You can do this by moving the guest to an air conditioned area and fanning him.
2. Remove as much of the guest's clothing as possible, while maintaining acceptable modesty.
3. Elevate the guest's legs approximately 12 inches.
4. As long as the guest is not nauseous, have him slowly drink cool water while you monitor his airway and level of consciousness.
5. Activate the EAS/EMS if the guest does not quickly improve.

Emergency Treatment for Severe Hyperthermia (Heat Stroke)

This is a life-threatening condition, and requires immediate action to save the guest's life.

1. Immediately remove the guest from the heat source. Fast cooling can make the difference between life or death. Seconds really count here!
2. Remove the guest's clothing, but try to maintain modesty.

3. Use whatever materials you have available to cool the guest's body. Several common ways to cool guests with hyperthermia are to soak towels in cool water and place them over the guest's body; place ice packs in his armpits and groin; pour cool water over his body and aggressively fan him—do whatever is necessary to rapidly cool the guest.

4. Establish an airway and provide rescue breathing or CPR if necessary. You can do this while others cool the guest.

5. Continue cooling the guest until he begins to shiver, or EMS personnel arrive.

6. Activate the EAS/EMS, because the guest will need advanced medical care.

Musculoskeletal Injuries

Musculoskeletal injuries are rarely life-threatening. Often, the best thing you can do is to help reduce the anxiety that guests commonly experience with a musculoskeletal injury, and keep him or her from moving the injured area.

Muscle, bone, and joint injuries share similar signs and symptoms, so it can often be difficult or impossible for you to determine the extent of the injury. Because of this, musculoskeletal injuries are managed using similar techniques. Occasionally, bone injuries can penetrate the skin, causing external bleeding and exposing the broken bone end.

Signs and Symptoms of a Musculoskeletal Injury

- Deformity or angulation of a body part
- Pain and tenderness
- Crepitus (bone ends grating)
- Swelling
- Bruising (discoloration)
- Exposed bone ends (open injury)
- Inability to use the affected area

Emergency Treatment for Musculoskeletal Injuries

1. Remember that the majority of musculoskeletal injuries are nonlife-threatening, and you should complete an initial assessment before giving care for them. The one exception to this rule is in the case of open bone injuries that are accompanied by massive bleeding. You should control this bleeding as part of the initial assessment.

2. Expose the affected area and look for bruising, swelling, deformity, or protruding bone ends.

3. Immobilize the injured area using a splint. You do not need a commercial splint to effectively stabilize the injured area, but can use items such as a rolled blanket or towel, a board, a magazine, or an uninjured body part.

4. You should not attempt to move the affected area, but splint it in the position you find it. Always place the splint so that the joints above and below the injury site cannot move. For example, if a guest has a forearm injury, place a splint that extends beyond both his elbow and his wrist.

5. The splint should be long enough and wide enough to properly stabilize the injury.

6. If the guest cannot move a limb, or has injured his head or neck, have him stay very still, and activate the EAS/EMS.

7. With the exception of open bone injuries, place a bag of ice over the affected area, elevate the splinted site, and wrap the area with ice and a compression (ACE) bandage.

Soft Tissue Injuries

Soft tissue injuries, or *wounds* as they are commonly called, are generally nonlife-threatening despite the blood and pain. Soft tissue injuries can range from a minor skinned knee (abrasion) or a bruise, to a major traumatic amputation.

When treating a soft tissue wound, you must be concerned with controlling bleeding and reducing the chances of infection. As with any situation where you might come in contact with a guest's bodily fluids, use body substance isolation (BSI) precautions prior to any contact with the guest.

Signs and Symptoms of Soft Tissue Injuries

Wounds are either internal (bruising) or external. Internal bleeding causes bruises to appear under the skin, and swelling is common. You can control internal bleeding with elevation, ice, and rest. If a guest is bleeding externally, quickly determine if the bleeding is coming from an artery. You can tell if it is, because the blood will be pumping (squirting). You must control arterial bleeding during your initial assessment. Do not try to determine if the blood is "bright red", it does not matter, blood is blood.

Guests suffering soft tissue injuries will frequently suffer other associated injuries involving the bones, muscles, or joints. These guests are usually experiencing severe pain that does not seem to fit the soft tissue wound. Remember to carefully conduct a focused physical exam on these guests.

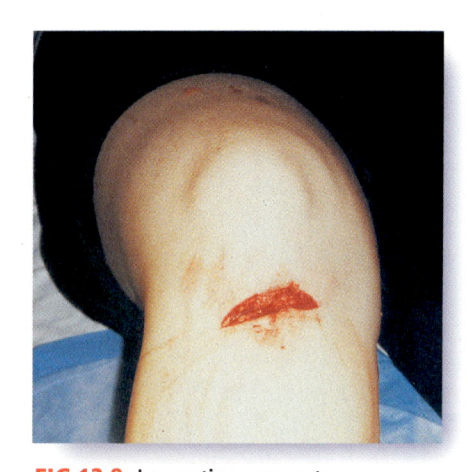

FIG 13.8 Lacerations are cuts produced by sharp objects.

Emergency Treatment for Soft Tissue Injuries

1. Take standard precautions; glove up!

2. Complete your initial assessment and determine if the bleeding (hemorrhaging) is arterial. Immediately apply direct pressure to the wound, and elevate it above the level of the guest's heart. As soon as you have one available, place a clean gauze or other clean material directly over the wound, and continue to apply pressure.

3. If bleeding continues and the gauze becomes soaked, apply additional gauze without removing the first.

4. Activate the EAS/EMS if bleeding continues, or if there are any deep wounds.

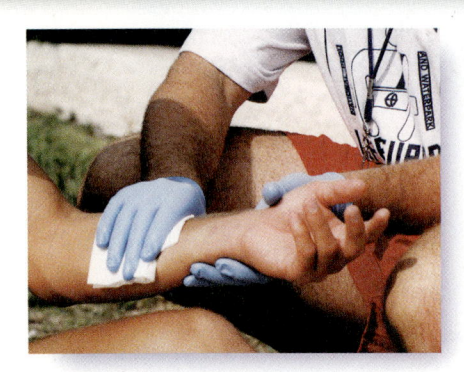

FIG 13.9a Direct pressure.

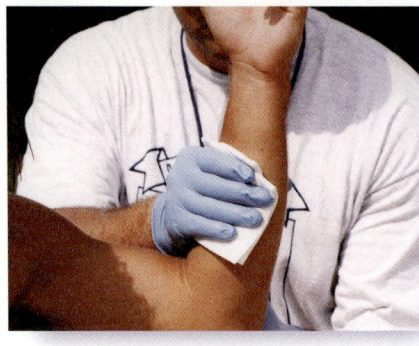

FIG 13.9b Elevation.

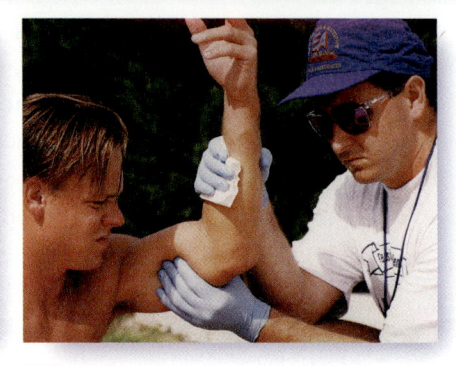

FIG 13.9c Direct pressure, elevation plus pressure point.

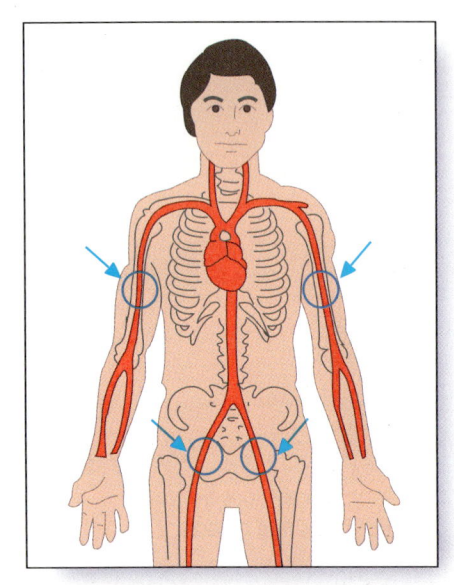

FIG 13.10 Major pressure points of the human body.

5. In most cases, direct pressure is all the action you will need to take for the first several minutes. If the wound is in the guest's arms or legs, and you cannot control the bleeding, apply firm pressure over the main pressure points while providing elevation.

Embedded Objects

If the wound includes an embedded object, leave the object in place. Stabilize the object until EMS personnel arrive. The simplest method of stabilizing an object is to use both of your gloved hands. The EMS professionals will decide the best method of stabilization and transportation.

Amputation

If the soft tissue injury involves an amputated part, complete an initial assessment and:

1. Provide direct pressure to the wound to control the bleeding.
2. Locate the severed part. If you find the part, place it in a clean, moist cloth (gauze).
3. Place the wrapped part in a plastic bag and seal it.
4. Keep the amputated part cool. Place the sealed bag on ice, making sure the part is not buried in, or in direct contact with the ice.
5. Activate the EAS/EMS. EMS personnel will transport the amputated part with the guest to the hospital.

Nosebleed

Nosebleeds are fairly common, especially in crowded places. At aquatic facilities, guests often suffer nosebleeds when they bump into each other. Begin caring for a guest with a nosebleed by directing the guest to provide self-care to control the bleeding. This will reduce your chances of coming into direct contact with the guest's blood. Also, help the guest limit the amount of blood that drains down his throat and into his stomach. This will lessen his chances of vomiting, which could block his airway.

Emergency treatment for nosebleeds should be as follows:

1. Follow BSI precautions: wear gloves.
2. Have the guest sit down and lean slightly forward.
3. Have the guest pinch his nostrils together at the bridge of his nose.

4. Have the guest maintain this pressure for at least 5 minutes. Then, have him slowly release the pressure, and determine if clotting has been successful. If bleeding continues, have the guest reapply pressure to his nostrils.

5. Activate the EAS/EMS if the bleeding cannot be controlled, or if the guest complains of any associated medical problems, such as another head injury.

Burns

The causes of burns are usually divided into three categories. **Thermal burns** are caused by contact with flame, super-heated air (steam), radiation (sun), scalding water, or any combination of these factors. **Chemical burns** occur after exposure to dry, liquid, or chemical gases. **Electrical burns** are caused by lightning, or by contact with electrical outlets or supply lines.

Burn Severity

Burns are classified according to the degree of tissue destruction. There are currently three distinct degrees or categories of burn injury: superficial, partial-thickness, and full-thickness. Burn victims may suffer all three levels of severity during an incident. If you encounter this situation, treat the area according to the highest severity level.

Signs and Symptoms of Burns

Superficial burns affect the outer layers of skin, usually turning the skin red and causing slight swelling. Superficial burns are often associated with sunburn, and can be very painful. If these burns cover a large portion of a guest's body, the guest should seek immediate medical attention. As a lifeguard, you will see many guests with superficial burns. Most of these burns will be minor, but some could be potentially dangerous. If you are not certain, activate the local EAS/EMS.

Partial-thickness burns damage deeper layers of skin, and cause blisters to form on the skin's surface. These blisters vary in size, and a single blister can sometimes cover a very large area of tissue. Movement usually causes the blisters to break, and the patient may complain of severe pain.

Full-thickness burns damage all layers of the skin, including muscle and bone. These burns can be multi-colored (black, red, gray, white), and cause little or no pain. This painless phenomenon results from the destruction of local nerve endings. However, the patient will experience extreme pain in the areas surrounding a full-thickness burn.

Emergency Treatment for Burns

For superficial (first-degree) burns, do the following:

1. Cool the affected area with cool water for up to 30 minutes. If the pain continues, suggest to the guest that she contact her personal physician.

For partial-thickness (second degree) burns, do the following:

1. After determining the cause of the burn and completing your initial assessment, cool the burned area.

2. Remove any jewelry or smoldering clothing.

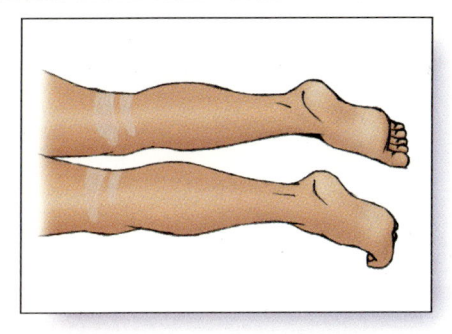

FIG 13.11a Superficial, or first-degree burn.

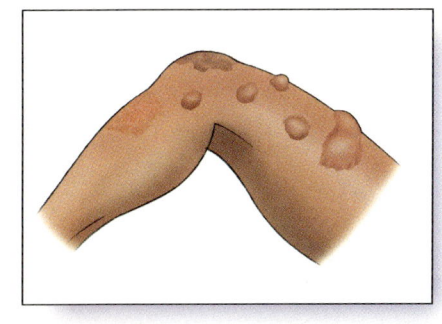

FIG 13.11b Partial thickness, or second-degree burn.

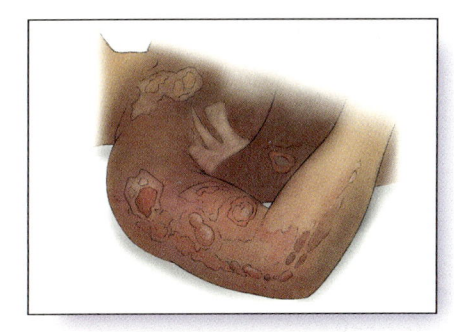

FIG 13.11c Full-thickness, or third degree burn.

3. Cover the burn area with dry, clean gauze, towels, or sheets. Do not apply pressure to blisters.
4. Provide supplemental oxygen therapy using high-flow oxygen.
5. Activate the EAS/EMS.

For full-thickness (third-degree) burns, do the following:

1. Conduct your initial assessment, and correct any immediately life-threatening problems.
2. Cover full-thickness burns with dry, clean gauze, towels, or sheets.
3. Quickly remove all jewelry in the burn area, and pay close attention to the guest's respiratory status.
4. Active the EAS/EMS—guests with full-thickness burns will be transported to the nearest hospital that has facilities to treat burn victims.

Chemical Burns

Chemical burns can produce all three degrees of burn damage. As in all emergency situations, first secure the scene and take precautions to protect yourself from coming in direct contact with the chemicals. If you are unsure of the exact nature of the chemical, *do not enter the scene.* Activate the EAS/EMS and wait for personnel to identify the materials and declare the scene safe.

If the scene is safe, be careful not to come in contact with the offending chemical. If the chemical was dry, quickly brush it off the guest using a cloth, and flush the area with water; then activate the EAS/EMS. Continue to flush the area until EMS personnel arrive.

Keep in mind that personal and team safety take priority during chemical or hazardous material emergencies. If you respond to an emergency involving chemicals or other hazardous materials, remember the old saying "Only fools rush in."

Electrical Burns

In many cases of electrocution, the superficial tissue damage you find during your initial assessment or focused physical exam may at first appear to be minor. Unfortunately, this external damage usually does not adequately reflect the serious tissue damage that may lie deep underneath the first layers of skin. With guests suffering from electrocution, always make sure the source of the electrocution has been removed. Once it is safe to enter the scene and approach the guest, conduct an initial assessment and correct any immediately life-threatening problems. Conduct a focused physical exam, and look for entrance and exit wounds caused by the electrocution.

External burns from electrocution should be treated similarly to full-thickness burns. Maintain the patient's ABC's and quickly activate the EAS/EMS.

Lightning

Victims of electrocution caused by lightning commonly suffer severe burns and are found pulseless and not breathing. Begin proper emergency care once you have removed the guest from the potentially unsafe area.

Never assume the power source is off! Always make sure that it is off before you move into the area. If you are unable to verify that the power is off and secured, wait to initiate care until the appropriate safety personnel arrive.

For guests suffering from a lightning strike who are pulseless and not breathing, you should begin CPR promptly. If an automated defibrillator is available, apply it to the guest as soon as possible.

Fainting (Syncope)

Fainting occurs when the flow of oxygen to the brain is temporarily disrupted. Guests may have early warning signs or symptoms of an impending fainting episode. These signs and symptoms include nausea, weakness, chills, abdominal pain, dizziness or headache. Fainting is rarely serious, and usually self-corrects after a few minutes. Guests who have fainted will usually describe their episode as beginning with a sensation of lightheadedness, then some nausea, followed by a temporary loss of consciousness. Guests who have fainted will often regain consciousness quickly after lying in a horizontal or flat position and allowing blood (oxygen) to return to their brain tissue.

Common Causes of Fainting

- Hyperventilation (rapid breathing)
- Hypoglycemia (low blood sugar)
- Heart problems
- Epilepsy
- Dehydration
- Blood loss
- Psychological stress

Emergency Treatment for Fainting

1. If a guest complains of "feeling like fainting," have him lie down on a flat surface. Lying on a flat surface can prevent him from incurring head or spinal injuries by falling if he becomes unconscious and falls without warning. If a guest has already fainted, look for signs of head and spinal injury, and treat him accordingly.
2. Elevate the guest's legs approximately 12 inches to help increase blood flow to his head, and monitor his ABC's.
3. If the guest vomits, roll him onto his side in the recovery position, and use manual suction as needed.
4. Loosen any restrictive clothing, and activate the EAS/EMS.

Seizures

Seizures are sudden, involuntary changes in a person's brain cell activity level, due to a massive electrical charge. These sudden changes can cause abnormal sensations, unusual behavior, muscle rigidity, or an altered level of consciousness. These conditions occur because the brain is sending mixed signals to the muscles, telling them to contract, relax, or do both at the same time.

Although there are many different causes of seizures, emergency treatment for them is very similar in most cases. Millions of people suffer seizures each year, so be prepared to appropriately treat the guest who has a seizure.

Never force anything into a guest's mouth if he is having a seizure.

Never attempt to restrain a guest who is having a seizure.

Never give a guest who is having a seizure anything to eat or drink.

Causes of Seizures

- Epilepsy
- Infection
- Alcohol intoxication
- Trauma
- Head injury
- Diabetes
- Stroke
- Drug overdose
- Tumor
- Fever
- Psychological stress
- Burns
- Pregnancy

Emergency Treatment for Seizures

1. Activate the EAS/EMS.
2. Remove any objects that may injure the guest.
3. Place a thin, soft object, such as a folded towel, between the guest's head and the floor.
4. Once the seizure subsides, carefully maintain an open airway.
5. Complete your initial assessment.
6. If you suspect a head or spinal injury, take the necessary precautions.
7. Quietly and calmly reassure the guest as she regains consciousness.
8. Monitor the guest's airway, be alert for vomiting, and suction as required.
9. Maintain normal body temperature.
10. Protect the guest's privacy.

Shock

Shock is defined as inadequate circulation of oxygenated blood to body tissues. Shock represents a severe condition that requires advanced care.

Hypovolemic (fluid loss) shock occurs when too much blood or other body fluids are lost from the circulatory system. Fluid loss generally occurs from vomiting, diarrhea, or burns, but it could also be caused by massive blood loss.

Anaphylactic shock occurs when the body has a severe allergic reaction to an offending agent, chemical, or toxin.

Signs and symptoms of hypovolemic shock

- Breathing difficulties
- Disorientation
- Nausea and vomiting
- Extreme thirst
- Cold, pale, moist skin
- Weakness

Emergency Treatment for Hypovolemic Shock

1. Immediately assess and manage the victim's ABC's.
2. Activate the EAS/EMS.
3. Complete a focused physical exam, paying particular attention to all bleeding wounds.
4. Maintain normal body temperature.
5. If possible, elevate the guest's legs approximately 12 inches.
6. If the guest is unconscious and does not have a spinal injury, place him in the recovery position.
7. If it is available, provide high-flow oxygen.
8. Suction the guest's airway as needed.

Signs and Symptoms of Anaphylactic Shock

- Respiratory wheezing
- Squeezing sensation in the chest
- Swelling in the airway
- Weak, rapid pulse
- Massive swelling
- Blueness around the mouth and lips
- Itching and burning of the skin
- Hives (large white and red spots)

Emergency Treatment for Anaphylactic Shock

1. Immediately assess and manage the guest's ABC's.
2. Do not be fooled if you observe minor signs of distress. Severe cases of anaphylactic shock can begin within minutes after exposure.
3. Activate the EAS/EMS.
4. If the allergic reaction is from a bee sting, locate the stinger and scrape it out. *Do not pluck out the stinger!* Plucking out the stinger can put pressure on the venom sac at the tip of the barb and push more venom into the skin.
5. Determine if the guest has medication for allergic reactions, and if he does, help him self-administer it.

Diabetic Emergencies

A person with diabetes must carefully regulate his blood sugar and insulin levels through a combination of medication, diet, and exercise. Keeping blood sugar and insulin levels in balance and under control can be difficult. Any significant imbalance between blood sugar and insulin levels can result in one of two types of diabetic emergencies: hypoglycemia (insulin shock) and hyperglycemia (diabetic ketoacidosis).

Hypoglycemia occurs when a person's blood sugar level is too low and his insulin level is too high. The symptoms of hypoglycemia can develop very rapidly. Hypoglycemia is usually caused by a person with diabetes

> **critical POINT!**
>
> If you are treating a conscious guest with a medical history of diabetes, and you are not sure which type of diabetic emergency you are facing, treat him as if he has hypoglycemia, and give him sugar. If hypoglycemia was the cause, once you have given the guest sugar, he may quickly improve. In cases of hyperglycemia, the guest's condition will remain unchanged, but the extra sugar will not be harmful.

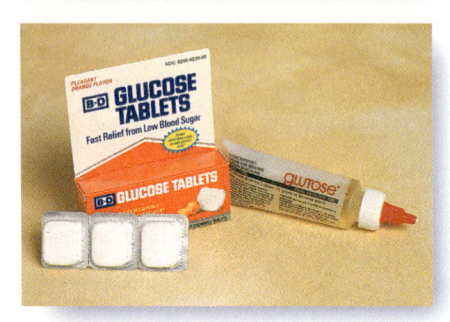

FIG 13.12 There are a variety of treatments for hypoglycemia.

taking too much insulin, eating at irregular intervals, or exercising (using energy) beyond normal levels. A person with hypoglycemia needs to quickly get sugar into his bloodstream to balance the effects of a high insulin level.

Signs and Symptoms of Hypoglycemia

- Diminished level of consciousness
- Rapid pulse
- Rapid breathing
- Profuse sweating
- Weakness
- Hunger
- Vision difficulties
- Numbness in all extremities

Emergency Treatment for Hypoglycemia

1. If the guest is conscious, he may be able to describe his specific treatment needs. He may also be able to tell when he last ate or took his medication.
2. Give the conscious guest, who is able to swallow, foods that contain a lot of sugar. Some foods that work well are soft drinks, fruit juices, or candy.
3. Activate the EAS/EMS.
4. Monitor the guest's ABCs until his symptoms subside or EMS personnel arrive.
5. If a guest is unconscious or unable to swallow, quickly activate the EAS/EMS.
6. Place the guest in the recovery position and monitor his airway. Carefully monitor the guest's airway to ensure that it remains clear. Suction as required, and watch for signs of vomiting.

Hyperglycemia occurs when a person's blood sugar level is too high and the insulin level in the bloodstream is too low. Unlike hypoglycemia with its rapid onset, hyperglycemia usually takes hours or even days to become a significant medical problem. The signs and symptoms of hyperglycemia usually develop slowly.

Signs and Symptoms of Hyperglycemia

- Drowsiness
- Confusion
- Fever
- Severe thirst
- Deep and rapid breathing
- Fruity breath odor
- History of frequent urination

Emergency Treatment for Hyperglycemia

1. Activate the EAS/EMS.
2. Assess and control the patient's ABC's.

Asthma Emergencies

Asthma is a chronic (long-term or ongoing) condition that constricts a person's breathing passages, causing periods of difficulty breathing. When a person experiences an asthma attack, the passageways to the lungs narrow, and airway tissues produce excessive amounts of thick mucous. Smaller airways full of mucous make breathing more difficult. In most cases, asthma is controlled with medication.

Asthma attacks can be caused by several factors, including infections, exercise, allergies, drug sensitivity, cold weather, second-hand tobacco smoke, and intense stress. Most asthmatics know how to avoid these factors, and are used to effectively dealing with their asthma. In other cases, a person may experience her first bout of asthma while attending your aquatic facility and be completely caught by surprise and unprepared. A prolonged or severe case of asthma can become life-threatening very quickly. Asthma attacks that do not quickly respond to basic treatment are dangerous. You should activate the EAS/EMS in all cases involving a guest who has asthma, or who has an asthma-like complaint.

Signs and Symptoms of Asthma

- Difficulty breathing
- Rapid, shallow breathing
- Spasmodic coughing
- Whistling or high-pitched wheezing
- Fatigue
- Stomach cramps, especially in younger children
- Anxiety

Emergency Treatment for Asthma

1. Activate the EAS/EMS.
2. Help the guest move into an upright or slightly bent forward posture.
3. Assist the guest in using her own prescribed medications (inhaler).
4. Provide oxygen (high-flow), if available.
5. Prepare the BVM and suction unit for possible use.

Poisoning Emergencies

The signs and symptoms of poisoning vary according to the substances involved. In poisoning emergencies, contact your regional Poison Control Center (PCC) as soon as possible. Write down the information the PCC gives you, and give it to the EAS/EMS teams when they arrive.

As with any potentially hazardous material, be careful not to come in contact with the toxic substances.

critical POINT

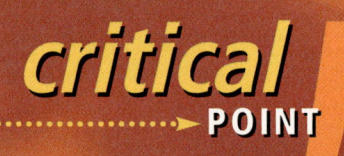

If you are not sure of the exact nature of the poison or toxin, do not enter the scene until it is declared safe by the appropriate authorities!

Quick Review

Reviewing Critical Steps in First Responder Emergency Care

- As a lifeguard, you are not a replacement for EAS/EMS professionals. You should activate the EAS/EMS as soon as possible after an incident occurs.
- You must be primarily concerned with your own safety in every rescue/emergency situation.
- Care begins with an initial assessment. You must control problems you find in the initial assessment before all other problems, with no exceptions!
- The focused physical exam begins at the head and ends at the toes, and is performed after the patient's airway, breathing, circulation, and major bleeding are controlled. This exam is completed by touching the body, looking for abnormal signs and symptoms, and asking questions regarding the injury or illness.
- Maintain spinal cord stabilization in all guests with a serious head injury, or significant mechanism of injury suggestive of a possible head or neck injury.
- Follow local emergency protocols if they differ from what you have learned in this manual.
- Practice all emergency care skills frequently.
- Document your emergency treatment immediately.
- After providing emergency care, and after you complete the proper documentation, return to your assigned duties.

General Signs and Symptoms of Inhaled Poisons

- Severe headache
- Nausea and/or vomiting
- Facial burns
- Burning sensation in the throat or chest
- Discoloration of the lips
- Difficulty breathing
- Coughing, bloody spit
- Altered consciousness
- Dizziness

Emergency Treatment for Inhaled Poisons

1. Activate the EAS/EMS.
2. Secure the safety of the scene.
3. Take BSI precautions.
4. Move the patient to safe surroundings where the air is clean.
5. Assess and manage the patient's ABCs.
6. Administer high-flow oxygen if it is available.
7. Perform CPR or rescue breathing as needed.

General Signs and Symptoms of Swallowed Poisons

- Nausea, abdominal cramps
- Vomiting
- Diarrhea
- Drowsiness
- Abnormal breathing
- Unusual breath or body odor
- Seizures
- Burns around the mouth and nose
- Hoarse voice
- Coughing, bloody spit

Emergency Treatment for Swallowed Poisons

1. Activate the EAS/EMS.
2. Take BSI precautions.
3. Assess and manage the patient's ABC's.
4. Suction the airway as needed, and place the patient in the recovery position to clear vomit and protect the airway.
5. Contact the regional poison control center, and identify what, how much, and when the poison was swallowed.
6. Follow the emergency care instructions given by the PCC staff.
7. Provide high-flow oxygen if it is available, and be prepared to use the BVM.

REVIEW QUESTIONS

1. (T) (F) Basic care skills, if not performed, could lead to additional injury and possible death.

2. (T) (F) Life-threatening emergencies are those that compromise a guest's airway, breathing, or circulation in any way, including those situations with massive bleeding.

3. (T) (F) As a lifeguard, your safety comes second to the guest's.

4. (T) (F) Guests can be spontaneously breathing and have no pulse.

5. (T) (F) Guests who are pulseless will not be breathing.

6. (T) (F) The first thing you should do is perform a focused physical exam.

7. (T) (F) In the focused physical exam you are checking the ABC's.

8. Match the sign/symptom with its type of burn:

   _____ Red skin, swelling, pain   a. Superficial

   _____ Blisters, extreme pain, and significant swelling   b. Partial-thickness

   _____ Deep bone injury   c. Full-thickness

9. Match the type of burn with the proper emergency treatment:

   _____ Place the injured area in cool water until the pain stops   a. Superficial

   _____ Focus primarily on maintaining the airway; cover with a dry clean dressing   b. Partial-thickness

   _____ Stop the burning process with sterile or clean water and cover with dry dressing   c. Full-thickness

10. Match treatment plans with the specific type of heat emergency:

    _____ Administer cool water and watch the patient   a. Mild hyperthermia

    _____ Open the airway and rapidly cool the body   b. Moderate hyperthermia

    _____ Administer cool water and elevate the legs   c. Severe hyperthermia

11. Matching:

    _____ Direct pressure   a. Skin flap injury

    _____ Elevation   b. Bruise

    _____ Pressure Points   c. Scrape

    _____ Contusion   d. First method used for controlling bleeding

    _____ Abrasion   e. Protecting yourself from contact with body fluids

    _____ Avulsions   f. Along with direct pressure, the second stage of controlling bleeding

    _____ BSI Precautions   g. Places around the body where an artery can be pressed against bone to slow the flow of blood.

12. (T) (F) Treatment for musculoskeletal injuries should only begin after problems found in the initial assessment have been properly cared for.

13. (T) (F) Bleeding that is "squirting with force" comes from the body's arteries, and must be controlled immediately.

14. (T) (F) To treat fainting without head or neck injury, you should monitor the guest's ABC's, look for any active bleeding, elevate the legs, and loosen restrictive clothing.

15. (T) (F) There are many different causes of seizures, and each must be treated differently.

16. (T) (F) Never force anything into the mouth of a seizuring person, attempt to restrain him, or give him anything to drink or eat.

17. The type of shock that occurs when the body has a severe allergic reaction is called _____.

18. (T) (F) If a guest has been stung or bitten by an insect and is exhibiting signs of an allergic reaction, you should immediately active the EAS/EMS.

19. (T) (F) When caring for external bleeding, you should apply pressure at a pressure point before direct pressure and elevation.

20. (T) (F) When treating a guest for hypovolemic shock, you should keep her warm, elevate her uninjured legs, and not overheat her.

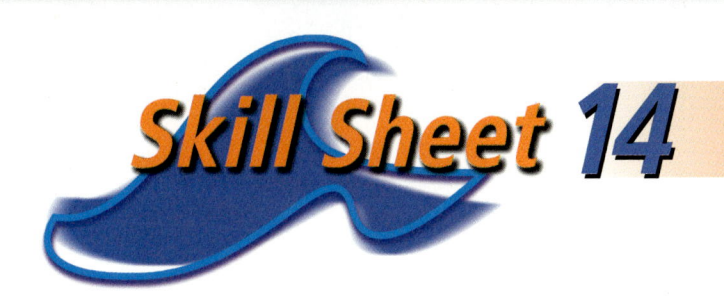

CHAPTER 13 • MEDICAL EMERGENCIES AND INJURIES   163

Skill Sheet 14

MEDICAL EMERGENCIES

1 Pressure point.

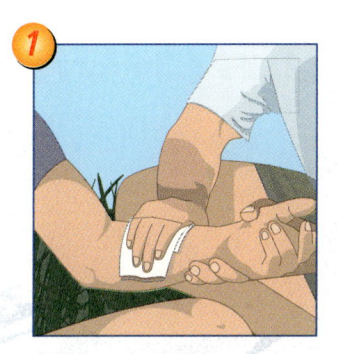

2 Assess and care for medical emergencies

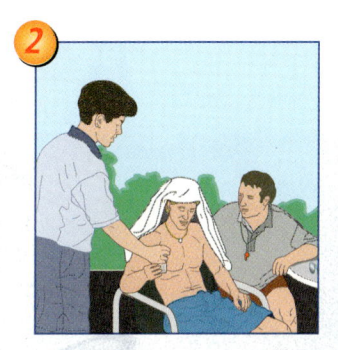

3 Take personal health and safety precautions

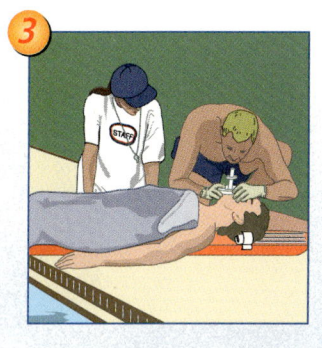

KEY POINTS:

- Stay calm.
- Assess and care for life-threatening conditions first.
- Conduct a focused physical exam only after all immediate life-threatening conditions are cared for.
- Remember BSI precautions.

CRITICAL THINKING:

1. How would you care for a guest who has severe bleeding, and is not breathing?

2. How would you care for a guest who is diabetic, states he feels faint, has eaten very little, and has been physically active at your facility?

Additional Responsibilities

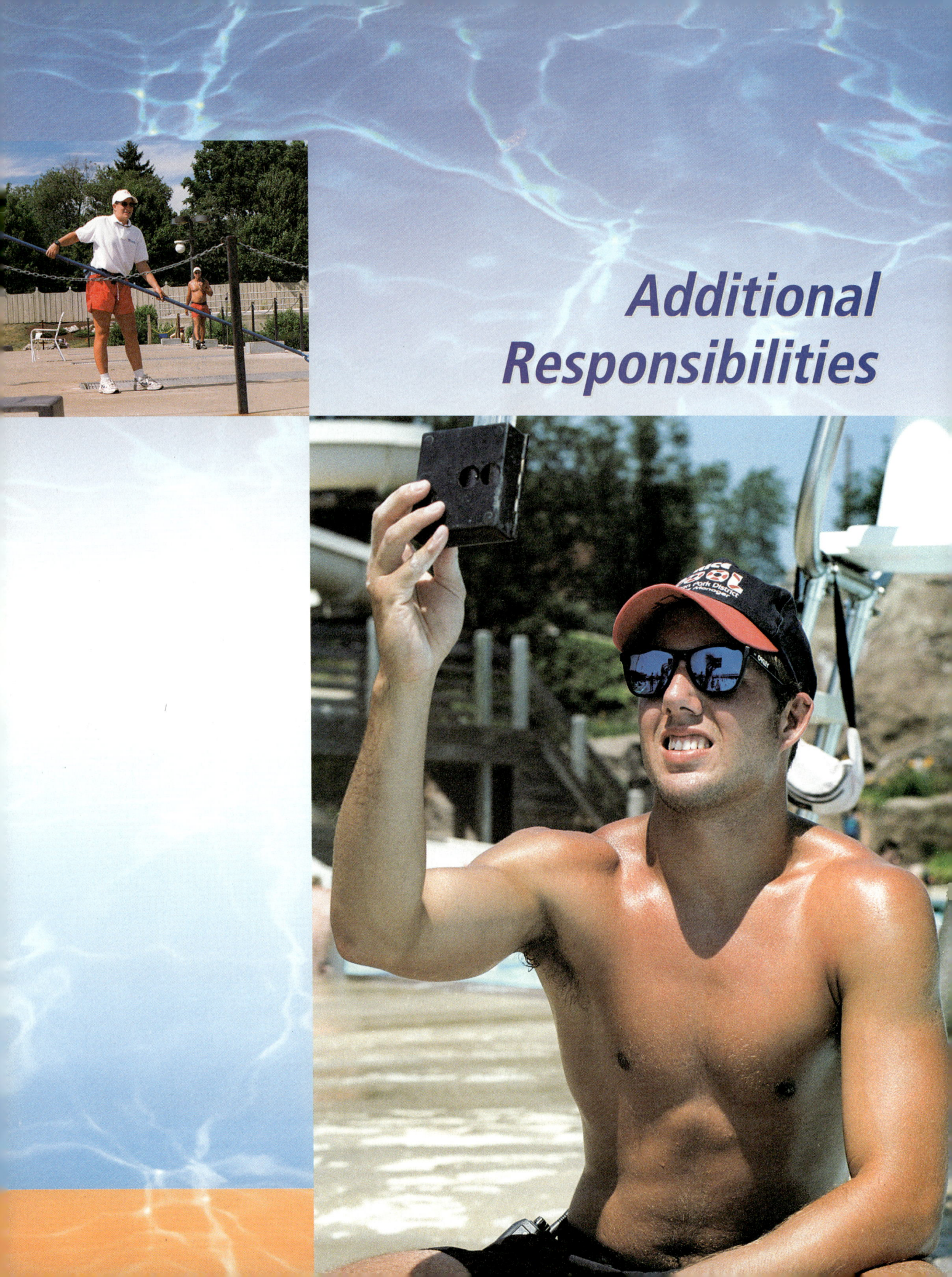

chapter 14

OBJECTIVES

After reading this chapter and completing the related course work, you should be able to:

1. Identify ways to enforce rules and maintain good guest relations.

2. Identify strategies for crowd control.

3. Explain the importance of paperwork and performing secondary duties.

4. Explain the importance of maintaining a high level of skill.

As a lifeguard, your main responsibility is the safety of the guests. Part of this responsibility depends on your ability to effectively deal with guests. You will have to manage and direct their actions, as well as provide protection for their health and safety.

RULE ENFORCEMENT

Enforcing rules as a lifeguard is often difficult because people come to your facility to enjoy themselves, and to get away from their daily pressures and problems. Just as society is governed by laws, your guests are governed by rules that are established for their health and safety.

Some rules that must be enforced and are common to all types of aquatic facilities are "Walk" or "No Glass on the Pool Deck." However, beyond these common rules, each facility will also have its own set of rules, specific to that facility. As a professional lifeguard, it is your responsibility to know all the rules of your facility, adhere to them yourself, and enforce them consistently. There are several important components of rule enforcement. These include:

- **Understanding and Explaining the Rules.** As a lifeguard, you should understand the reason for a rule and be able to explain it to guests. You may find that once you have explained a rule to someone, enforcing it will be easier. Your goal is to prevent injuries and drownings. If the guests understand why certain actions are not safe, they are less likely to repeat them.

    For example, instead of saying, "Sir, you can't bring that bottle in here," you might try saying, "Excuse me sir, glass containers are not allowed on the pool deck. If it breaks, it is dangerous because the pieces are almost impossible to find and remove."

    This is positive and more effective, and will help guests see you as a professional. Also, whenever possible, make eye contact with the guests. Particularly when you are talking with children, they are often more responsive if you make eye contact with them

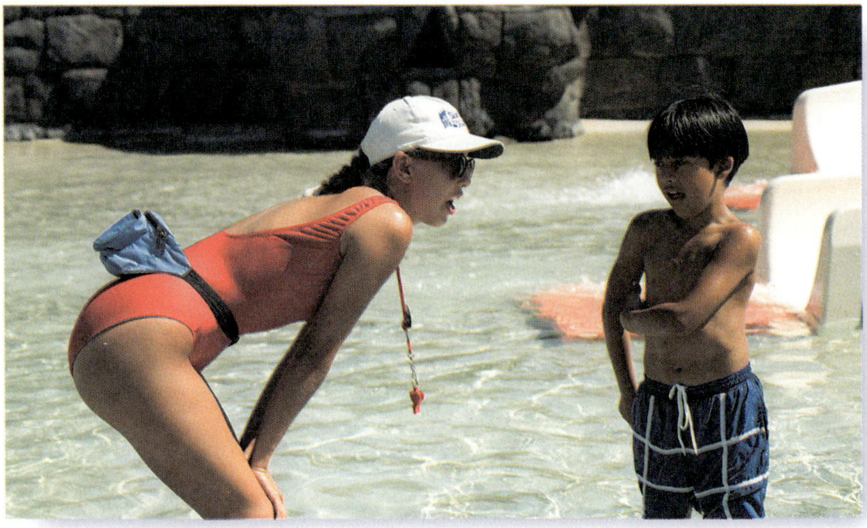

FIG 14.1 Talking to a child.

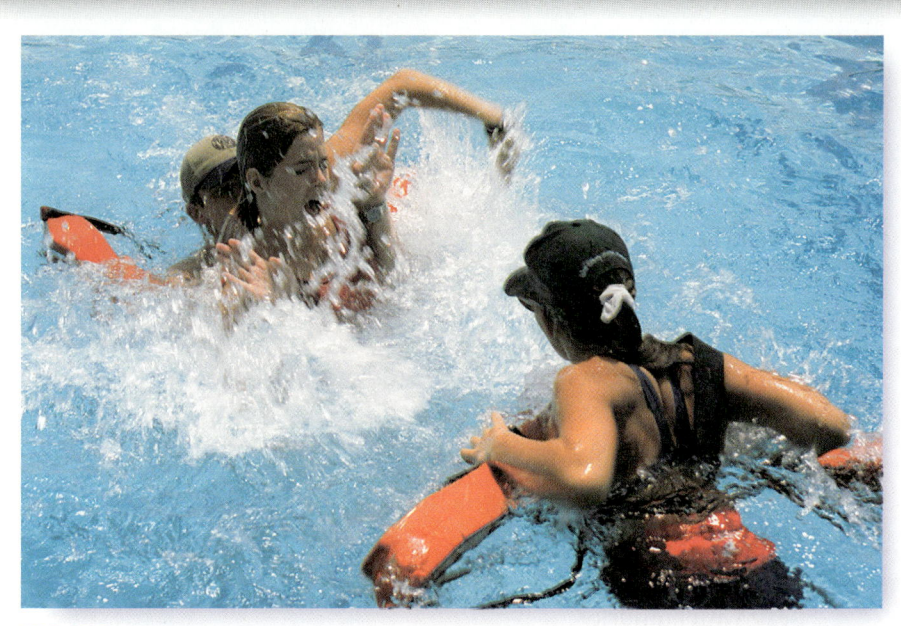

FIG 14.2 Inservice training keeps you test-ready.

- **Be Consistent When Enforcing Rules.** Being consistent means enforcing the same rule, in the same way, every time. If you correct guests' actions today, you should correct the same action in the same way tomorrow.

- **Enforce Rules Uniformly**. Uniform rule enforcement means that if two different guests are violating the same rule, you must stop both of them. Remember, the rules apply equally to all of your guests.

- **Use a Positive Approach.** When you make corrections, use a positive approach whenever possible. For example, instead of saying: "Don't run" say, "Please walk."

- **Remember the "Golden Rule."** The golden rule of excellent guest service is to treat guests like you would like to be treated—with respect.

- **Know Where the Rules Are Posted.** The posted rules are a backup authority for you. Know where they are posted and refer guests to them when necessary. In larger facilities such as water parks, rules are posted in several locations. There may also be specific rules for each attraction. As a professional lifeguard, it is your responsibility to know the rules for all of the attractions at your facility and in your area of responsibility.

- **Refer Problems to Your Supervisor.** If children keep violating a rule, have them sit for a few minutes. Sometimes a "time-out" will solve the problem. If the problem persists, or if an older guest argues with you about a rule, do not hesitate to seek assistance from your supervisor. Whether that supervisor is a head lifeguard, assistant manager, or a manager, it is part of his or her job to help you with rule enforcement, and enable you to maintain the 10/20 Protection Rule. You cannot allow yourself to be distracted from your zone.

CROWD CONTROL

During an emergency, it may be necessary for you to control large numbers of guests simultaneously to maintain order. Examples are a weather emergency, or any emergency in which groups of people need to be moved or directed. You should practice your Emergency Action Plan so that you are always prepared for such an incident. Know what your responsibilities are for different events and situations, and where all the access and exit points are for your facility. It may sometimes be necessary to evacuate the area or open a path so that Emergency Medical Personnel can reach an injured guest.

If you need to control a crowd:

- Keep calm
- Speak loudly and clearly
- Give precise, simple directions
- Speak with authority

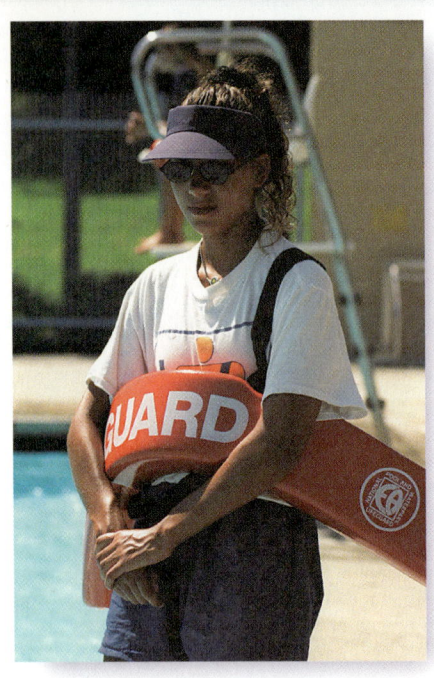

FIG 14.3 Be attentive to your guests so you will be ready to move or direct them quickly when the need arises.

PAPERWORK

Another responsibility you will have as a lifeguard is to complete reports and maintain records. Each facility will have records and reports that are specific to the operation of that facility.

These include:

- Attendance records
- Sign-in sheets
- Maintenance schedules
- Daily work schedules
- Lifeguard rotations
- Pool chemistry
- Weather conditions
- Inservice training records
- Incident reports

Incident reports are among the most important records/reports you will complete. Every rescue requires careful documentation. The documentation must be completed as soon as the incident has been resolved. Use the incident report forms supplied by your facility, making sure to fill in each section completely. These forms may become legal records in the future, and adequate documentation will minimize problems at that time.

RELATED DUTIES

Aquatic facilities often require lifeguards to perform duties not directly related to the two primary responsibilities: preventing aquatic incidents and providing rescue and emergency care. These additional duties will vary depending on the facility; it is the responsibility of your employer to provide you with a complete job description. Read the job description carefully. It is very important that you clearly understand your duties and responsibilities before you begin work. These related duties are performed during times when you are not responsible for watching patrons. They may include:

- Locker room attendance
- Front desk attendance
- General facility maintenance

MAINTAINING YOUR SKILLS

As a National Pool and Waterpark Lifeguard, you will sign a License Agreement stating that you will maintain your skills at "test ready" levels at all times. The skills you learn in this course will require constant review and practice. The inservice training conducted at your facility will help you maintain your skill level, but it is up to you to be sure that your observation, rescue, and emergency care skills are at "test ready" levels at all times.

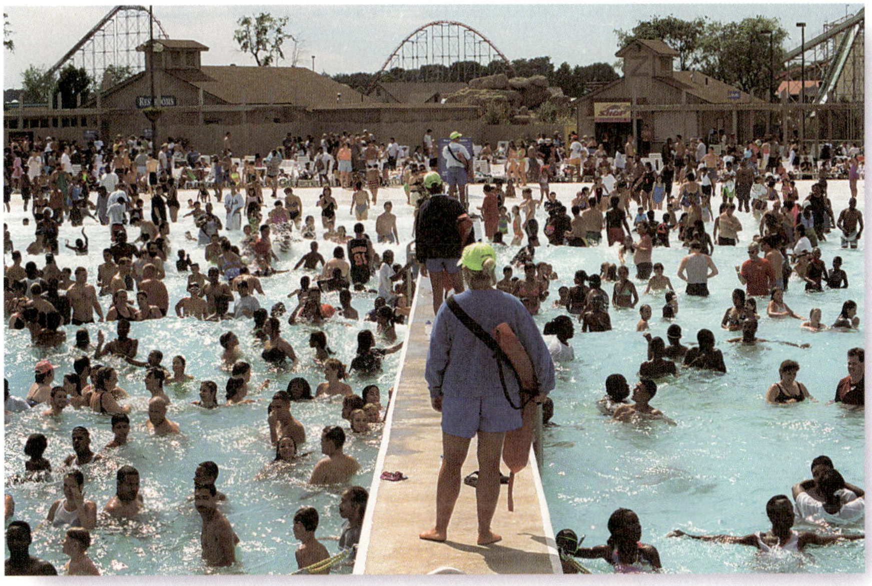

FIG 14.4 As a lifeguard, your observation, rescue, and emergency care skills should be maintained so that you are ready to help any guest at anytime.

REVIEW QUESTIONS

1. List three components of proper rule enforcement:

   a. _____

   b. _____

   c. _____

2. What is the Golden Rule?

3. List three things that will help you control a crowd:

   a. _____

   b. _____

   c. _____

4. (T) (F) Only rescues that involve CPR need documentation.

5. Working as a lifeguard means that you:
   a. Should expect to participate in regular in-service training.
   b. Might have to perform related duties at your facility.
   c. Will be expected to maintain professional standards.
   d. All of the above.

CHAPTER 14 • ADDITIONAL RESPONSIBILITIES   171

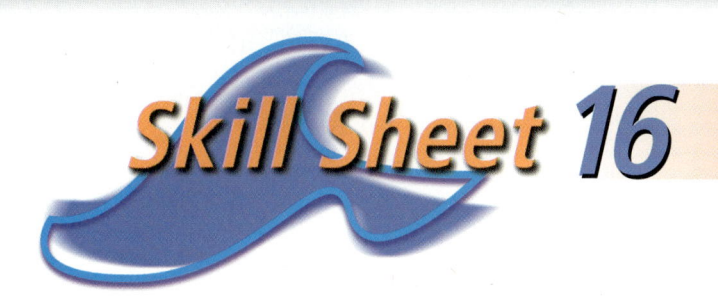

Skill Sheet 16 — LIFEGUARD RESPONSIBILITIES

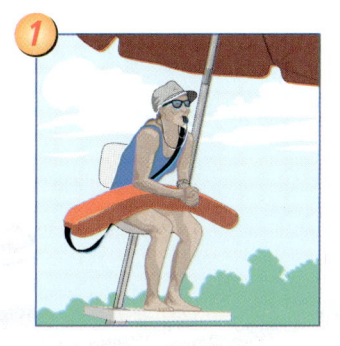

1. Professional image and surveillance.
2. Guest relations.
3. Rule enforcement.
4. Crowd control.
5. Paperwork.
6. Related duties.
7. Maintain skill level.

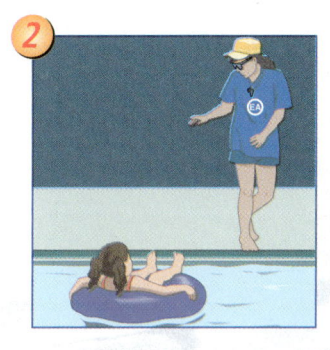

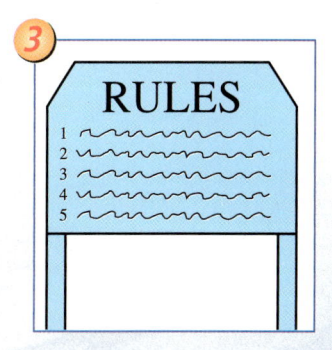

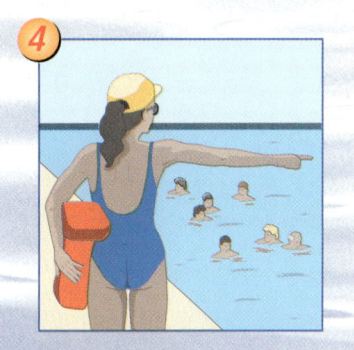

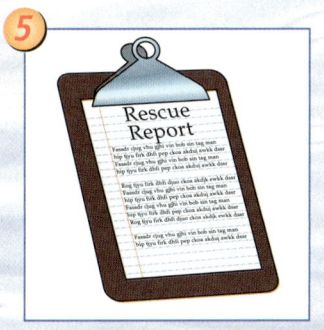

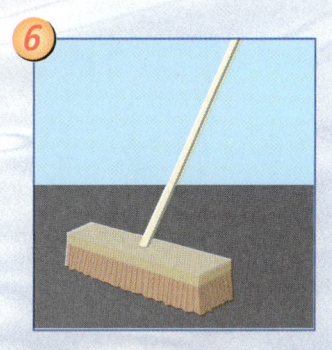

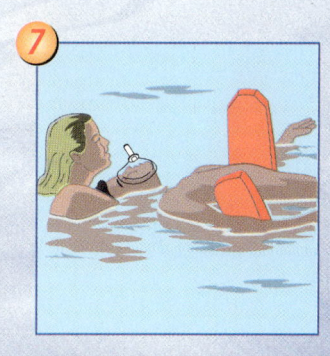

KEY POINTS:

- Be courteous and kind to guests and fellow staff.
- Remember the Golden Rule.
- You can make a difference and save lives.

CRITICAL THINKING:

1. How would you handle an irate guest?
2. What is the best way to enforce a rule?
3. What types of non-lifeguarding related duties do you think you may have to do?

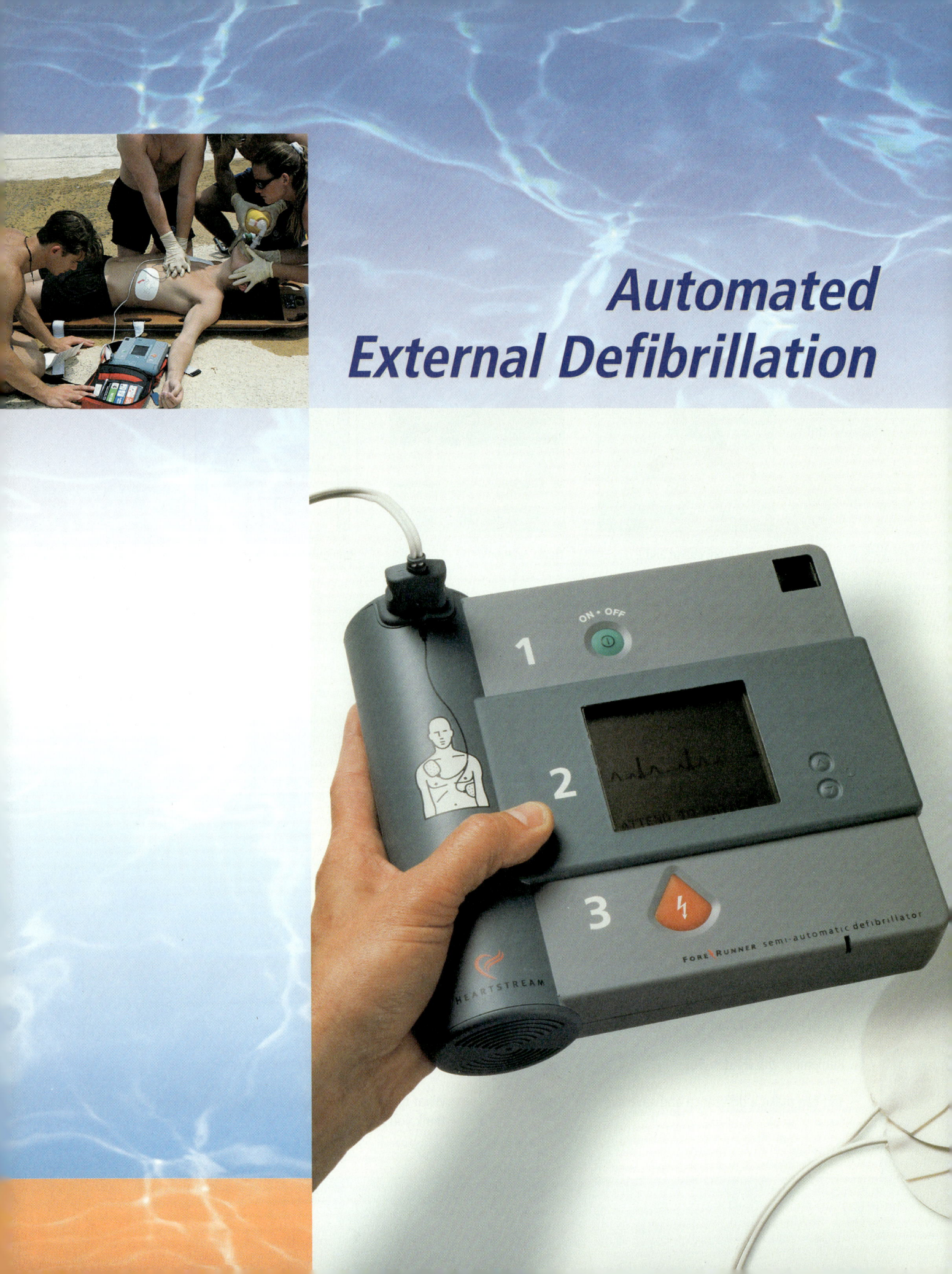

Automated External Defibrillation

chapter 15

OBJECTIVES

After reading this chapter and completing the related course work, you should be able to:

1. Explain the value of early defibrillation in the Chain of Survival.

2. Describe the electrical system of the heart.

3. Describe ventricular fibrillation and ventricular tachycardia.

4. Describe the general steps involved with the use of any automated external defibrillator (AED).

5. Explain the protocol for the operation of an AED.

6. Demonstrate how to use an AED.

Sudden cardiac death remains an unresolved public health crisis in the United States. More than 300,000 people die annually from sudden cardiac death. These deaths occur at home, at work, and during recreation. As you learned in previous chapters, a guest who suffers cardiac arrest needs prompt CPR and more advanced care. A guest's chance of survival is dramatically improved through early defibrillation and CPR. This combination has the potential to save thousands of lives each year. But or this to occur, time is the critical element. For every minute defibrillation is delayed, the chance of successful resuscitation is reduced by 10%! For this reason, lifeguards must be prepared to administer defibrillation as part of their care for a guest in cardiac arrest.

THE CHAIN OF SURVIVAL

The Chain of Survival recognizes the importance of early defibrillation. It consists of four links:

- Early access
- Early CPR
- Early defibrillation
- Early advanced cardiac life support

Early Access

Early Access is the activation of the EMS system by calling 9-1-1 or another local emergency number. This allows the necessary personnel to arrive early and provide professional treatment.

Early CPR

CPR supplies the minimum amount of oxygen to keep the brain and heart alive for a few extra minutes. CPR "buys time" until a defibrillator and more advanced personnel can arrive.

Early Defibrillation

This is the critical factor, because defibrillation provides a chance of restoring the heartbeat. In the past, physicians or paramedics would defibrillate the heart after they analyzed the heart rhythm on a monitor. With the development of automated external defibrillators (AEDs),

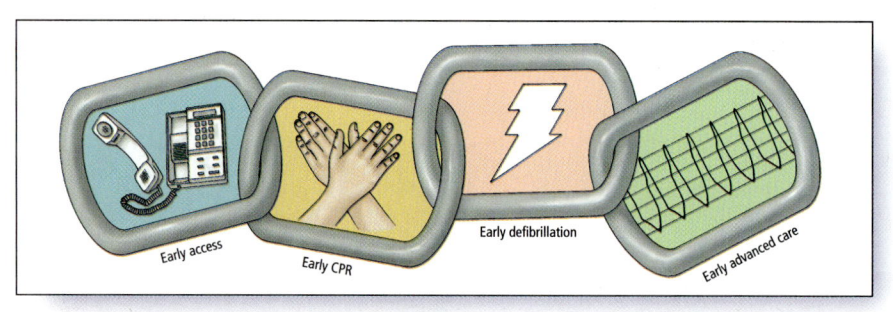

FIG 15.1 The four links in the chain of survival.

it is now possible for anyone to take appropriate action to defibrillate a heart. When applied to a guest in cardiac arrest, an AED automatically analyzes the heart rhythm, determines the need for a shock, and advises you how to proceed to deliver the shock by simply pushing a button.

Early Advanced Cardiac Life Support (ACLS)

ACLS involves the administration of medications and other advanced skills by specially trained medical personnel, most often paramedics, nurses, or physicans. Although defibrillation may initially correct the guest's problem, he or she is not likely to survive without more advanced care.

HOW THE HEART WORKS

The heart is an organ that has four chambers: two on the right side and two on the left side. Oxygen-deficient blood from the body enters the right side of the heart and is pumped to the lungs, where the waste products are removed and oxygen is received. This oxygen-rich blood is returned to the left side of the heart. Because of the workload that the heart must perform, it needs an abundant supply of oxygen. It gets this oxygen through its own vessels, the coronary arteries. The heart also pumps oxygen-rich blood to all parts of the body, to satisfy the needs of other organs.

The electrical system of the heart controls the rate that the heart beats and the amount of work the heart performs. In the upper right chamber of the heart, there is a small collection of special pacemaker cells. These pacemaker cells emit electrical impulses that cause heart muscle cells to contract in a coordinated manner. An impulse is emitted about 60 to 100 times a minute. When the heart functions in this normal manner, the heart rhythm is referred to as normal sinus rhythm.

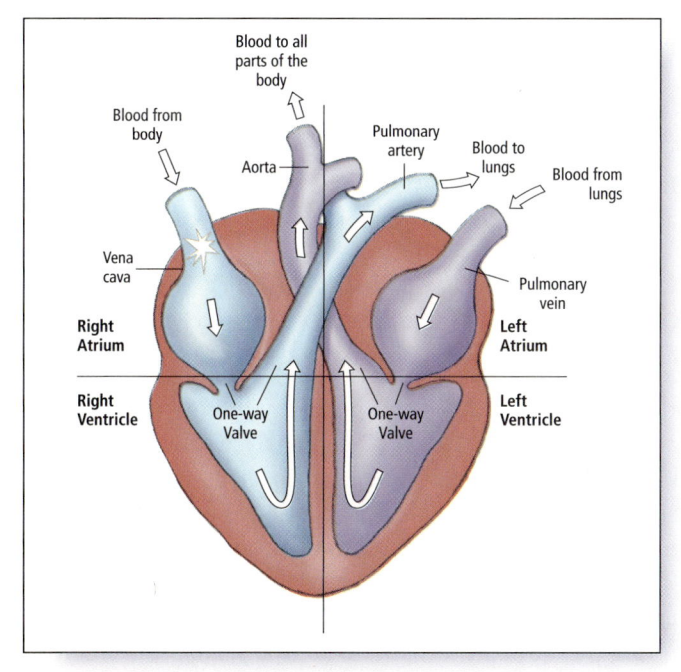

FIG 15.2 The four chambers of the human heart.

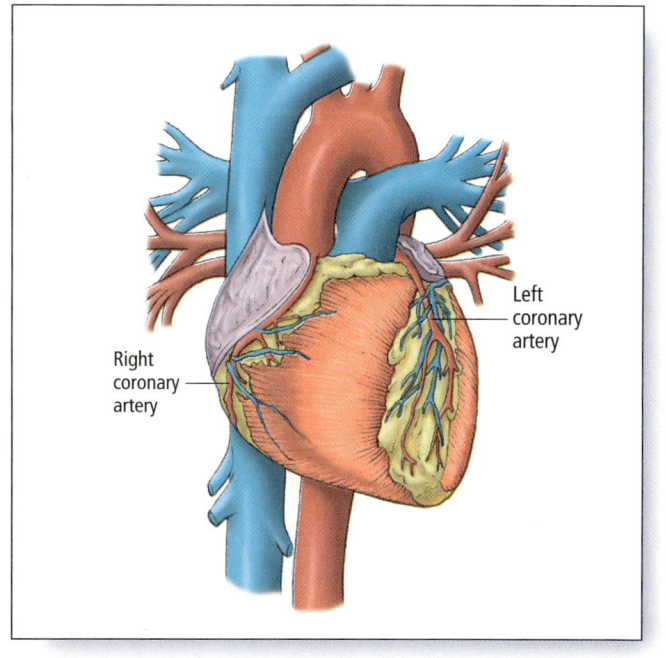

FIG 15.3 Coronary arteries of the heart that supply oxygen to the heart muscle.

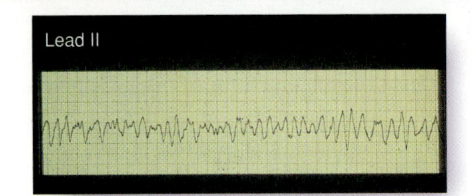

FIG 15.4 An example of an ECG tracing showing the abnormal heart rhythm ventricular fibrillation.

WHEN THE HEART FAILS

Sometimes the electrical system suddenly malfunctions. When this occurs, the result can be a life-threatening heart rhythm known as **ventricular fibrillation (V-fib)**. This abnormal rhythm is the most common cause of sudden and unexpected cardiac arrest in adults. About 75% of all sudden cardiac arrest patients are initially in ventricular fibrillation.

The organized wave of electricity that causes the heart muscle to contract and relax in a regular fashion is lost when the heart is in ventricular fibrillation. When that occurs, the chambers of the heart quiver (fibrillate); the heart cannot pump blood and the pulse cannot be detected.

A second potentially life-threatening electrical problem is known as **ventricular tachycardia (V-tach)**, in which the heart beats too fast to effectively pump blood. Depending on its severity, a pulse may or may not be present.

When the heart stops beating, the blood stops circulating, and all oxygen and other nourishment to the body is cut off. This is called *clinical death*, the start of the dying process. Without immediate intervention, death is certain.

The time factor is crucial. After 8 to 10 minutes of arrested circulation, damage may be so extensive that survival is no longer possible. This is called *biological death*. As the graph in Figure 15-5 shows, the chances of survival fade away with each passing minute of untreated cardiac arrest. The benefit of adding defibrillation to your resuscitation protocols is unquestioned.

DEFIBRILLATION

The definitive treatment for ventricular fibrillation is the delivery of an electric shock, known as **defibrillation**. This will momentarily stop all electrical activity in the heart. Then, the electrical impulses of the special pacemaker cells will take command of the heart muscle activity and produce a coordinated heart beat that will circulate blood throughout the body. It often takes more than one electrical shock to produce this effect on the heart. In some cases, shocks will not be successful due to severe heart muscle damage or other underlying factors.

AUTOMATED EXTERNAL DEFIBRILLATION

An automated external defibrillator (AED) is a device that replaces the need for hand-held defibrillator paddles and heart rhythm interpretation by higher trained medical personnel. An AED can analyze the heart's rhythm and signal the need to administer the electric shock (defibrillation) needed to convert the heart's abnormal electrical activity back to a rhythm that will generate a pulse. This makes early defibrillation by minimally trained personnel possible.

There are several different AEDs on the market. Regardless of the AED manufacturer, the principles for AED operation are the same for each type, but displays, controls, and options vary. Some models have screens that display the heart rhythm as well as visual and verbal prompts. Others have a screen displaying only visual prompts, and some have no screen at all. AEDs also have recording devices that store the guest's heart rhythm, shock data, and other information about the device. Some even record the voices of the rescuers for later playback. All AEDs are attached to the guest by a cable connected to two adhesive pads placed on the guest's chest. The purpose of the pad and cable system is to send the electrical signal from the guest's heart into the device for analysis, and secondly, to deliver the electric shock to the guest.

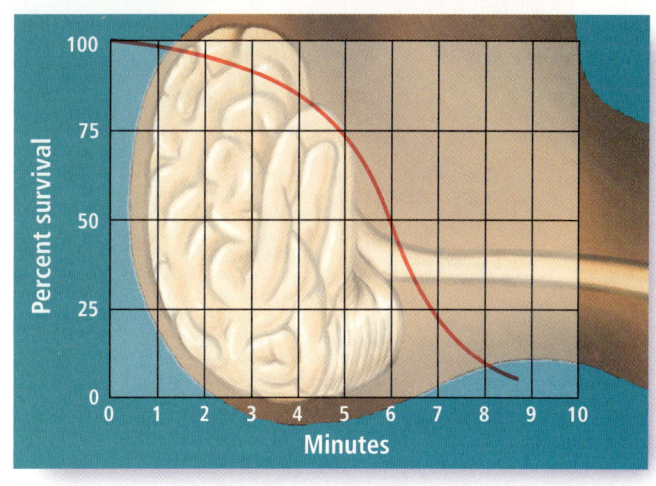

FIG 15.5 A guest's chance of survival decreases with each minute that passes without treatment.

GENERAL AED USE

As a lifeguard, you must become thoroughly familiar with the operation of the equipment you will use at your aquatic facility. Even with manufacturer differences, the basic operation of any device still follows the same four steps:

1. Turn the power on.
2. Apply the electrode pads.
3. Initiate analysis of the rhythm.
4. Deliver a shock as indicated.

Proper use of an AED involves practicing the following elements until they can be performed smoothly:

- Assess the safety of the scene and maintain control of the guests.
- Assess the guest's situation.
- Provide CPR until an AED is available.
- Follow specific AED protocols.

A successful AED operator can integrate these elements under stress. This can only be accomplished by thorough and repetitive training. The actual use of an AED is simple, but integrating the other elements in a smooth manner can sometimes be difficult, especially if your team has not rehearsed the steps.

Heartstart® 911 LIFEPAK® 500 VivaLink®

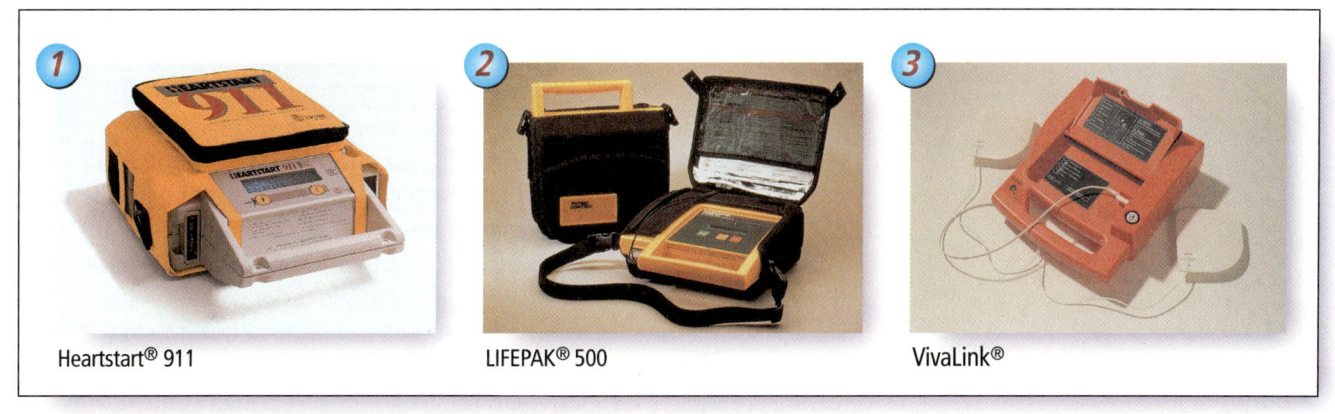

FIG 15.6 Examples of AEDs: 1) Heartstart® 911 2) LIFEPAK® 3) VivaLink®.

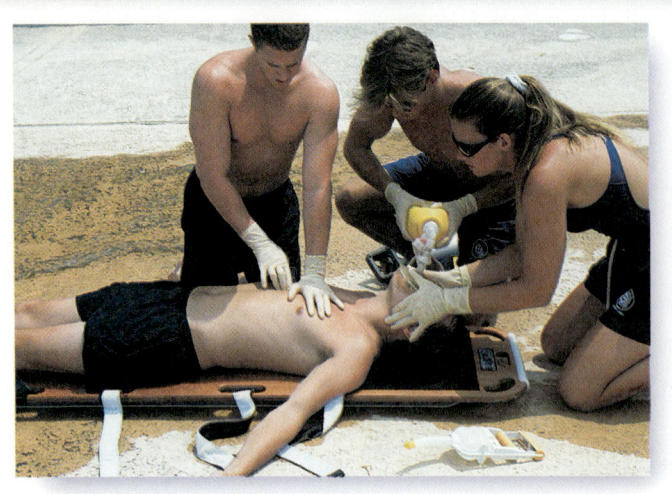

FIG 15.7 If the guest does not have a pulse, begin CPR until an AED is available.

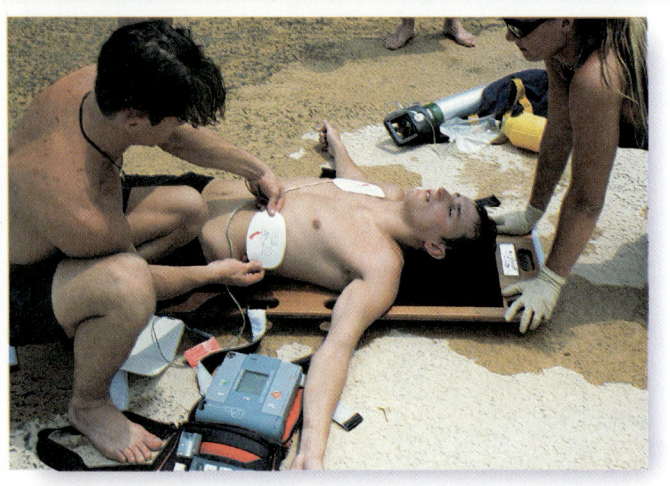

FIG 15.8 The pad and cable system pick up electrical signals for analysis.

MEDICAL DIRECTION

Upon successful completion of this program, you will have the skills necessary to effectively operate an AED. However, this program cannot authorize you to provide this treatment to guests. Defibrillation with an AED can only be administered under the authority of a physician. You will be operating under the physician's medical license when performing these skills. He or she will dictate the exact procedures and protocols you must follow for operation at your facility.

SCENE SAFETY AND CONTROL

Before approaching a guest, you must ensure that it is safe to do so. The scene must be assessed for possible dangers that could jeopardize your safety. To safely operate the AED, the guest rescued in the water must be placed on land, several feet away from the water. To prevent direct contact with the guest's blood or other bodily fluids, body substance isolation (BSI) precautions must be observed.

Cardiac arrest scenes can be chaotic. They often involve distraught family members and numerous bystanders. Bystanders may have some training and may offer their assistance. These people can be helpful as you begin your assessment and treatment of the guest. There will also be bystanders with or without training who may be a hindrance, as they crowd to see what is going on.

To ensure safe and fast assessment, application, and use of the AED, you must quickly gain control of the scene. Your actions in the first few minutes of an incident can determine how well scene control is maintained. In most cases, simply acting in a calm and professional manner will organize those present. Delegation of simple tasks will also give bystanders something to focus on. Tasks can include helping with CPR (if you need additional help, and you feel comfortable with their skills), directing additional responders to the location, and crowd control if necessary.

GUEST ASSESSMENT

The initial steps include identifying guests to whom you will apply the AED. These are the same steps you learned previously for CPR:

1. Determine unresponsiveness.
2. Check airway, breathing, and circulation (pulse).

AED PROTOCOL

In order to attach the AED to the guest, he or she must meet **ALL** of the following criteria:

- At least 8 years old
- Unresponsive
- Not breathing
- No pulse

When two lifeguards are present, one assesses the guest and begins CPR if necessary. The other lifeguard operates the AED. If you are alone and have the AED nearby, assess the guest, apply the AED, and proceed with the protocols prior to initiating CPR.

As an Ellis & Associates lifeguard, you will be trained to use an AED to help save lives. This device has been designed for safe operation around wet environments, when basic safety precautions are followed. These precautions include:

- Removing the guest completely from the water and moving at least two feet from the water's edge.
- Placing the guest on a backboard to ensure that he is not lying directly on a wet deck.
- Drying the guest's chest with a towel.

Always follow the directions provided by the AED voice prompts and screen!

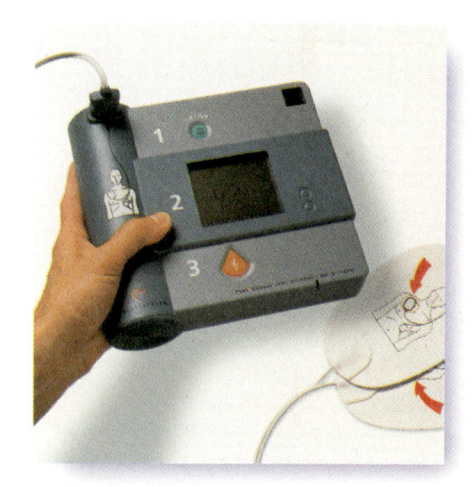

FIG 15.9 Heartstream ForeRunner® AED.

With the guest properly prepared, follow these specific steps to use an AED:

1. Turn the unit on by depressing the green on/off button on the device. At this point, voice and screen prompts guide you through the remaining steps.

2. Open the package containing the defibrillation pads and attached cable. Remove the backing and attach the pads to the guest's bare, dry chest as indicated by the illustration on the pads. Excessive body hair on the chest will interfere with adhesion and conduction and must be shaved off where the electrodes will be placed. (A razor is provided with the kit.) Insert the free end of the cable into the designated slot in the AED.

3. Stand clear of the guest and allow the AED to automatically analyze the heart rhythm. This takes at least five seconds.

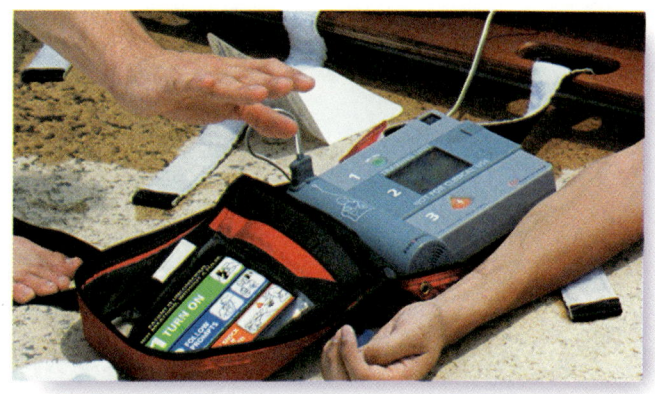

FIG 15.10a When the AED arrives, begin by turning it on, and then listening for instructions.

4. If a shock is indicated, you will be prompted to push the appropriate button. Make sure no one is touching the guest or any conductive material in contact with the guest. This can be accomplished by shouting loudly, "I'm clear! You're clear! Everyone's clear." Once it is safe to do so, press the shock button to deliver the electrical charge

5. Once the shock is delivered, the AED will re-analyze the rhythm and advise how to proceed. This could include delivering additional shocks or evaluating the guest for the presence of a pulse and performing one minute of CPR if the guest is pulseless.

6. After the third shock in a series, perform one minute of CPR.

7. After one minute of CPR, the AED will advise you to stand clear of the guest while it re-analyzes the heart rhythm.

Any time the AED detects a non-shockable rhythm during analysis, it will advise you to check the guest's pulse and begin CPR if pulseless. After one minute of CPR, it will advise you to stand clear of the guest while it re-analyzes the heart rhythm. Your local protocols will dictate how many sets of shocks can be administered prior to the arrival of EMS personnel.

If the Guest Regains a Pulse

If the guest regains a pulse at any time, follow your local basic life support treatment protocols. Do not turn off or remove the AED from the guest. These guests most often require oxygen, ventilation, and suctioning of the airway. You must recheck the guest's pulse and breathing periodically. Guests who have been successfully defibrillated can go back into V-fib and become pulseless again. Stand clear and allow the AED to automatically detect this problem and resume where it left off.

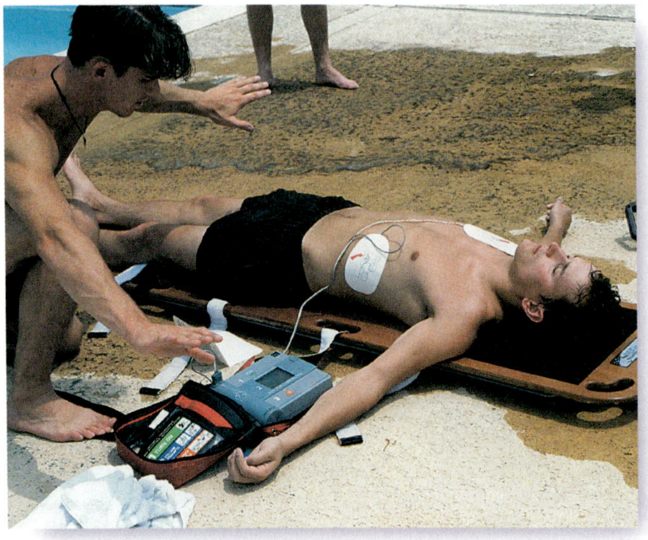

FIG 15.10b Dry off the guest's chest, apply pads, and stand clear to avoid any electrical charge.

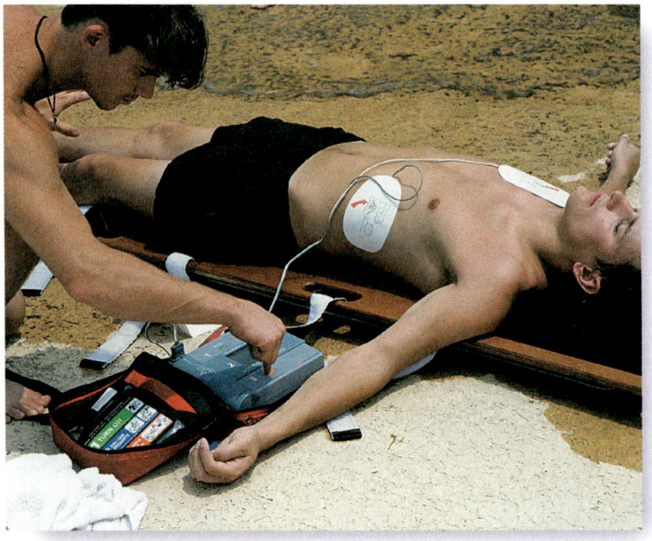

FIG 15.10c After analyzing the rhythm, the AED will advise if there is a need to administer a shock.

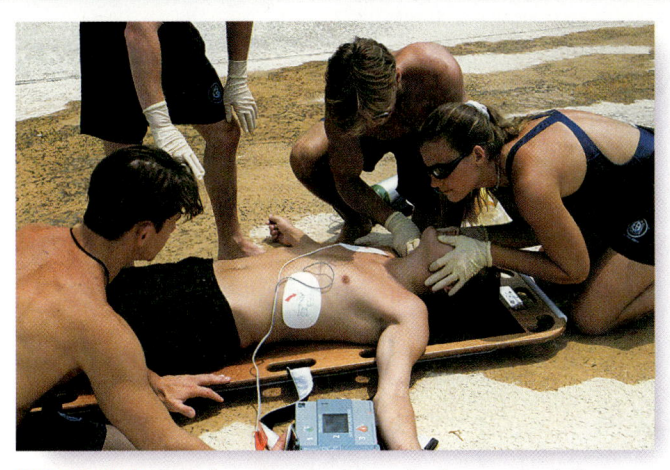

FIG 15.10d If the "no shock" advisory is given, recheck the guest's breathing and pulse.

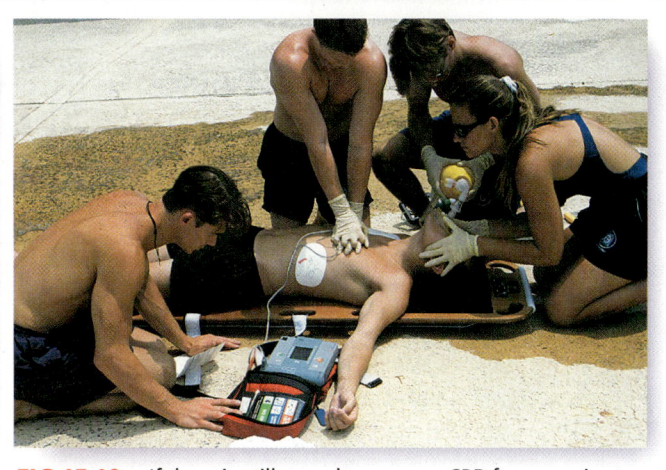

FIG 15.10e If there is still no pulse, resume CPR for one minute and then reanalyze.

Transferring Care

Upon arrival of EMS personnel, a concise report should be given regarding the incident and resuscitation efforts. Some AED screens also provide the following information:

- Elapsed time the device has been on
- Number of shocks delivered
- Current heart rhythm
- Heart rate (if applicable)

Prior to leaving the scene, EMS personnel will switch over to their own defibrillator. It is important to restock the AED with another package of electrode pads and to return it to its normal location.

Documentation

Documentation provides a permanent record of your actions during the incident. The written documentation should be a detailed account of your objective findings: assessment findings, treatment provided, and the guest's response to treatment. The form to be used will be provided by your facility. This documentation may become a legal document and a permanent part of the guest's medical record. Additionally, some AEDs have recording devices which store important information that can be reviewed later. If problems are identified, protocols or training may be changed to improve the level of care being provided to guests.

AED MAINTENANCE

Minimal time is needed to perform daily maintenance on your AED:

- Verify that it is ready for use by turning it on and evaluating its status.
- Ensure that all supplies, such as pads, spare battery, and razor are available and that expiration dates on packaging have not expired.
- Refer to your AED "Use Log" for weekly, monthly, and after-each-use maintenance tasks.

182 PART 3 • LIFEGUARD FIRST RESPONDER

AUTOMATED EXTERNAL DEFIBRILLATOR
Daily/Shift Inspection Checklist

Serial# _____ Date _____ Time _____

Model # _____ Inspected by _____

	Pass	Fail

Item:
Exterior/Cables:
Nothing stored on top of unit
Carry case intact and clean
Exterior/LCD screen clean and undamaged
Cables/connnectors clean and undamaged
Cables securely attached to unit

Batteries:
Unit charger is plugged in and operational (if applicable)
Fully charged battery in unti
Fully chaged spare battery
Spare battery charger plugged in and operational (if applicable)
Valid expiration date on both batteries

Supplies:
Two sets of electrodes
Electrodes in sealed packages with valide expiration dates
Razor
Hand towel
Alcohol wipes
Memory/voice recording device—module, card, microcassette
Manual override—module, ke (if applicable)
Printer pater (if applicable)

Operation:
Unit self-test per manufacturer's recommendation/instructions
    Display (if applicable)
    Visual indicators
    Verbal prompts
    Printer (if applicable)

Attach AED to simulator/tester:
    Recognizes shockable rhythm
    Charges to corect energy level within manufacturer's spefications
    Delivers charge
    Recognizes nonshockable rhythm
    Manual override system in working orger (if applicable)

Signature _____

FIG 15.11 Example of an AED maintenance chart.

SPECIAL SITUATIONS

There are some types of guests who will require additional steps before applying the AED. The following list of special considerations outlines these different types of guests and how to deal with them.

Children and Infants

AED's are not designed or tested to interpret heart rhythms or administer energy for children. The current guidelines for emergency cardiac care recommend that AEDs not be used for guests under 8 years old.

Medication Patches

Some guests wear an adhesive patch containing medication that is absorbed through the skin. These patches need to be removed and the skin wiped clean prior to beginning CPR or applying the AED. If an electrical current is passed through a pad, sparking and burns may occur. In addition, you can absorb some of the medication if it comes in contact with your skin; be sure to use BSI precautions.

Pacemakers

Pacemakers use electrical impulses to correct problems with the heart's normal electrical rhythm. Pacemakers are usually placed just underneath the skin on the upper left side of the chest and can be visualized or felt after exposing the chest. Avoid placing the pads over or near the pacemaker as it can absorb or reflect some of the energy, thus decreasing the chance of a successful defibrillation.

Implantable Defibrillators

Some guests have small automatic defibrillators placed in their body. They are usually found just underneath the skin in the upper abdomen and can be visualized after exposing the guest's abdomen. They are about the shape and size of a deck of cards. As with the pacemaker, avoid placing electrodes over or near the unit. If the unit is firing (visible twitching of the guest), allow it to stop before applying the pads.

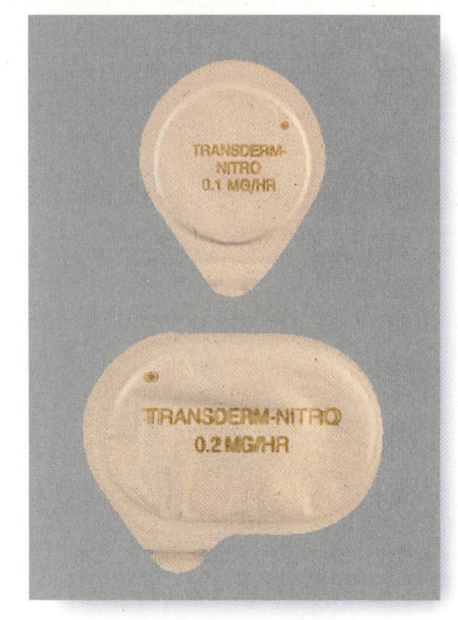

FIG 5.12 Medication patches must be removed before beginning CPR or applying the AED.

REVIEW QUESTIONS

1. Which link in the Chain of Survival is the most critical in restoring a normal heart rhythm following a cardiac arrest?
   a. Early access
   b. Early CPR
   c. Early defibrillation
   d. Early ACLS

2. The most common initial abnormal heart rhythm in a person undergoing cardiac arrest is:
   a. Normal sinus rhythm
   b. Ventricular tachycardia
   c. Ventricular fibrillation

3. List the four general steps involved in the operation of any AED.

   a. _____

   b. _____

   c. _____

   d. _____

4. A guest has collapsed in the locker room. He is unconscious, not breathing, and has no pulse. If an AED is immediately available, your first step is to:
   a. Perform one minute of CPR.
   b. Apply the AED.
   c. Call 9-1-1 or your local emergency number.
   d. Perform the Heimlich Maneuver.

5. After delivering the first three shocks, what is the next step?
   a. Administer three more shocks.
   b. Check pulse, and if absent, do one minute of CPR.
   c. Check breathing.
   d. Call 9-1-1 or your local emergency number.

6. Which of the following guests should have the AED applied? Assume all guests are not breathing and do not have a pulse.
   a. 15-year-old male found submerged in a pool.
   b. 60-year-old female found in the locker room.
   c. 10-year-old weighing 90 pounds.
   d. 6-year-old weighing 80 pounds.

7. (T) (F) Treatment differs if a guest is found to have an implantable defibrillator or pacemaker.

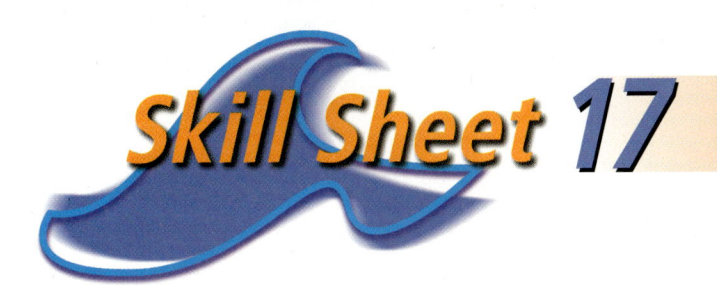

CHAPTER 15 • AUTOMATED EXTERNAL DEFIBRILLATION

Skill Sheet 17

USING THE AED

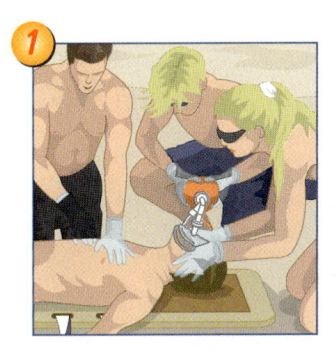

1. Unresponsive, no breathing, no pulse. Perform CPR until defibrillator is available.

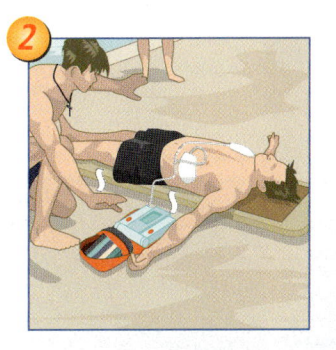

2. Turn power on. Attach pads to guest's chest and cable to AED.

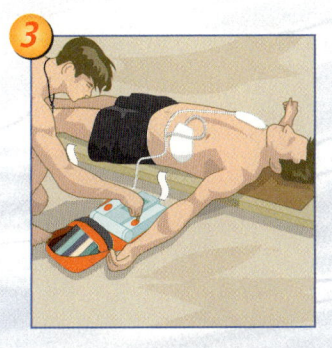

3. If shock is indicated, clear guest. Press to shock. Await analysis and follow prompts.

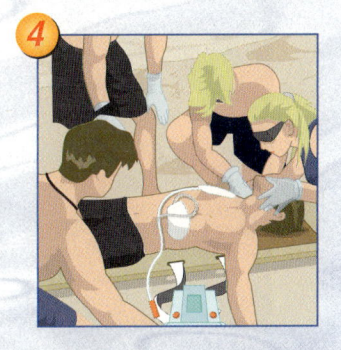

4. If shock not indicated, check pulse. If no pulse, do CPR for 1 minute. Re-analyze and follow prompts.

KEY POINTS:

- Apply the AED as quickly as possible to any guest who is unrespnsive, not breathing, and pulseless.

- Follow the same four general steps for using any AED.

- Anytime an AED gives a "no shock" advisory message, check the guest's pulse. If pulseless, perform one minute of CPR as re-analyze.

CRITICAL THINKING:

1. A child has been removed from the water. He is unresponsive, not breathing and pulseless. No one is available to tell you his age or weight. You think he is about 9 years old, but uncertain abou; his weight. What do you do?

2. Following the delivery of a shock, the AED analyzes sand advises "no shock" needed. You check the pulse, and there is one present. What do you next?

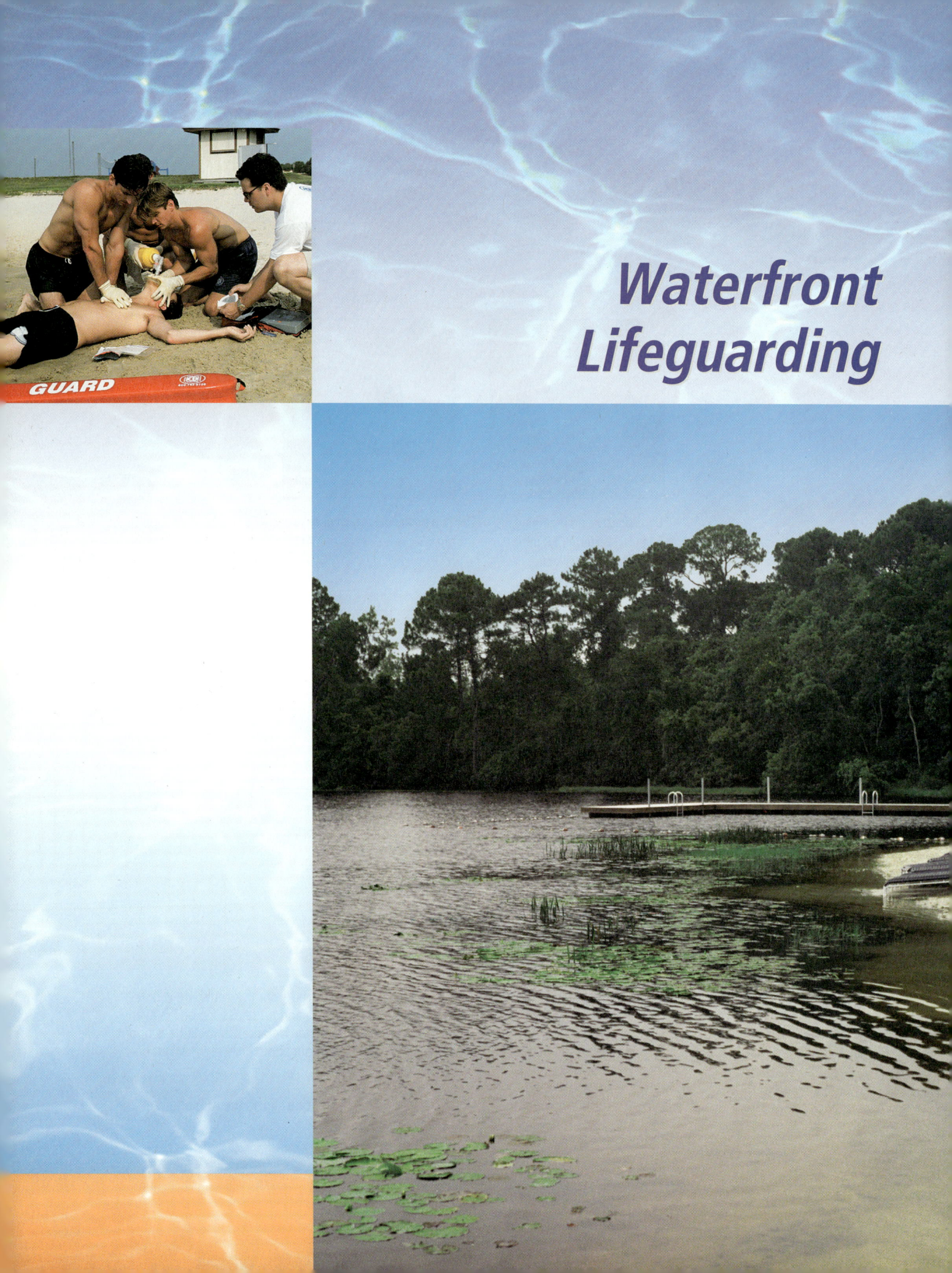

Waterfront Lifeguarding

chapter 16

SIXTEEN

OBJECTIVES

After reading this chapter and completing the related course work, you should be able to:

1. Describe how your surveillance technique of a waterfront differs from that of a pool.

2. Describe how the equipment used for lifeguarding a waterfront differs from the equipment used for lifeguarding a pool.

3. Demonstrate how to use a rescue board to rescue a conscious or unconscious guest.

Common Causes of Incidents in Waterfront Environments

- Holes or sudden drop-offs that guests might step into.
- Areas where water depth is unknown, where diving accidents could occur.
- Cold water, causing shock.
- Currents that guests are unable to handle.
- Waves washing guests onto rocks.
- Wind that may cause a guest to be hit by flying objects (sand, rocks, etc.).
- Novice or non-swimmers falling off piers, rock jetties, or inner tubes.
- Items obscured by the sand or water, such as broken or sharp bottles or cans that guests might step on.
- Guests' inability to swim.
- Swimmers pushing and dunking each other.
- Guests entering water at unguarded beaches.
- Untrained persons attempting rescues.
- Careless or poor boat handling by novice boaters.
- Guests being on board non-seaworthy crafts.

Open-water facilities such as lakefronts, resorts, camps, and other non-surf areas present challenges you will not normally find when you are lifeguarding a pool. The general principles of lifeguarding are the same, but each open-water facility is unique and may require some facility-specific training.

It is important to keep in mind that while the lifeguarding skills presented in earlier chapters apply to waterfront as well as to pool settings, there are several instances where you will need to modify your technique or use slightly different equipment to maintain open-water safety and effectively manage rescues. These modifications to technique and the different equipment used in open-water facilities are the topics that will be discussed in this chapter. By having this information, you will be aware of your options and can choose the most effective rescue method in your lifeguarding situation.

One of the largest differences between lifeguarding open-water areas and lifeguarding pools is the modification of the 10/20 rule. Because of the greater distance you will be responsible for in an open-water environment, the recognition and rescue rule for open-water facilities is 10/3 minutes. 10/3 stands for recognition in 10 seconds, and rescue in 3 minutes or less. This means that lifeguard coverage must be sufficient to allow you to reach any part of your zone within 3 minutes. It is crucial for you to maintain the 10/3 minute rule while guarding open-water areas, because in addition to dealing with the common difficulties of guests, there are the added hazards of the natural environment.

PREVENTING INJURIES THROUGH PROPER SURVEILLANCE

As a proactive lifeguard, you must constantly scan your zone to prevent incidents from occurring needlessly. Some of the actions you can take while scanning, which will lessen the chances of harmful incidents occurring, are to: caution the overambitious swimmer about the dangers of swimming too far from shore; warn guests not to swim in unguarded or restricted areas; and tactfully, but firmly, inform rule-violators of the actions you or your supervisor will take on behalf of your facility if they continue to disregard the rules. It is also very important that you develop an awareness of activities outside your lifeguard zone that may affect the safety of guests in your zone.

Inspecting Your Facility

You and the other lifeguards at your open-water facility should conduct frequent and regular safety inspections of both the immediate area (beach, shoreline, and shallow water) and your equipment. While conducting your inspection, you should carefully survey your entire area for sharp or potentially tainted objects such as broken glass, rocks, and litter; check the lifeguard stands for hidden objects that could injure you as you come down from the stand; inspect docks for loose or rotting wood and weak or frayed anchor lines; and assess shallow water for sharp objects, depressions, and obstructions. Inspect your equipment daily for cleanliness and make sure that it is in good working condition and in the correct location. Always report damaged or missing equipment immediately to your supervisor.

CHAIN OF COMMAND

All open-water facilities will have one or more supervisors, and your responsibilities will be defined by your facility's chain of command. There may be several layers to the chain, such as aquatic coordinator, aquatic supervisor, facility supervisor, and head lifeguard. Some chains may include staff such as park rangers, security guards, swimming and boating instructors, and concession-stand employees.

You should familiarize yourself with all of the staff at your facility until you know their names, titles, and responsibilities, and the way each of their positions relates to the others. In an emergency, it will be crucial for you to know whom to contact. It is essential that you (and the other staff members) report any problems to your supervisor, so that he or she is aware of them.

WATERFRONT RESCUES

When you are lifeguarding at an open-water facility, begin your rescue attempt by climbing down from the lifeguard stand, taking all of your equipment with you. Since there may be a considerable distance between you and a distressed guest, it will usually be best to use rescue watercraft or a rescue board to reach him rapidly. If you do not have either of these items available, and you must make a swimming rescue, you will have

> **critical POINT**
> For every injury, there is a cause, and for every cause, there is a preventive measure. Taking precautions can prevent a minor incident from developing into a major one.

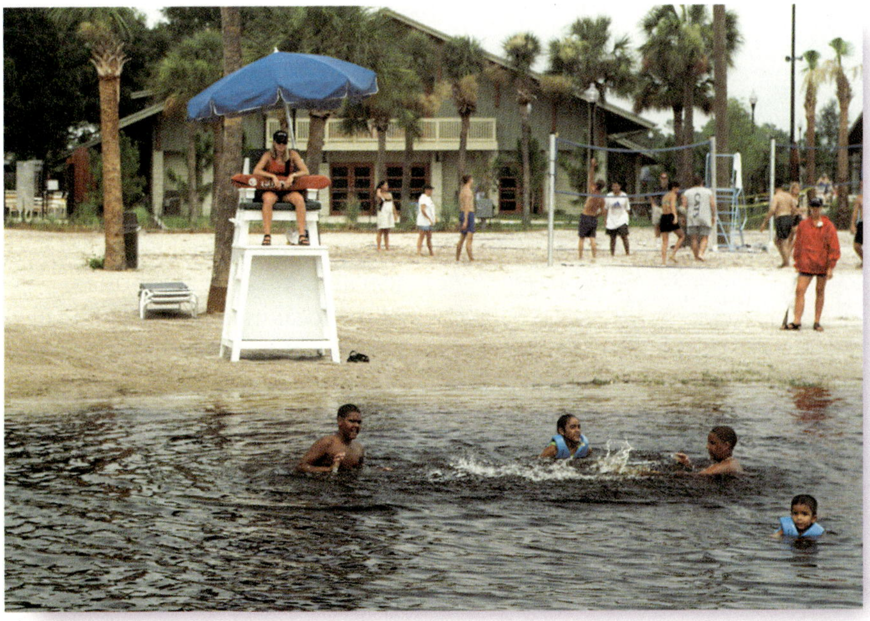

FIG 16.1 Lifeguarding a waterfront.

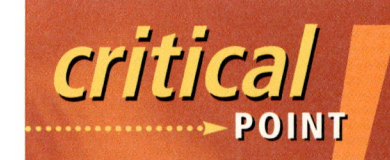

greatest efficiency if you trail your rescue tube behind you as you swim, rather than swimming with it in front of you as you would in a pool. Evacuate the swimming area until another lifeguard is available to cover the your zone—only attempt a rescue alone if no assistance is immediately available.

CLEARING THE BEACH

When you go off duty, clear the swimming area, announce that the lifeguards are now off duty, and give the time when supervised swimming will re-open.

IDENTIFICATION AND SAFETY CHECKS

It is important to identify and communicate with large groups that visit your facility. Discuss your facility's rules and regulations with group leaders and guests. Some facilities may have rules, such as requiring swimmers to take a shallow water swim test before allowing them to enter deep water.

WATERCRAFT

If your waterfront facility uses watercraft for rescues, it will be important for you to learn to use them correctly in various rescue situations, and in risky weather conditions. Practice until your skill level meets your facility's standards and you are familiar with the watercraft's safe use guidelines.

As an open-water lifeguard, one of your responsibilities may be to patrol your zone from the water. Although each facility will have some different rules and regulations, usually all watercraft are subject to them equally. As you patrol, check to see that the edges of your zone are clearly marked so that safety limits are obvious to watercraft operators. Your facility can also post signs at boat launch areas to warn boaters of the "swimmers only" sections of the water prior to launching their boats.

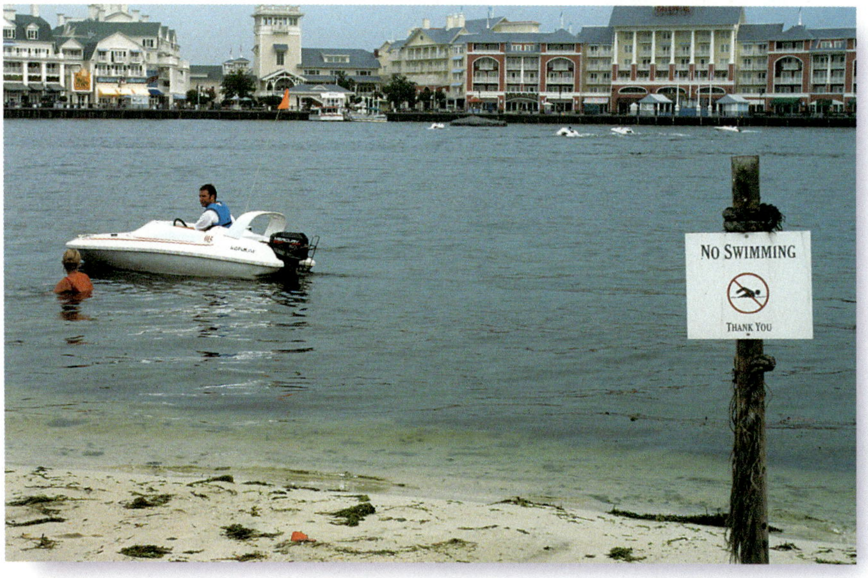

Open-water speed limits are usually set by the authorities of the local municipality, and fall between 8 and 35 miles per hour (mph); they also can be accompanied by a "no-wake" policy. The watercraft speed at your open-water area will determine the safety zone you must maintain between boaters and swimmers. You should discuss this with your supervisor, who may be responsible for patrolling the lake for

FIG 16.2 As you patrol, scan the edges of your zone from your watercraft to ensure safety for your guests.

speeding and safety violations, to avoid confusion. Usually, lifeguards and park rangers respond first, and, if necessary, they contact local law enforcement officers for reinforcement.

Your rescue watercraft should be equipped with the following items at all times:

- Coastguard approved P.F.D.'s
- Full tank of gas
- Two-way FM radio system
- Fire extinguisher
- Rescue tube
- First aid kit
- Anchor and line
- Oxygen unit
- Bailer
- Emergency blanket

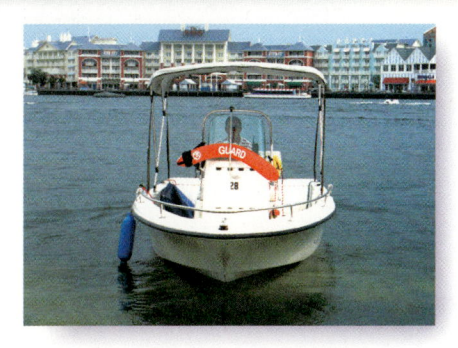

FIG 16.3 Watercraft are used at many facilities for water rescues and patrols.

If there is enough storage space, and you are certified and authorized to dive in the area with a partner, it could be helpful to keep scuba gear on board.

DOCKS

There are three common types of docks used for swimming, boating, and fishing. Most open-water facilities distinguish among these three areas, and use each only for its designated purpose, to help eliminate unsafe conditions for guests.

NOTIFICATION SYSTEM

One of the most common means of alerting swimmers to current water and weather conditions is the **flag system**. Flags should be placed in a central location, along with directions to educate guests on their purpose. The lifeguard or waterfront supervisor monitors the water and weather conditions, and directs the placement of the correct flag.

- A **green flag** means the beach is open, and water and weather conditions are safe for swimming.
- A **yellow flag** means that swimmers should exercise caution because weather and water conditions are changing, and are being monitored by the lifeguards.
- A **red flag** means no swimming, and the area is (being) closed because water and weather conditions are dangerous.

WEATHER

Weather conditions are a day-to-day concern for open-water facilities. The risk of weather-related problems is best addressed by a comprehensive plan that monitors weather daily.

The most common weather concerns for open-water lifeguards are thunderstorms and lightening strikes. Thunderstorms can be very unpredictable, and can cause swimming conditions to deteriorate dangerously within minutes. The best course of action to prepare for lightning is to develop an individual waterfront policy that encompasses safe shelter not only from lightning, but from the other natural elements that often accompany it, such as hail, high winds, and tornadoes.

It is the lifeguard's responsibility to scan the sky for impending thunderstorms, and to provide guidance to the facility's guests for their safe departure from the area. Many open-water swimming areas are in heavily forested locations, making visual assessment difficult. A possible solution to this situation may be coordinating a hazardous weather warning system with local law enforcement personnel. If you notice thunder or lightning near the facility, inform your supervisor immediately. Depending upon the severity of the weather, the facility may need to be closed.

Another weather danger involves high wind that results in large crashing waves, hypothermia, and swimmer fatigue, and will negatively affect your ability to respond to a distressed guest within 3 minutes.

On some waterfronts, fog may obscure buoy markers, and watercraft may inadvertently enter a restricted area. Fog may also jeopardize your ability to scan your zone effectively. If fog becomes too dense for effective scanning, it may be necessary to close your zone. If you observe that the fog is becoming a problem, you should immediately inform your supervisor.

Other weather factors that you should be aware of include: water temperature, visibility, and water level. Cold water can quickly cause hypothermia, which endangers both the judgment and endurance of swimmers. Water visibility can change overnight as a result of a storm, and water levels may fluctuate considerably with rainfall. These factors will affect a rescue, so you need to keep them in mind.

Severe Weather Conditions

Your facility will have procedures for you to follow during severe weather conditions, and learning these procedures will be part of your initial training. If a tornado warning is issued by the National Weather Service for your county, your facility manager will immediately announce to guests via the public address system that the beach will close due to impending severe weather and that they must vacate the water immediately. In addition, guests will be asked to seek shelter.

POTENTIAL HAZARDS

Changing Water Conditions

Water and weather conditions at open-water facilities can fluctuate daily. The water can range from being very calm some days to being very active other days. If you are experiencing a day with a lot of wave action and the waves are high enough that you are losing sight of swimmers, adjust your observation techniques by standing on the guard tower. If you decide that conditions are too dangerous to swim, let your supervisor know, so that he or she can make the judgment about whether to close the facility.

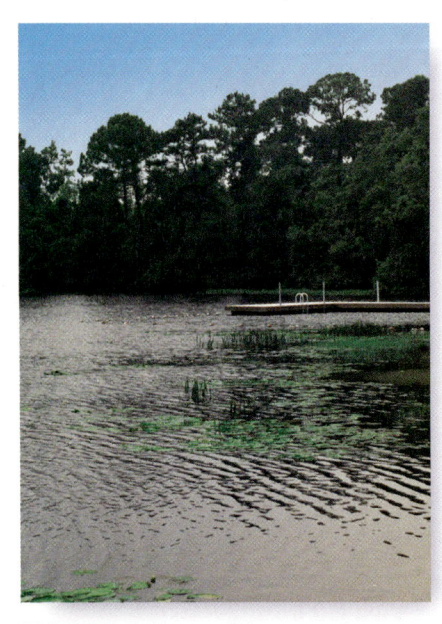

FIG 16.4 Water conditions can change quickly from calm, as seen in this photo, to tubulent, almost without warning.

Aside from the danger of waves, unusually heavy or light rainfall can also be dangerous, as they can change water depth and currents. As the summer season progresses, water depth can decrease and become too shallow for diving.

Underwater plants are another hazard. Underwater plants can present risks to swimmers by limiting both your and their visibility, and entangling them. Some open-water facilities actually harvest underwater plants in or near designated swimming areas, to reduce the growth and danger.

Water Temperature

Water temperature can be deceptive to swimmers, as it may be warm on the surface, but much colder as the depth increases. Water temperature is usually colder in early summer than it is later in the season. You can help swimmers avoid hypothermia by alerting them to cold water conditions and watching them carefully for signs and symptoms of hypothermia. Cold water becomes a serious concern for swimmers and lifeguards during a rescue. If you must conduct a rescue in very cold water, you may want to wear a wet suit to minimize the effects of cold water on yourself. As with pool rescues, avoid personal risks. If you become a victim yourself, you cannot help the initial victim.

Water Visibility

In calm water areas, visibility is usually best in the early morning. Under some conditions, visibility can be reduced to less than one foot. Stirred-up sediment, bad weather, and plant growth can all contribute to create a visibility-blocking cloud during a submerged guest rescue, or during a missing person search. Because of this, it is important to clear the swimming area to maintain as much visibility as possible during the rescue operation.

Bottom Conditions

As a lifeguard, you should be aware of items that can be potentially harmful to both yourself and guests, such as rocks, glass, and fishing lines and hooks; you should remove or have these items removed from the area whenever they are found.

Many lakes have natural conditions that cause silt to build up, in some cases as deep as four feet. Silty lake bottoms are dangerous because they can hinder search and rescue efforts. As part of your facility's training, you should rehearse rescue operations during all types of conditions.

Refuse and Contaminants

At some waterfronts, lifeguards are responsible for clearing the beach of trash and debris. It is important to keep the beach clean, because the cleaner it is, the less there will be to attract animals and water fowl invaders. Another potentially contaminated factor to watch for and report to your supervisor is runoff from roadways and storm drains during heavy rain storms.

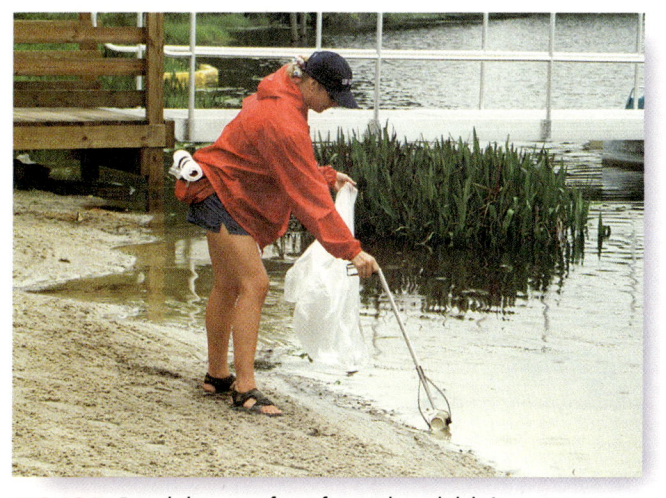

FIG 16.5 Patrol the waterfront for trash and debris.

Wildlife and Parasites

If there is a large population of water fowl, lily pads, millfoil, and algae on the lake, the possibility of parasites and/or swimmer's itch exists. Many waterfront areas have adopted policies to prohibit the feeding of ducks and geese, so that the birds will leave the area and limit liability to swimmers.

RESCUE EQUIPMENT

Waterfront lifeguards use some of the same equipment that pool lifeguards use, as well as some additional equipment that is specialized for open-water use. As part of your ongoing responsibilities, you should inspect all equipment daily, to ensure that it is in rescue-ready shape, and in the proper location. You should record the condition of safety equipment daily. Equipment your facility may include the following:

- Searching devices, such as masks, fins, and snorkels.
- Communication devices, such as whistles, megaphones, radios, a PA system, and a telephone.
- Rescue devices, such as rescue tubes, backboard, first aid equipment, lifejackets, watercraft, rescue boards, and scuba equipment.

Equipment must be reliable and easily accessible in an emergency. If equipment has been damaged or stolen, report it to your supervisor immediately. Lifeguards need to know how to use all equipment at their facility. If there is some equipment you are unfamiliar with—a public address system, for example—let your supervisor know that you need instruction in its use.

Rescue Tubes

Rescue tubes can support up to 700 pounds, and are extremely durable and easy to use. Because of this versatile durability, rescue tubes are recommended for use at waterfront settings. Rescue cans are much more difficult to use than rescue tubes, and are designed mainly for conscious guests.

Rescue Boards

Many open-water facilities station a lifeguard on a rescue board at the perimeter of a swimming area during times when the facility is crowded. A lifeguard on a rescue board can reach a distressed swimmer efficiently because a large area of water can be covered quickly. In a rescue situation, it is important to know how to handle yourself, the rescue board, and the guest in distress effectively.

Portable First Aid Kits

A portable first aid kit is very useful when you need assistance immediately, and are far away from first aid stations or other help.

Mask, Fins, and Snorkel

Masks, fins, and snorkeling equipment can be helpful for searching the bottom of the swimming area during your facility inspection, and also in guest recovery situations. As with other equipment, you must become proficient in its use before you are involved in a rescue situation.

Scuba Equipment

You may sometimes need scuba equipment to search the bottom of the swimming area, especially in deep lakes. Scuba diving involves a special training course, and you should not use scuba gear if you are untrained. Check with your supervisor to see if your facility has a cooperative agreement with a local scuba shop, or fire and rescue response team, for diver assistance in emergencies.

Binoculars

Binoculars are standard equipment for larger lakes and recreation areas. They make it possible for lifeguards to recognize problems in the distance.

Megaphone and Radio Usage

Megaphones are often used for communication during crowded, noisy times, and two-way radios are often the standard communication equipment used in large beach areas. Radio systems are designed to provide quick and effective communication among personnel in different locations during an emergency.

Telephones

Telephones will always be located at open-water facilities in an accessible location. Telephones are emergency units and must be accessible at all times. Pay telephones must be accessible to your guests so you can keep your telephone available for emergencies.

POLICIES AND PROCEDURES

Each waterfront area will have its own policies and procedures for opening and closing, ensuring water safety, responding to emergencies, and maintaining beach security. These policies and procedures will list responsibilities of various personnel. Your original training at the facility should include the lifeguard's responsibilities and the reporting system. The development of risk management and accident protection plans are a management responsibility, but you should know your own duties and responsibilities for the supervision of patrons and rule enforcement.

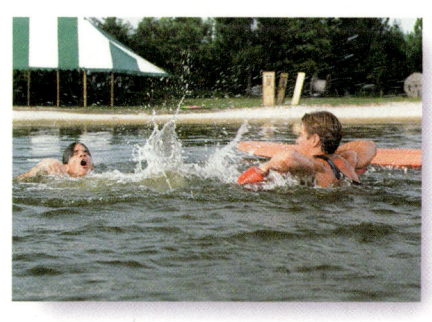

FIG 16.6 Active guest rescue at waterfront.

10 Second/3 Minute Rule

The *10 second/3 Minute Rule* is applied with the same principles as the pool and waterpark 10/20 Protection Rule. The size of the designated open-water area should reflect the ability of each of the staff on duty to scan his or her assigned area every 10 seconds, and reach and recover a victim within a maximum time of 3 minutes.

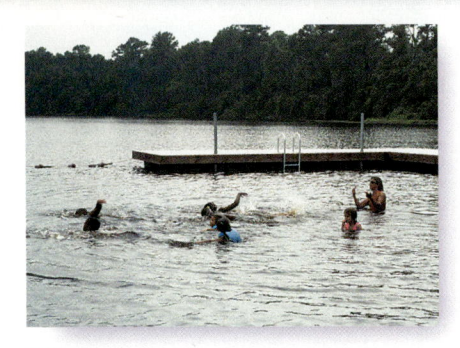

FIG 16.7 Guests within designated swimming area.

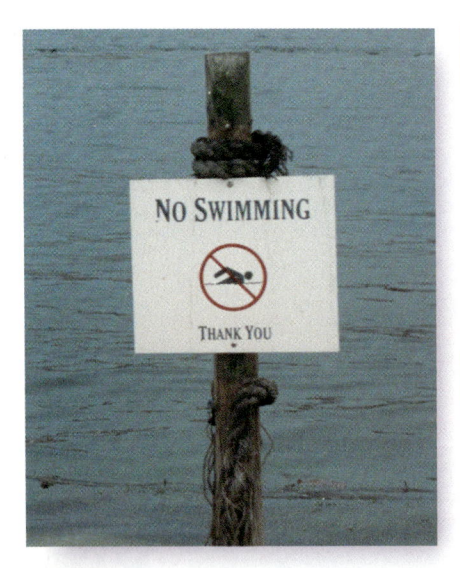

FIG 16.8 Refer guests to the posted rules whenever necessary.

SAFE SWIMMING AREAS

It is your responsibility to keep guests within the designated swimming areas, and your zone should be well-marked so that you can call the guests' attention to buoy markers or signs, if you need to. If there are hazards within the swimming area, you should caution guests about those areas, and make certain they are marked with hazard signs. In some facilities, if these hazards are not removable, you may be posted near them.

SIGNAGE FOR GUESTS

Your facility should have signs posted to inform guests of rules and warnings. These rules and warnings need to be specific to your individual waterfront area. You may need to call a guest's attention to a particular sign or warning, as you caution him regarding hazardous behavior. If it is apparent that a guest does not understand a warning sign, you should inform your supervisor.

EMERGENCY RESPONSE

You need to know your role and be ready to respond appropriately in emergency situations. Knowing your role includes being familiar with your facility's emergency action system (EAS), and your waterfront's layout. EAS plans differ depending upon the size and shape of the facility, the number of lifeguards and other staff on duty, available equipment, and the relationship with local EMS personnel.

STAFF RESPONSIBILITIES IN EMERGENCIES

Lifeguards' responsibilities will vary from facility to facility. You may have specific responsibilities to conduct safety checks. Certainly in an emergency you will need to activate your EAS. Be sure that you understand your responsibilities in guest safety and in your facility's emergency response system. If a guest reports to you that someone is missing, you must report to your supervisor at once, and/or activate the emergency action system.

Emergency Action Systems have been discussed in other sections of this text. Such systems for waterfronts are very facility-specific, and you will be trained in the system for your waterfront during pre-season and in-service training sessions throughout the season. It is your responsibility to retain competency in the various aspects to which you will be assigned. In particular, if you will be doing boat rescues, you need to practice regularly, so that in an emergency you can react quickly and with competence. For example, patrol boat rescues may require you to run the boat to waist-deep water, vault in, row to the guest, drop anchor, ship oars, pull the guest into boat, and then return to shore. Other facilities may have you perform the rescue and begin care in the water until other rescuers arrive in a watercraft. These and other procedures will be covered in your facility training.

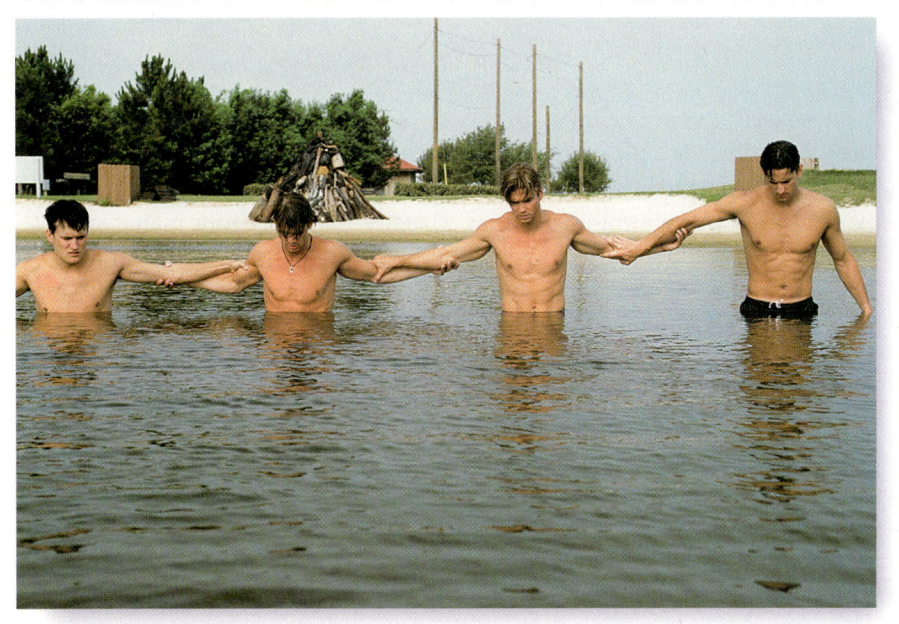

FIG 16.9 Walking line search team.

Missing Guest Search

If you suspect that a missing guest is submerged, there are two search skills that you may use to find him. These skills are the snorkeling swim search and the walking line search.

You may perform the *snorkeling swim search* when you a guest is submerged in deep water. This type of search is coordinated with a rescue team by performing surface dives, and then realigning on the surface to repeat the process. You can modify this procedure based upon your environment and staff input. The rescue swimmers should be utilized to find a victim within three minutes.

You may perform the *walking line search* when the water is shallow enough to walk in, but too murky for you to see the bottom. This procedure may require the assistance of all staff members and possibly some guests. To begin this procedure, position all rescue participants in a line, linking arms with each other. The line should move forward in unison, under your direction, or under the direction of the designated line leader. The line members conduct the search by stepping forward with a sweeping motion of their legs. The line should be utilized to find a victim within 3 minutes.

Violent Incidents

You must handle violent incidents very carefully. If violence occurs at your waterfront, try to keep your distance physically while intervening verbally. Your first action should be to see to the physical and emotional safety of the guests. You can help ensure the guest's safety by warning them to stay away. Lifeguards should not physically confront violent or potentially violent guests, but allow law enforcement officials to take restraining measures and document the problem. You should collect data for the law enforcement officials, such as a description of the person and his watercraft or land vehicle.

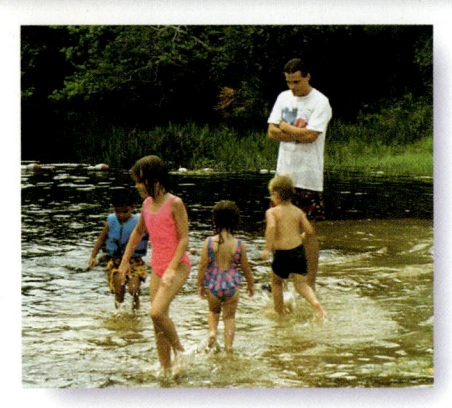

FIG 16.10 Camping groups can present special challenges.

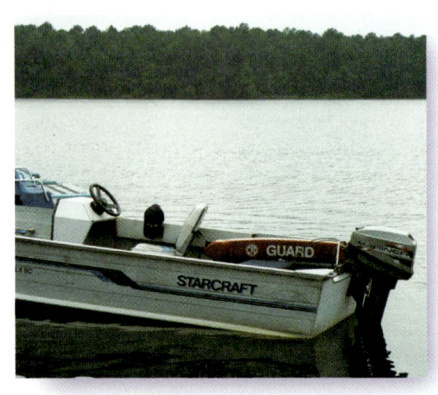

FIG 16.11 Lifeboats should only be used by lifeguards for patrolling or training sessions.

LIFEGUARDING THE AQUATIC CAMP

Your waterfront may be used for day or other camping groups. Your responsibilities as a lifeguard remain essentially the same, although you may be asked to help conduct swim skill screening prior to children's participation in swimming activities. Usually, the waterfront manager will conduct such tests, and assign children to specific groups. You may be asked to conduct periodic "buddy checks" for campers, or to explain the rules and safety considerations to them.

Waterfront Equipment Skills

Boatmanship

The lifeboat can be the most important part of your equipment at some waterfronts. Your responsibilities in the lifeboat are the same as they are on shore and in lifeguard stands. Your alertness in the lifeboat will coincide, and cooperate, with the alertness of the lifeguard on shore. This will guarantee that no time or effort will be lost in emergencies. If one lifeboat is out of position for any reason, the adjacent lifeboats should cover its area until the boat has returned. During active patrol, the stern should face the shore to permit an unobstructed view of the swimmers. Lifeboats must only be used by lifeguards, and only for the purpose of patrolling or conducting in-service training sessions.

If your facility uses boats for rescue, your initial training, as well as follow-up inservice sessions, will include practice using such craft. If you are inexperienced in rowing, you should practice the techniques described here. Rowing a boat for pleasure can look deceptively easy; rowing rescue craft demands practice. Expertise in rowing can make the difference between a rapid, effective rescue and a slow and inefficient one. In other words, it can make the difference between life and death for a drowning person.

When you are rowing a boat, take a position in the exact center of the seat, and place your feet on the foot rest. Bend your legs slightly until you are comfortable. Properly equipped boats are furnished with a stretcher that you can adjust to the desired distance. Keep your back straight and shoulders square.

Grip the oars as close to the ends of the handles as possible; place your fingers over the top and your thumbs underneath. You should never place your thumbs over the ends of the handles because you can injure yourself. Hold the oars with your wrists straight, and make sure the blade of each oar is perpendicular to the water's surface.

To start the stroke, bend forward from your hips, with your arms extended straight ahead. Raise your arms, dip the blades gently into the water, and pull. In the first part of the stroke, pull with your back and shoulders. Finish the stroke by bending your elbows and pulling with your arms, bringing your body upright. Your stroke should be steady, firm, and even. As your arms pull against the oars at the finish and you bring your body upright, the natural spring of the oars adds a final "kick" to the stroke, increasing propelling power and aiding in the recovery. Do not reach too far forward at the beginning of your stroke, and do not extend it too far at the end. These movements increase the length of the stroke, but at these extremes the stroke has little propelling force.

When you are using long-handled oars, the handles tend to collide on recovery unless one handle is brought back slightly in advance of the other. With unusually long-handled oars, this also may be necessary on the stroke, but there is less danger of the oars colliding because of the angle at which the oars make the stroke. In a boat with ample "freeboard," that is, one in which the gunwales are high enough above the water level, it usually is possible to pull the oars in parallel movements without danger of their colliding.

You may also use alternate arm movements to stroke. As one arm is stroking, the other is recovering. The stroke and recovery of each oar is accomplished with the same technique as previously described, except that your body remains stationary and you control the oars entirely with your arms. Consequently, your strokes are short and rapid. This method is frequently used for rest and relief after a long period of rowing. The chief value of this method is in locations where careful steering is necessary. When watching for hazards or approaching a dock, the oarsman can look back over his shoulder while stroking rapidly, and can direct the boat by pulling longer and harder on one oar.

Rescue Board

The rescue board is a valuable piece of equipment for the open-water lifeguard. It can serve as a platform from which you observe the swimming area, or as a rescue device that can cover great distances very quickly.

Performing a Rescue

Entry into the water may be accomplished in several different ways, depending on your environment. Ellis & Associates recommend that you enter the water directly with the rescue board, and approach the distressed swimmer from the water, as opposed to running down the beach with the rescue board.

To maintain consistency and to continue to provide protection, you will be required to have a rescue tube with you even when you are using a rescue board. You can accomplish this by wearing the rescue tube strap over your shoulder, and allowing the rescue tube to drag behind you while you are paddling toward the guest.

When you enter the water, hold the board on the sides around its midpoint for stability. When you reach waist-deep water, mount the board with either a prone/lying position, or a kneeling position. It is critical to practice your initial entry and boarding, to master the balance you need.

When paddling the rescue board, there are two types of positions you may use: the kneeling position, or the prone position. It is important that you practice maintaining balance and stability in both positions. The prone position is preferred because it maintains a low center of gravity. Once in position on the rescue board, use a butterfly or crawl stroke to get to the guest.

Approach the guest from the side, bring your rescue tube to a holding position, and dismount from the board. Gain control of the rescue tube before

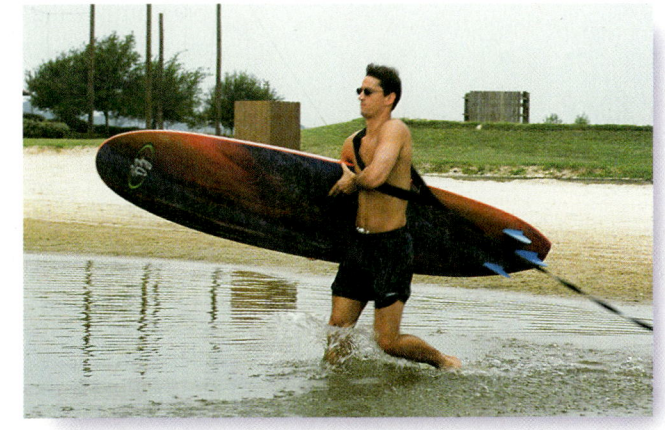

FIG 16.12 Enter the water with your rescue board and rescue tube.

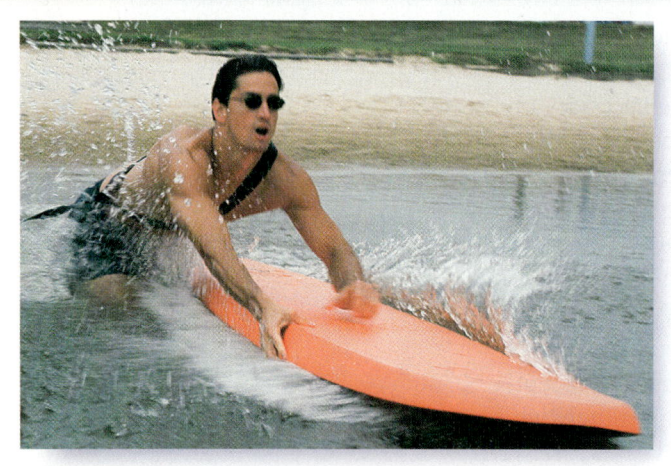

FIG 16.13 When you reach waist-deep water, place yourself in a prone position on the rescue board.

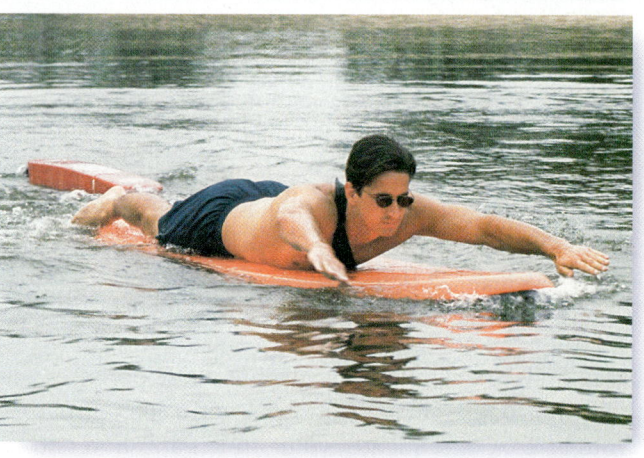

FIG 16.14 Paddle out to the guest.

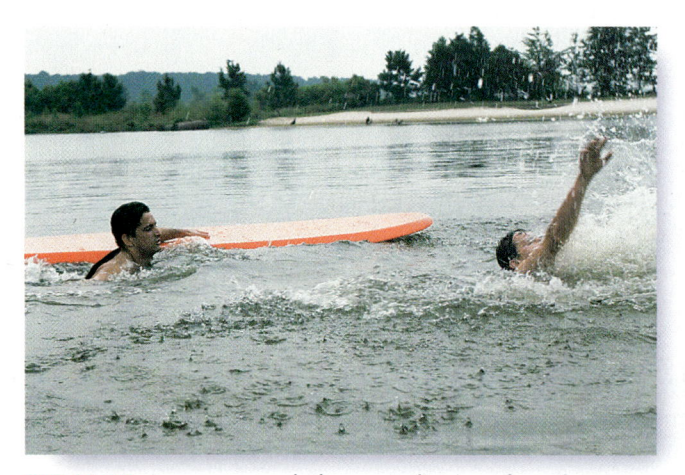

FIG 16.15 As you approach the guest, dismount from the rescue board.

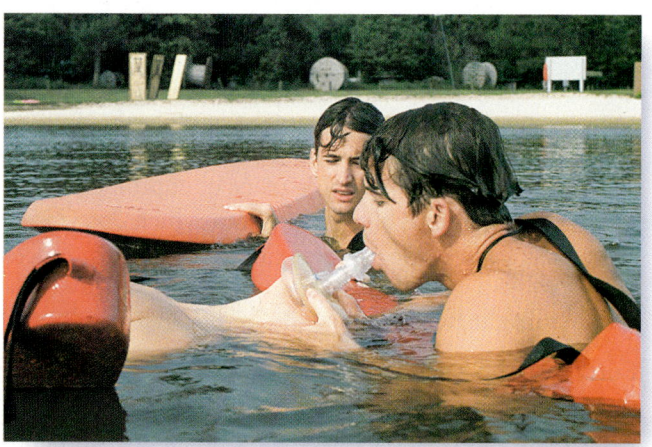

FIG 16.16 Begin to provide care until a second lifeguard arrives to assist you.

attempting to rescue the guest. Execute the necessary rescue. Bring the guest back to safety, either by swimming with him using the rescue tube, or by using the rescue board.

If the guest is unconscious, summon additional assistance and begin the Heimlich Maneuver. If the guest does not begin to breathe, begin rescue breathing while moving toward the shore. A second lifeguard can extend an additional rescue tube, recover your rescue board, and paddle to shore, towing you and the guest if necessary. A second option for you to use is to roll the unconscious guest onto the rescue board, mount the board, and paddle to the shore. However, this will delay the initial care of clearing the airway and providing oxygen. This skill requires significant practice and can only be accomplished on a large, wide rescue board, capable of supporting both you and the unconscious guest.

Once you reach the shore, drag the guest away from the water and continue to provide care. Once you have practiced and developed proficiency in the use of rescue boards, you will find that board rescues are both faster and easier than distance swimming rescues.

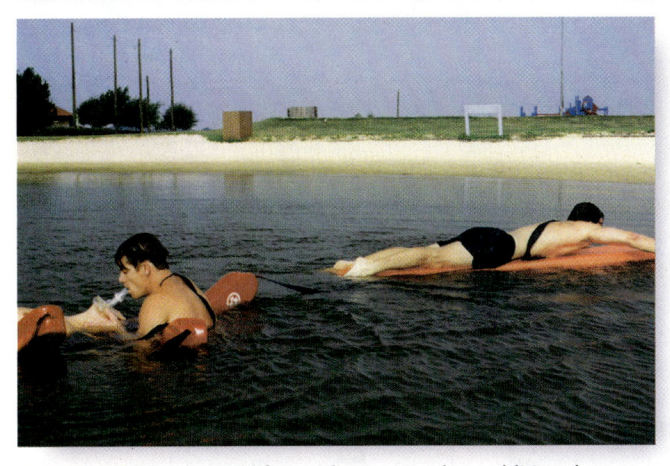

FIG 16.17 The second lifeguard can extend an additional rescue tube, recover your rescue board, and paddle you into shore.

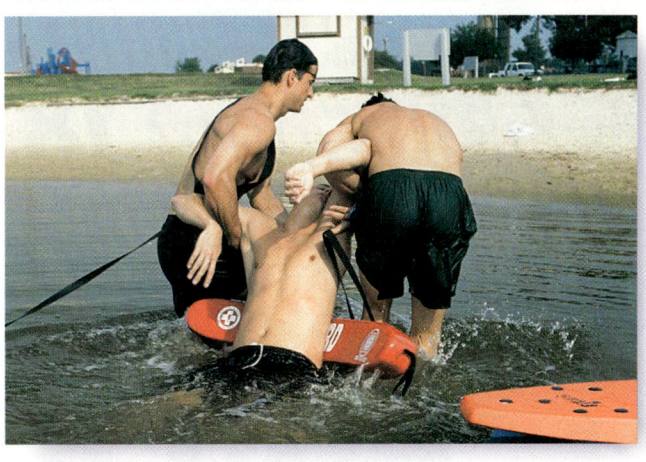

FIG 16.18 Once you reach the shore, drag the guest away from the water and continue to provide care.

REVIEW QUESTIONS

1. List four common causes of incidents at waterfront facilities:
   a. _____
   b. _____
   c. _____
   d. _____

2. What is the purpose of the flag system? What does each flag signify?

3. In flat-water areas, what time of day is visibility usually the best?

4. List several natural environmental hazards that make it so crucial for you to maintain the 10/3 Protection Rule while you are lifeguarding at an open-water facility.

5. Give two examples of rescue equipment used at open-water facilities, but not at pools and waterparks:
   a. _____
   b. _____

6. Identify three weather factors that you should be aware of as a waterfront lifeguard.
   a. _____
   b. _____
   c. _____

7. Identify and describe the two search techniques you will use if you suspect that a missing guest is submerged.
   a. _____
   b. _____

Skill Sheet 18

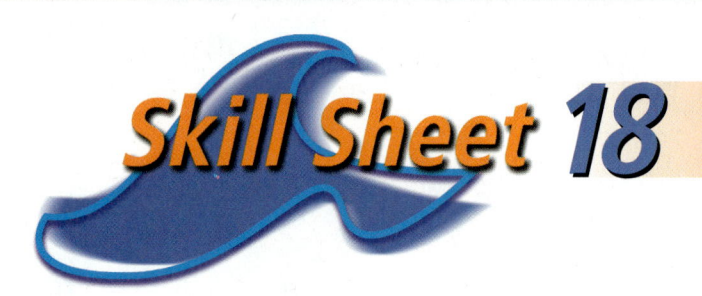

WATERFRONT LIFEGUARDING

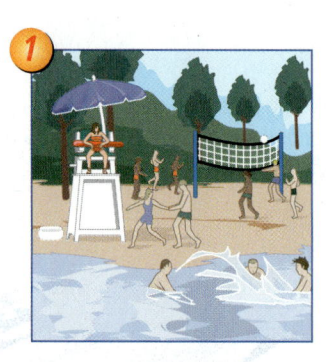

1. Lifeguarding the aquatic camp.

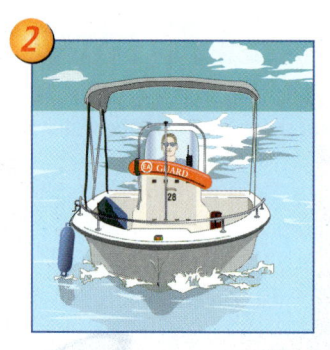

2. Practicing and maintaining your skill level with your facility's watercraft will be essential to the success of your rescue incidents.

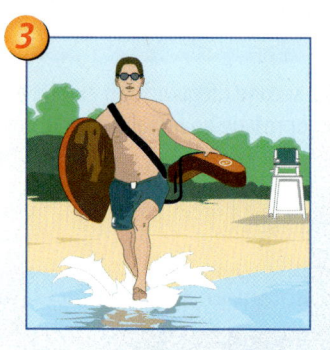

3. Enter the water holding your rescue board around its mid-point for stability.

KEY POINTS:

- Know the common causes of incidents at waterfront facilities.
- Carefully inspect your facility.
- Be aware of how environmental changes can impact your facility.
- Practice using your rescue devices frequently.

CRITICAL THINKING:

1. How would you quickly organize a team of lifeguards to reach for a missing child?
2. How would you get the attention of a swimmer who is out beyond the designated swimming area at your facility?

part FOUR 4

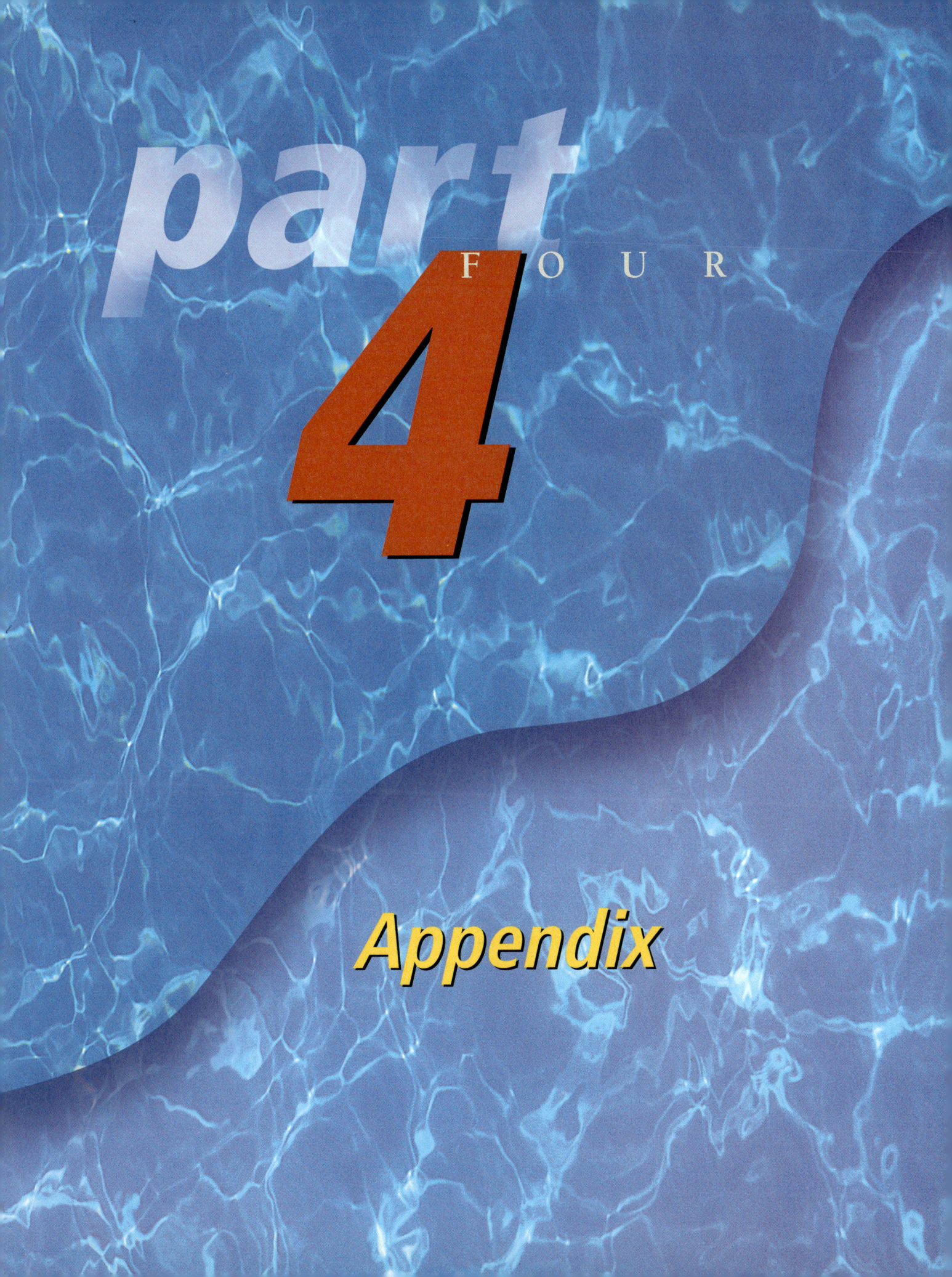

Appendix

Appendix A

Sample Rescue Flow Chart: PASSIVE GUEST

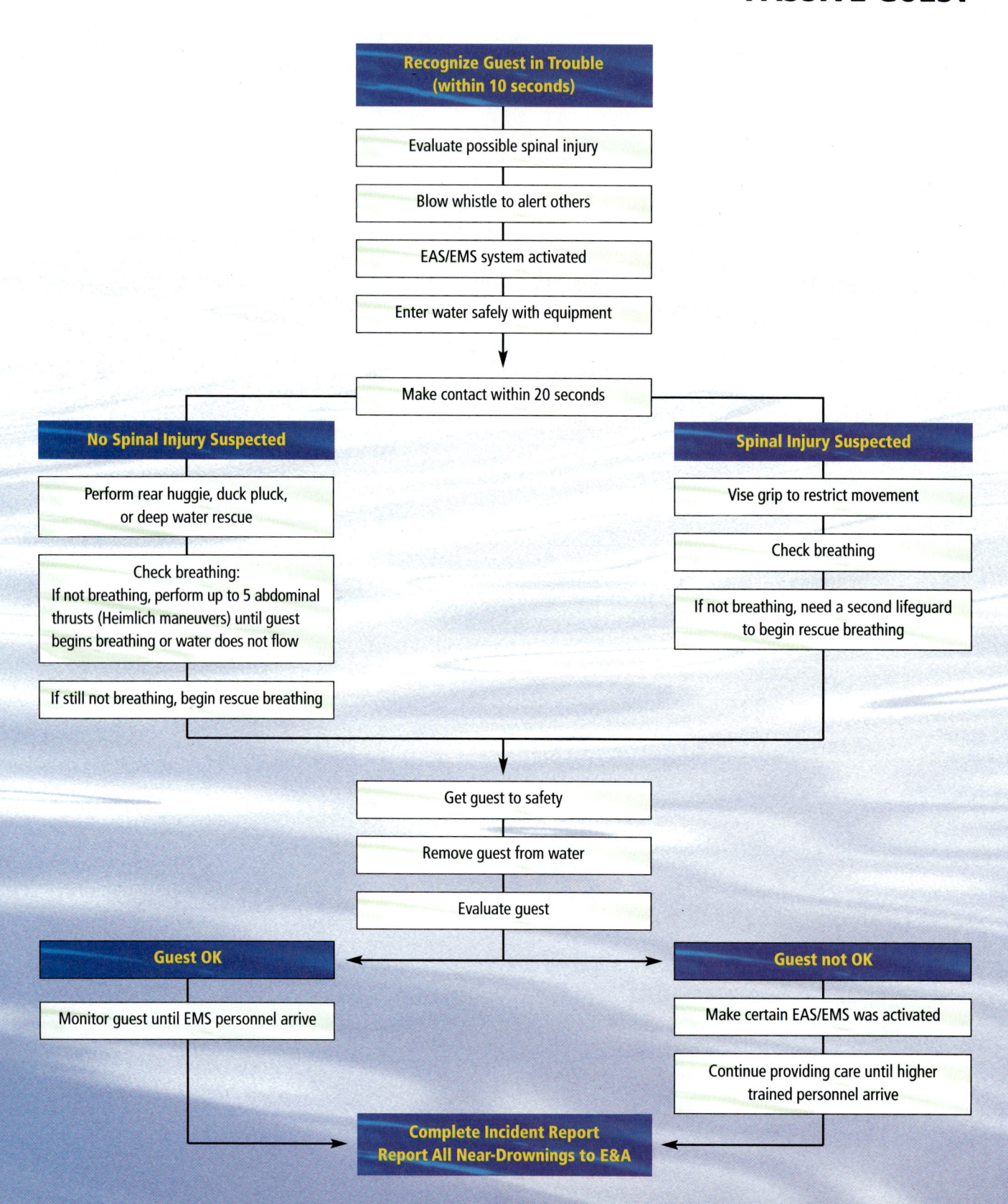

Recognize Guest in Trouble (within 10 seconds)
↓
Evaluate possible spinal injury
↓
Blow whistle to alert others
↓
EAS/EMS system activated
↓
Enter water safely with equipment
↓
Make contact within 20 seconds

No Spinal Injury Suspected
- Perform rear huggie, duck pluck, or deep water rescue
- Check breathing: If not breathing, perform up to 5 abdominal thrusts (Heimlich maneuvers) until guest begins breathing or water does not flow
- If still not breathing, begin rescue breathing

Spinal Injury Suspected
- Vise grip to restrict movement
- Check breathing
- If not breathing, need a second lifeguard to begin rescue breathing

↓
Get guest to safety
↓
Remove guest from water
↓
Evaluate guest

Guest OK
Monitor guest until EMS personnel arrive

Guest not OK
- Make certain EAS/EMS was activated
- Continue providing care until higher trained personnel arrive

Complete Incident Report — Report All Near-Drownings to E&A

Sample Rescue Flow Chart: ACTIVE GUEST

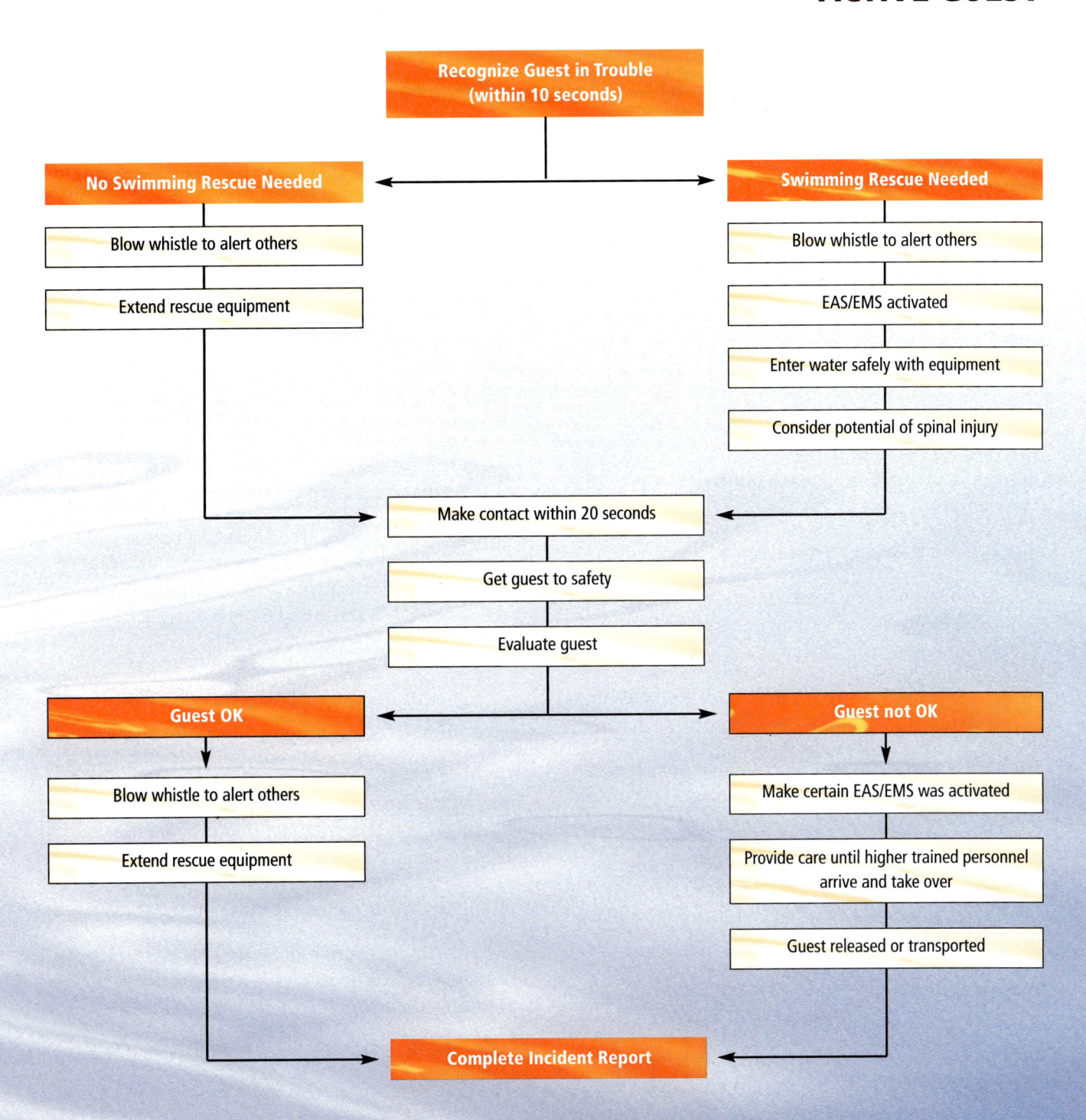

Recognize Guest in Trouble (within 10 seconds)

No Swimming Rescue Needed
- Blow whistle to alert others
- Extend rescue equipment

Swimming Rescue Needed
- Blow whistle to alert others
- EAS/EMS activated
- Enter water safely with equipment
- Consider potential of spinal injury

- Make contact within 20 seconds
- Get guest to safety
- Evaluate guest

Guest OK
- Blow whistle to alert others
- Extend rescue equipment

Guest not OK
- Make certain EAS/EMS was activated
- Provide care until higher trained personnel arrive and take over
- Guest released or transported

Complete Incident Report

Appendix B
Glossary of Key Terms

10/20 second protection rule. Allowing a lifeguard 10 seconds to recognize an aquatic emergency and another 20 seconds to perform a rescue and begin care.

10/3 minute protection rule. Allowing a lifeguard 10 seconds to recognize an aquatic emergency and 3 minutes to perform a rescue and begin care.

Abdominal thrust. Pushing upward on the abdomen to remove a foreign body obstruction and open the airway.

Abrasion. An open wound from a scrape that damages the surface of the skin.

Airway management. Keeping open the passage through which air goes into the lungs.

Anaphylactic shock. A type of shock that occurs when the body has a severe allergic reaction.

Approach stroke. Any combination of leg kicks and arm movements that allow you to make the fastest forward progress in the water.

Assist. To help a distressed swimmer while being able to maintain the 10/20 Protection Rule in the zone.

Audit. The process through which lifeguards are held accountable for maintaining their skills and professionalism at "test-ready" levels at all times.

Automated external defibrillator (AED). A device that analyzes the heart's rhythm and signals the need to administer an electric shock (defibrillation) to a patient in cardiac arrest.

Avulsion. An open wound with a portion of the skin or tissue torn away from the body.

Backboard. A rigid board with straps to secure the body and a device to secure the head. It is used to remove a guest with a suspected spinal injury from the water while minimizing the movement of the body and the head. It is also used without straps to quickly and safely remove an unconscious guest from the water.

Backboarding. The process used by two or more lifeguards to remove a guest with a suspected spinal cord injury from the water without further injury to the spine.

Bag-valve-mask (BVM). A device with a face mask attached to a bag with a reservoir, and connected to oxygen, that is capable of delivering 90% supplemental oxygen to a patient.

Biological death. The point when body cells and systems begin to die, and survival is no longer possible; usually occurring 8 to 10 minutes after circulation stops.

Bloodborne pathogen. Viruses or other disease organisms that are carried by the blood.

Body substance isolation. Articles of clothing and other devices that are worn by rescuers to limit or eliminate direct contact with a patient's potentially infectious blood or other bodily fluids.

Cardiac arrest. The point in time when the heart has stopped pumping blood and functioning.

Cardiopulmonary. Referring to the heart (cardio) and lungs (pulmonary).

Cardiopulmonary resuscitation (CPR). A combination of chest compressions and rescue breathing used to help sustain oxygen to the brain via the lungs until EMS arrives. It is used for someone who is not breathing and does not have a pulse.

Cervical. The area of the spinal column most susceptible to injury, because it has the least amount of protection—the neck.

Clinical death. The exact point in time when the heart stops beating.

Coccyx. The tailbone and last 3 t0 4 vertebrae of the spine.

Compact jump. An entry into the water from a height keeping the rescue tube up under the armpits, feet flat, knees slightly bent. It is designed to minimize the risk of injury to the lifeguard while allowing for speed in initiating a rescue.

Crowd control. Giving directions or controlling the behavior of a large group of people at one time.

Deep water rescue. A rescue in which the guest in distress is below arm's reach.

Defibrillation. The delivery of an electric shock to a patient in cardiac arrest, that will momentarily stop all electrical activity in the heart, thus allowing the pacemaker cells to produce a coordinated heart beat.

Diligence. The attention and care expected and required of you by your facility.

Dehydration. Loss of water in the body.

Disability. A condition that takes away the normal ability to do something.

Distress. Being unable to maintain a position on top of the water, or being unable to make progress to safety without assistance.

Distressed swimmer rescue. A rescue for a guest who has shown an inability to remain upon, or return to, the surface of the water.

Drowning. Death caused by A) a fluid in the lungs or B) a laryngospasm.

Dry drowning. Asphyxiation, or suffocation, resulting from a laryngospasm. Water droplets irritate the epiglottis, which closes over the glottis preventing air from entering the air passage; there is no water in the victim's lungs.

Duck pluck. A rescue technique used to bring a person who is just under the water to the top, using a rescue tube.

Emergency action system (EAS). The integration of all the people, equipment, and plans involved in dealing with an emergency, such as aquatic staff, EMS response team, bystanders, facility administrators, etc.

Emergency action plan (EAP). A plan written for a specific facility and type of emergency that outlines step-by-step emergency procedures and responsibilities.

Emergency medical system (EMS). Trained personnel who respond to an emergency when you call 911 or your local emergency number.

Epiglottis. A cartilage behind the tongue which works like a valve over the windpipe.

Extension assist. When you help a guest reach safety by extending a body part, pole, rescue tube, or other device.

Extrication. Removal of a nonbreathing guest from the water, whom you do not suspect of having a spinal cord injury.

Feet first surface dive. A method of propelling the body toward the bottom, feet first, by pushing the water upward with the arms.

Flag system. System by which centrally located colored flags are used to alert guests and guards of changing weather conditions.

Foreign body. An object that causes an obstruction or blockage of a person's airway.

Front drive. A rescue technique used when a guest is actively in distress on top of the water, performed with a rescue tube.

Golden Rule (of guest relations). Treat people like you would like to be treated.

Guest relations. The way in which you treat and respond to guests at your facility.

HBV. A virus carried in the blood (bloodborne) that causes Hepatitis B, an incurable disease that affects the liver and is potentially life-threatening.

Head-tilt/chin-lift. Tilting the head back while lifting the chin to open the airway of an unconscious person.

Heat cramps. Cramps in the muscles caused by loss of water and salt from the body due to overexposure to heat.

Heat exhaustion. A heat-related illness that is caused by loss of significant amounts of fluid from perspiration. The symptoms include profuse sweating; fatigue; cool, pale, sweaty skin; nausea/vomiting.

Heat stroke. A life-threatening rise in body temperature due to overexposure to heat and breakdown of the body's temperature control system. It is a life-threatening condition.

Heimlich Maneuver. The technique of clearing a nonbreathing patient's blocked airway by providing him or her with abdominal thrusts.

Hemorrhaging. Massive bleeding.

High risk. Conditions or characteristics that make it more likely for an accident or incident to happen.

Hyperthermia. Heat related emergencies that occur when a person spends too much time in a hot environment, without taking in enough fluid to maintain the body's equilibrium.

Hypothermia. A loss of body heat.

Hypovolemic shock. Inadequate circulation of oxygenated blood to the vital organs, as result of the body's attempts to recover from severe injury or trauma.

Hypoxic convulsions. Due to lack of oxygen in the brain, persons may appear rigid or stiff, may jerk violently, and/or froth at the mouth.

Impairment. A condition that takes away from the strength or quality of being able to do something.

Inservice. Training received after obtaining a lifeguard license and becoming employed at an aquatic facility.

Insulin shock. A condition when a diabetic has to much insulin and / or too little sugar.

Intervertabral discs. Circular cushions of cartilage that separate the vertebrae.

Jaw-thrust. A method of opening the airway in patients with suspected neck injuries.

Laceration. A soft tissue open wound that has a ragged or torn edges.

Larynx. The upper part of the trachea (windpipe) where the vocal cords are located.

Liability. Being legally responsible.

Lifeguard first responder. A lifeguard or aquatic professional who is responsible for activating the EMS when a life-threatening emergency occurs, and managing with appropriate care until help arrives.

Life-threatening. An injury or condition that could cause loss of life if specific care is not given.

Lumbar. The lower back area.

Mechanism of injury. The means by which the incident occurred, which the first responder should gather for his or her incident report, or for the EMS provider's report.

Musculoskeletal. The muscle and bone systems of the body.

Near drowning rescue. A rescue for an individual who has become unconscious during an immersion incident.

Post incident stress. The emotional, psychological, and physical stress that can occur after an individual had been involved in a traumatic experience.

Primary survey. Examining or checking a person to see if they have any life-threatening conditions.

Professional image. Giving the impression of responsibility, authority, friendliness, and competency to guests at your facility by the way you look and act.

Protected lakefront. An area of open water that has been sectioned off by buoys, ropes, docks, or boats to control access by guests.

Pulse. The verification of a beating heart, achieved by feeling the blood expand and contract in the arteries.

Puncture wound. A wound with little bleeding, caused by a sharp pointed object piercing and entering the skin.

Qualifying questions. Questions asked of an injured guest to determine the possible cause, symptoms, and severity of their injury.

Rear huggie. A rescue technique used for a guest who is on the surface of the water facing away from the rescuer. The technique can be used on an unconscious or conscious guest, and is always performed with a rescue tube.

Recovery position. The maneuver used to turn a patient onto his or her side, so gravity will aid in moving the tongue off of the back of the throat, thus allowing both the passage of air and the drainage of fluids.

Rescue. Any situation where you enter the water to aid a guest in distress.

Rescue tube. A piece of rescue equipment that is always kept between the guest and a rescuer. It is usually made of vinyl-dipped foam for buoyancy, and has a body strap and line.

Respiratory arrest. When breathing suddenly stops.

Risk management. Reducing the likelihood of an accident by controlling the factors that make the situation high risk.

Rotation. The system you employ each time you leave your post and are relieved by another lifeguard.

Sacrum. The pelvic area.

Scanning. Moving the eyes across the surface and along the bottom of the zone, within the 10/20 protection rule.

Seizure. Sudden involuntary changes in the activity level of brain cells usually due to disease, trauma, or overdose / chemical reactions.

Shock. A collapse of circulatory function caused by severe injury, blood loss, or disease.

Silent drowning. A drowning caused by several physical conditions such as a heart attack or stroke, where the surface of the water shows no signs of struggle.

Skin cancer. A cancer caused by sun exposure.

Snorkeling swim search. This is performed when a guest is submerged in deep water. This type of search is coordinated with a rescue team by performing surface dives.

Special event. Any activity that is different from the normal daily routine at a facility.

Special facility. Any facility determined by Ellis & Associates to have features that require lifeguards to have specialized training. Examples may include facilities with wave pools, multiple slides, etc.

Spine. A column of 33 vertebrae that extend from the base of the head to the tip of the coccyx (tailbone).

Spinal Cord. A group of nerve tissue that carries messages from the brain to the rest of the body. It runs through and is protected by the vertebrae.

Squeeze play. A technique similar to the vice grip, used to stabilize a standing or sitting guest who is displaying the signs and symptoms of a spinal injury.

Sun protection factor (SPF). This indicates the level of protection a sunscreen product gives from ultraviolet rays.

Spinal column. The cord of nerve tissue extending through the center of the spinal column.

Spinal injury. Injury to the spinal cord usually caused by a blow to the head, neck, or spine. The compression or severing of the cord can cause paralysis or death

Sprain. Tearing of ligaments from muscles.

Standard of care. The skills and care which would normally be known and done by others working as lifeguards.

Strain. Tearing of tendons or muscle.

Thoracic. The middle back area.

Trough. The low part between two waves.

Two-lifeguard rescue. When two lifeguards work together, combining the front drive and the rear huggie into a "sandwich," to obtain a larger degree of control over difficult guests.

Ultra violet rays (UV). A type of radiation from the sun that produces harmful effects on the body, such as skin cancer.

Variance. Written approval to modify any National Pool and Waterpark Lifeguard Training Program or Ellis & Associates, Inc. policy or procedure.

Ventricular fibrillation. A life threatening rapid and disorganized heart rhythm, the most common cause of sudden and unexpected cardiac arrest in adults.

Ventricular tachycardia. An abnormal heart rhythm that causes the heart to beat too fast to effectively pump blood.

Vertebrae. The bones and segments composing the spinal column.

Vise grip. A rescue technique used to prevent further injury to a guest who is suspected of having suffered a spinal injury.

Walking line search. This is performed when the water is shallow enough to walk in, but too murky for you to see the bottom. This procedure may require the assistance of all staff members.

Wet drowning. Drowning caused by fluid in the lungs.

Zone. The area a lifeguard is responsible for scanning and maintaining the 10/20 or 10/3 Minute Protection Rules.

Index

A

ABC assessment, 146
Accountability, 4
Active guest rescue, 205
Advanced Cardiac Life Support (ACLS), 175
Airway management, 146
    See also Foreign body airway obstruction (FBAO) management
Amputated part, 152
Anaphylactic shock, 156-157
Approach stroke, 43
Arterial bleeding, 151
Asphyxiation, 17
Assessment, emergency, 145-147
Assist, 32
    extension, 40-41
Asthma emergency, 159
Audit, 6-7
Automated External Defibrillation (AED), 174-185
    Chain of Survival, 174-175
    children and infants, 183
    criteria for use, 179
    and heart rhythm, 175-176
    and implantable defibrillator, 183
    maintenance, 181-182
    operation, 177-181
    types of, 176-177
    See also Cardiopulmonary resuscitation (CPR)

B

Backboarding, 97-99
    spinal injury, 108-114
    team, 113-114, 119
    two-lifeguard, 110-112
Back-up lifeguard, 29, 30, 32
Bag-valve-mask (BVM), 56-59
Basic airway management, 54
Bee sting, 157
Binoculars, 195
Biological death, 17, 176
Bleeding, 146, 151-153
Boatmanship, 198-199
"Bobbing", 15
Body Substance Isolation (BSI), 92
Bottom condition, 193

Breath holding, involuntary, 16
Breathing. *See* Rescue breathing
Burn, 153-155

C

Cardiac arrest, 16-17
Cardiopulmonary resuscitation (CPR), 17, 76-89
    ABC assessment, 146
    adult, 76-80
    chest compressions, 78-80
    child, 82-83
    cycle, 79
    and disease transmission, 76
    flow chart, 88-89
    foreign body airway obstruction, 80-84
    infant, 83-84
    review, 86
    spinal injury, 116
    two-lifeguard, 79-80, 87
    See also Automated External Defibrillation; Rescue breathing
Cardiovascular system, 65-66
Cervical region, 105
Chain of command, 189
Chain of Survival, 174-175
Chemical burn, 153-154
Chest compression
    adult, 78-79
    child/infant, 82-83
Child
    and AED, 183
    CPR/FBAO, 82-83
Chin-lift, 54
Choking, 81
Clinical death, 16-17, 176
Coccyx, 105
Code system, 32
Communication, 29-32
Compact jump entry, 42-43
Crowd control, 168, 178
Cylinder, oxygen, 68-69

D

Death
    biological, 17, 176
    clinical, 16-17, 176

Deep water rescue, 128-132
Defibrillation. *See* Automated External Defibrillation (AED)
Diabetic emergency, 157-159
Diligence, 12
Disease transmission, 76
Distressed swimmer rescue, 42
Dock, 191
Drowning, 15-18
    and oxygen supply, 66-67
    stages of, 15-17
    types of, 17-18, 67
Dry drowning, 17-18, 67
Duck pluck, 122-125

E

Early Access, 174
Electrical burn, 153-155
Embedded object, 152
Emergency. *See* Medical emergency
Emergency Action System (EAS), 28-29
    activating, 144, 174
    hand signals, 31
    rescue vs. assist, 32
    and supplemental oxygen, 71-72
    waterfront, 196
    whistle signals, 30
Emergency stop button (E-stop), 30
Emotional risk, 137-138
Employer accountability, 4
Enhanced airway management, 55
Epiglottis, 16
Extension assist, 40-41
Extrication procedure
    backboarding, 108-114
    nonspinal, 97-99, 101

F

Fainting, 155
First aid. *See* Medical emergency
Flip-over, 45
Focused physical exam, 147
Foreign body airway obstruction (FBAO) management, 54-55, 80-84
    child, 82-83
    complete, 81-82
    infant, 84
    partial, 80

Front drive, 44-45, 49
Front huggie, 45
Full-thickness burn, 153

G

Golden Rule, 5, 167
Green flag, 191
Guest
  accountability, 4
  assist, 40
  recognition of distress, 14-15
  relations, 5
  rule enforcement, 166-167
  types of, 18-19

H

Hand signal, 31
Head immobilizer, 112
Head injury, 147-148
Head-tilt/chin-lift, 54
Health risk, 136
Heart, 175-176
Heat-related emergency, 148-150
Heimlich Maneuver, 81, 93-94
  deep water, 130
Hyperglycemia, 157-159
Hyperthermia, 148-150
Hypoglycemia, 157-158
Hypothermia, 109, 114
Hypovolemic shock, 156-157
Hypoxic convulsion, 16

I

Incident report, 168
Infant
  and AED, 183
  CPR/FBAO, 83-84
Injury. See Medical emergency
Insulin shock, 157-158
Internal bleeding, 151
Intervertabral disc, 104

J

Jaw displacement, 54

K

Ketoacidosis, 157-159

L

Legal risk, 138-141
Lightning, 154-155, 192
Location, high risk, 19
Logroll technique, 107, 108
Lumbar region, 105

M

Manual suction device, 59-61
Mechanism of injury, 147
Medical emergency, 144-163
  asthma, 159
  burns, 153-155
  diabetic, 157-159
  fainting, 155
  focused physical exam, 147
  head injury, 147-148
  hyperthermia, 148-150
  initial assessment, 145-146
  musculoskeletal injury, 150-151
  poisoning, 159-160
  seizure, 155-156
  shock, 156-157
  soft-tissue injury, 151-153
  steps in emergency care, 160
  See also Spinal injury
Medication patch, 183
Megaphone, 31, 195
Missing guest search, 197
Mouth-to-barrier rescue breathing, 95-96
Musculoskeletal injury, 150-151

N

Near-drowning Rescue, 42
Nosebleed, 152-153

O

Overarm vise grip, 109
Oxygen. See Supplemental oxygen
Oxygen cylinder, 68-69

P

Pacemaker, 183
Paperwork, 168
Partial-thickness burn, 153
Passive guest rescue, 204

Physical exam, 147
Poisoning emergency, 159-160
Pole extension, 40-41
Pressure regulator, 69
Professionalism
  image, 5
  legal risks, 139
Public address system, 32
Pulse, 145, 146
Push-away, 45

R

Radio, 32, 195
Rapid extrication procedure, 97-99
Rear huggie, 46, 50
  nonbreathing guest, 93-94
Recognition of distress, 14-15
Recovery position, 54
Red flag, 191
Report, 168, 181
Rescue, 32, 41-51
  ABC assessment, 146
  active victim, 205
  approach stroke, 43
  compact jump entry, 42-43
  deep water, 128-132
  Distressed swimmer, 42
  duck pluck, 122-125
  equipment, 194-195
  extrication procedure, 97-99
  front drive, 44-45, 49
  Near-drowning, 42
  on-deck care, 99
  passive victim, 204
  rear huggie, 46, 50, 93-94
  reports, 168
  waterfront, 189-191, 199-200
  See also Two-lifeguard rescue
Rescue board, 194, 199-200
Rescue breathing, 54-61
  airway management, 54-55
  bag-valve-mask, 56-59
  manual suction device, 59-61
  resuscitation mask, 55-56, 69
  spinal injury, 116
  and supplemental oxygen, 56, 67
  in water, 95-96
  See also Cardiopulmonary
    resuscitation (CPR)

Rescue tube, 33-34, 194
  deep water rescue, 128-130
  extension assist, 41
Respiratory system, 16, 66
Response category, 146
Responsibility, 144-145, 166-171
Resuscitation mask, 55-56, 69
Risk
  emotional, 137-138
  health, 136
  legal, 138-141
Rotation, lifeguard, 20-25
Rowing, 198-199
Rule enforcement, 166-167

S

Sacrum, 105
Scanning, 12-14
  and rotations, 20-25
  waterfront, 188
Scuba equipment, 195
Seizure, 155-156
Shock, 156-157
Sign, waterfront, 196
Signal, 36
  hand, 31
  two-lifeguard rescue, 47-48
  whistle, 30
Silent drowning, 17
Snorkeling swim search, 195, 197
Soft-tissue injury, 151-153
Speed slide, 114-115
Spinal injury, 104-119
  backboarding, 108-114
  composition of spine, 104-105
  CPR, 116
  NPWLTP position statement, 104
  signs and symptoms, 105, 147-148
  speed slides, 114-115
  squeeze play, 115-116
  vise grip, 106-109, 118
Splint, 150-151

Squeeze play, 115-116
Superficial burn, 153
Supplemental oxygen support (SOS) system, 64-73
  cardiovascular and respiratory systems, 65-66
  design of, 69-70
  maintenance, 70-71
  and rescue breathing, 56, 67
  system components, 68-70
  use of, 71-72
Syncope, 155

T

Team lifeguarding, 29, 30, 32
  backboarding, 110-114, 119
Telephone, 32, 195
Temperature, water, 193
10/3 Minute Protection rule, 10, 188, 195
10/20 Protection rule, 10
  rescue vs. assist, 32
  scanning, 20, 25
Thermal burn, 153
Thoracic region, 105
Thunderstorm, 192
Time, high risk, 20
Tongue obstruction, 54
Trash, 193
Tube, rescue, 33-34, 194
  deep water rescue, 128-130
  extension assist, 41
Two-lifeguard rescue, 47-48, 51
  CPR, 79-80, 87
  nonbreathing guest, 94-96
  rapid extrication procedure, 97-99
  spinal injury, 110-112, 119
2-way radio, 32, 195

U

Unconsciousness, 16
Universal Distress Sign of Choking, 81
Universal Precautions, 92

V

Valve, oxygen cylinder, 68-69
Ventilation. *See* Rescue breathing
Ventricular fibrillation (V-fib), 176
Ventricular tachycardia (V-tach), 176
Vertebra, 104
Violence, 197
Vise grip, 106-109, 118
Visibility, 193
Vomiting, 60-61, 148

W

Walking line search, 197
Water condition, 192-193
Waterfront lifeguarding, 188-202
  chain of command, 189
  equipment, 194-195, 198-200
  flag system, 191
  hazards, 188, 192-194
  missing guest search, 197
  rescues, 189-191, 199-200
  safe swimming areas and signs, 196
  scanning, 188
  10/3 Minute Protection Rule, 188, 195
  violence, 197
  watercraft, 190-191
  weather conditions, 191-192
Wet drowning, 17, 67
Whistle signal, 30
Wildlife, 194
Wound. *See* Soft-tissue injury

Y

Yellow flag, 191

Z

Zone, 11
  emergency back-up, 29, 30